CHIROPRACTIC RADIOGRAPHY
AND
QUALITY
ASSURANCE
HANDBOOK

Russell L. Wilson

CRC Press
Boca Raton   London   New York   Washington, D.C.

Acquiring Editor:	Liz Covello
Project Editor:	Susan Fox
Cover design:	Dawn Boyd

Library of Congress Cataloging-in-Publication Data

Wilson, Russell L.
    Chiropractic radiography and quality assurance handbook / by
Russell L. Wilson.
        p. cm.
    Includes index.
    ISBN 0-8493-0785-6 (alk. paper)
    1. Radiography--Quality control Handbooks, manuals, etc.
2. Spine--Radiography--Quality control Handbooks, manuals, etc.
I. Title.
    [DNLM: 1. Chiropractic--methods Handbooks. 2. Radiography-
-methods Handbooks. 3. Bone and Bones--radiography Handbooks.
4. Posture Handbooks. WB 39 W752c 1999]
RZ251.R33.W55 1999
616.07'572--dc21
DNLM/DLC
for Library of Congress   99-26555
                                                         CIP

No claim to original U.S. Government works
International Standard Book Number 0-8493-0785-6
Library of Congress Card Number 99-26555
Printed in the United States of America 1 2 3 4 5 6 7 8 9 0
Printed on acid-free paper

The Author

Russell Wilson has been a Registered Radiologic Technologist since 1970. He received his training in the United States Navy. He has worked in this field continuously since leaving the Navy in 1973. He has 17 years of experience in management of medical imaging departments and radiology quality assurance programs.

Russell Wilson has been an instructor of radiographic technology at Palmer College of Chiropractic West since 1994. He is married and has one daughter.

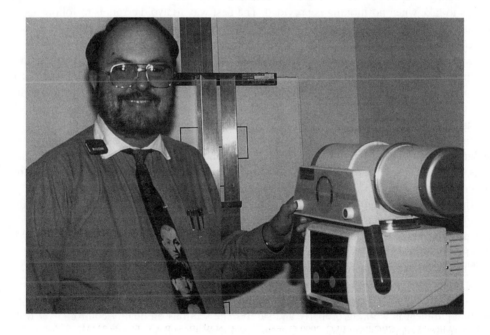

Preface

This book was designed to provide students of skeletal radiography with a positioning text that demonstrates the positioning on equipment they are likely to see in clinical experience. Almost all of the radiographs used as illustrations in the book were taken by chiropractic interns at Palmer College of Chiropractic–West. The illustrations demonstrate an important point. Chiropractic interns and chiropractors can produce high-quality radiographs using modern radiographic equipment. In many cases, these images are superior to what is turned in at hospitals and large medical clinics.

The early chapters cover the basics of radiography, processing films, and safety. A sequence of steps to take when positioning is provided. The best way to avoid errors is to follow a step-by-step format. Positioning is presented in two formats. A quick reference chart is provided that can be used to study for tests and put in the X-ray room of an office. The chart covers the main details of the views, including film sizes, recommended identification placement, tube angulation, and basic positioning. Note that some colleges recommend different or larger film sizes. The illustrated section provides detailed step-by-step instruction covering how to position the patient and what needs to be seen on the film. It is the author's hope that this will provide the student with the most convenient method to learn the concept of positioning for quality radiography.

The chapters covering extremity radiography are much more extensive than most skeletal radiographic positioning texts. Chiropractic can produce miracles in the treatment of joint and sports injuries. These chapters provide the positioning tools that will help in diagnosing and treating extremity injuries.

There is no substitute for hands-on experience. The student should spend as much time as possible in the positioning lab, getting familiar with the tools of radiographic positioning. Confidence is gained only through repetition and practice. I was as nervous as any student the first time I had to demonstrate how to position a view in training.

I have been an advocate of the performance of quality control in radiography for nearly 30 years. Radiographic quality assurance and quality control are mandated by all medical facilities that perform mammography. It works. The best way to have consistently good radiography is to ensure that all equipment is working properly and safely. The sections on quality control cover tests that do not require expensive equipment to monitor equipment operation.

A special thanks goes to the California Department of Radiologic Health for establishing a standard of good practice for radiography. This standard is used as the backbone of the quality control section of this text. Ms. Rebecca Lem, R.T(R), wrote an excellent home study program for the American Society of Radiologic Technologists. This guide is used as one of the reference materials for the processor quality control chapter.

Russell L. Wilson, R.T(R), C.R.T.

Acknowledgments
and Dedication

A special thanks and dedication go to my students at Palmer College of Chiropractic–West. There is no greater joy for a teacher than to see students produce films that one is proud to submit to the D.A.C.B.R. Their work provides the illustrations in this book.

I also want to thank the college for providing a curriculum that allows the time and resources to teach students of chiropractic how to position the views in this text. The encouragement from my superior and other instructors provided the drive to complete this book.

Dr. Teresa Whitney, D.C., was such a help in proofreading the text. There are things that the computer cannot fix and the author fails to see.

A special thanks goes to my daughter, Stephanie Wilson, for playing the patient for many of the illustrations. Her patience with Dad during this project is greatly appreciated. It was probably the toughest community service a teenager could experience. Others who helped by posing as patients are Benjamin Glass, D.C., Stuart Bickel, D.C., and Shannon Whandler, D.C.

Both Linda, my wife, and Stephanie, my daughter, deserve a special reward for putting up with me during this 3-year project.

Contents

Chapter **1**

Basic Radiography Concepts and Principles

The first three sections of this chapter review some of the key properties of radiographic image production. The first section discusses the equipment and accessories needed to produce consistently high-quality radiographs. It also covers shielding and some recommendations on room design. The second section is a review of radiation physics principles that impact image quality. The third section introduces the elements of a technique chart and discusses more physics.

The remaining sections of the chapter explore the darkroom and film processing. The first time a student enters the darkroom, it can very intimidating. There are some important safety issues for working near and with processing chemicals. There are environmental issues about the handling of used processing solutions, which is also covered in this chapter. Samples of the Material Data Safety Sheets for Developer and Fixer are included. Later in the Quality Control chapter (Chapter 21), mechanical sections of an automatic film processor are covered.

1.1 Chiropractic Radiographic Equipment and Accessories

The radiographic equipment and accessories needed to properly perform chiropractic radiography should be as modern as the doctor can afford. The greatest positioning skill will not overcome the limits of old and poorly maintained equipment. The chiropractor should consider the age and body habitus of potential patients. One must also consider if one is intending to do radiographic studies other than basic limited spinal radiography. Chiropractic radiography is more difficult to do compared to generally recumbent medical radiography. The patient will be much less stable. The patient will also be farther away from the film so loss of resolution due to increased object to film distance will impact the film quality. Good erect radiography requires top-quality equipment and very precise positioning of the patient.

The X-ray Machine

One of the greatest deterrents of good image quality is patient motion. If limited to a single-phase machine, one is twice as likely to get motion on the film than when using a high-frequency or three-phase machine. This is due to the single-phase unit being less efficient and having limited selection of mA and time selection. Because the typical lateral view of the lumbar spine has an optimum kVp of 90 kVp, it is not uncommon to have exposure times well in excess of 1 second. For long exposure times, even involuntary body motion such as peristalsis can result in a repeated film.

It is difficult to keep older equipment in proper calibration. If one wants to use 30 mAs for a film, the exposure should be the same on the large or small focal spot, and from mA station to mA station. As the X-ray tube ages, tungsten is built up on the window of the tube. This adds filtration to the beam and reduces contrast on the film. The filament will be the first part of the tube to show age. This impacts the geometric detail of the film.

When first setting up an X-ray department, have a physicist or other qualified person test the equipment before paying for it. This is extremely important with used equipment or when buying a practice. Used X-ray units that are not high frequency or three phase should definitely be evaluated before purchase. It might be better to wait until the practice grows and buy new equipment rather than install someone's obsolete equipment.

The grid in the film holder or Bucky must not be overlooked. One will need at least 103 lines and a 10:1 ratio to do adequate-quality spinal radiography. Make sure that it is installed perpendicular to the central ray. Many units in offices get grid cut-off because the grid is not properly aligned to the tube. Also make sure that the focal distance of the grid is consistent with the studies that will be done in the office.

One should have a Non-Bucky film holder for the erect film holder. The lateral cervical spine should never be taken using the grid at 72 in. SID; one is overexposing the patient by 5 times compared to the use of the Non-Bucky film holder. That overexposure also reduces the life of the X-ray tube.

There will be occasions when erect radiography is not practical, particularly with elderly or handicapped patients. A mobile X-ray table can be a very valuable part of the X-ray equipment. The alternative may be to put the patient on the floor to do recumbent studies. Examinations such as lumbar oblique view are best done recumbent. With any lordotic curve, it is impossible to get the lumbar spine in the same plane when doing obliques erect. For obese patients, the adipose tissue will roll away from the spine when X-rayed recumbent.

The basic X-ray room should include a three-phase or high-frequency generator, a Bucky with a 10:1 or better grid, and a mobile X-ray table (see Figure 1.1). The room must be shielded to 7 feet above the floor. The controls must be shielded and have a leaded glass window to observe the patient during the study. The equipment should be serviced according to manufacturer recommendations. A systematic quality assurance program should monitor the performance of the equipment.

The Film and Cassettes

Each component must be matched to the other components. All brands of film are not created equal. Film brands cannot be switched from one type of cassette and screen to another without the potential for grave problems. Some screens generate a blue/green spectrum of light, while others produce a green spectrum. If the film is not matched to the light spectrum of the screens, the potential for significant overexposure to the patient can result. The Relative Speed Value (RSV) is used to establish the exposure parameters of a given screen and film combination. It works very similar to the speed system used for photographic film.

The standard of the radiographic community for general radiography is a 400 speed screen and film combination. These are generally green-spectrum systems. This is a relatively high speed and low exposure system. All film manufacturers make this speed. The quantum mottle or noise on the film is acceptable and it will provide good detail for general Bucky-type work. Some manufacturers make a relatively good 800 speed system; it is noisier than the 400 speed system. There are systems as high as 1600 but the noise or grainy image makes them of limited value. A

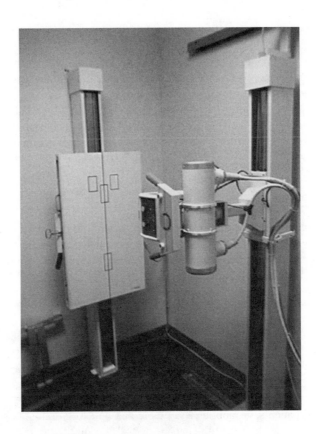

FIGURE 1.1
Basic X-ray unit.

very high-speed screen and film combination is not a substitute for a more powerful X-ray machine. If planning to use a blue-sensitive system, such as "high speed" or" high speed plus" (200 speed) for general radiography, one can reduce exposure and exposure times with a 400 speed system.

Do not attempt to do small extremity work without a dedicated extremity cassette system. The 80 speed Kodak Lanex Fine system uses the same film as the 400 speed Lanex Regular system. This makes their use very practical. Some of the extremity systems use single emulsion film that increases inventory costs. The 400 speed systems are too fast for hand, ankle, foot, and phalange studies. The kVp used with 400 speed systems is usually way too low and the contrast so poor that it is difficult to avoid overexposure. With extremities, one also needs finer detail that is not available with the 400 speed system.

The Kodak Lanex Cassette System provides very good screen contact and consistent image quality using Kodak and other manufacturers' film. They do not last forever. In 10 years of use, they will start to crack at the hinges. Proper care of the cassettes is very important to get full useful life from them. (See Figure 1.2.)

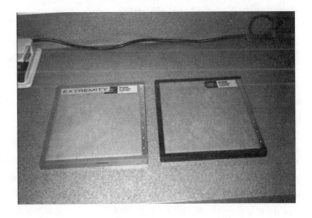

FIGURE 1.2
Cassette types.

Accessories and Radiation Protection

Obtain some positioning sponges and lead blockers. They will make it easier and more comfortable to position the patient. Anatomical and view lead markers must also be used. One can get by with just right and left markers and an arrow.

Gonad protection must be provided. This should include a half-apron of 0.5 mm lead rating. All aprons should be tested at least annually for holes and leaks. If one plans to take films on children or take stress films, lead gloves and a full-coat apron will be needed for one's own protection.

Compensating Filters

Full spine radiography should not be attempted without compensating filters, such as those manufactured by Dr. Ralph Nolan. These filters will also improve thoracic and lumbar spine studies. The gonad protection system that is part of Nolan's system is also one of the best on the market. (See Figure 1.3.)

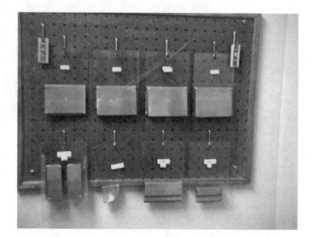

FIGURE 1.3
Filter rack.

Processing and Dark Room

One also needs a reliable film processor, an I.D. camera to print the patient information on the film, a safelight in the darkroom suitable for the film being used, silver recovery with secondary containment for the used fixer, fresh water and drain for the processor, and a means to exhaust the dryer heat. A cool, dry place to store film is also very important.

Quality Control

To monitor the film processor, one should have a thermometer, a densitometer, and a sensitometer. Without processing quality control, one will not be able to determine what is causing inconsistent image quality. The X-ray company will blame the processor, and vice versa. Significant volumes of film are quickly wasted and many needless repeated films are necessary if one does not monitor the processor.

Other necessary test equipment includes a screen contact test wire mesh. The cassettes should be tested semi-annually. Screen cleaning solution that is designed for the specific type of screen used should be used monthly. A piece of 14 in. × 17 in. × 2 in. Lucite is very useful to check for grid alignment, and a step wedge is useful for output testing. The more that one is able to monitor, the less one needs to spend on needless repairs; you will be able to detect problems before they degrade the images.

A chapter on quality control (Chapter 21) is included in this book.

Using the Universal X-ray Units

The Universal X-ray Corporation equipment in the Palmer College Clinics is state-of-the-art high-frequency radiographic equipment. High-frequency generation is the most efficient X-ray generator available, providing the lowest dose and fastest exposure times possible in the office environment.

The Control Panel

The AP-700 in Room One (Figure 1.4) has the technical factors for most of the spinal positions programed into the generator. By selecting the body region and view and entering the patient measurement, the generator will select the exposure factors stored for that body size. To enter the measurement, highlight the size by pressing the arrow above size. Use the up and down arrows to the right to enter the measurement. Use the technique chart to determine filtration.

The CP-700 or MP-700 generator has arrows under the exposure factors. These arrows are used to enter the technical factors from the technique chart. At some facilities, these units have automatic exposure control (AEC). With AEC, an ion chamber reads the exposure and terminates the exposure automatically. The optimum kVp is put into the control panel. The mAs is set higher than normal to allow the unit to stop the exposure. Density on the film is adjustable on the control panel. The ion chamber must also be selected. AEC is very useful for very large or muscular patients.

Radiation exposure is a two-step process for most X-ray machines. With Universal, the Prep button is pressed first. Prep will bring the rotor up to speed and set the potentials on the tube. A green light on the control panel will indicate that the machine is ready for exposure. While continuing to depress the Prep button, also push the Exposure button. The exposure light will come on and an audible tone will indicate the actual X-ray exposure. Hold both buttons down until the tone stops. The most common mistake made by students is lifting the exposure button too soon. This will reduce the mAs below the desired factors. The AP-700 will let one know what the exposure time will be before the film is taken. The MP or CP type unit indicates the actual exposure time after the exposure is made. It is important to have confidence in the equipment and hold the exposure buttons down until the exposure is completed.

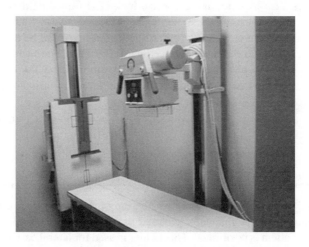

FIGURE 1.4
X-ray unit.

Tube Stand and Collimator Controls

The tube stand has two electromagnetic locks. They are controlled by individual buttons. With Universal units, when the button is depressed, the lock unlocks until the button is released. With other manufacturers, the lock will remain unlocked until the button is depressed again.

The vertical lock allows one to raise or lower the tube. For upright radiography, this is how the central ray or tube is centered to the patient. For recumbent radiography, the vertical lock sets the SID.

The horizontal or longitudinal lock is used to set the SID for upright radiography. The universal units have a light on the Bucky that activates when the tube is at 40 in. or 72 in. from the Bucky. For recumbent radiography, the horizontal lock is used to center the tube to the patient.

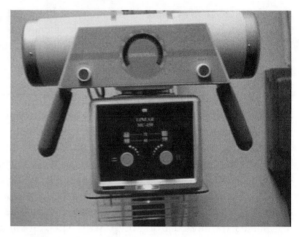

FIGURE 1.5
X-ray tube.

The tube stand (see Figure 1.5) also has two handles that are used to angle the tube. For upright radiography, the tube is set at 90° to get it perpendicular to the upright Bucky. To set tube angles, one must subtract the desires angle for caudal tilts. For cephalad angles, add the desired angle to 90°. For recumbent radiography, the tube is set at 0°.

There are three controls for the collimator. The lamp button turns on the collimator light and the film centering light. The light is used to set the field of exposure. The crosshairs are used to set the horizontal and vertical central ray alignment. Where the crosshairs cross is the central ray. There are also two knobs that are turned to restrict or open the lead shutters in the collimator. There are windows where the size of the field can be viewed for 40 in. and 72 in. These numbers must be within 5% accuracy by state and federal law. Use these numbers to set film size. Remember that one should never expose the patient to a field larger than the film size.

The Bucky

The Bucky has a tray, a grid, and a vertical lock. The film should always be locked horizontally into the center of the Bucky tray. When using AEC, it must also be centered vertically. The grid is protected by the front cover. The center line of the cover can be used to help center P-A views. The Bucky is raised or lowered with the vertical lock control button and handle. With a 14 in. × 3 in. Bucky, the tray can be positioned in the top or bottom of the Bucky. Put the tray in the top for spinal, chest, and upper extremity views. The bottom position is used for lower extremities. The tray is removed to install a 14 in. × 36 in. cassette.

Always remember to push the Bucky tray in before shooting the film using the Bucky. Also make sure the film is locked into the center of the Bucky tray.

The Non-Bucky Holder

The Non-Bucky film holder attaches over the top of the Bucky. It is used to take non-grid upright views. The film should be manually centered to the beam and the collimation restricted to the film size before the patient is positioned. This holder is used for lateral cervical spine views taken at 72 in.

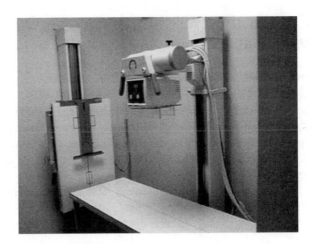

FIGURE 1.6
X-ray unit with table.

The Mobile Table

The mobile table is used for recumbent radiography. It is important to center the table to the central ray and lock the wheel locks. Check the center after the patient is placed on the table to see if it moved. If the table is not centered, the beam will not be centered to the table Bucky. Grid cut-off or the anatomy missing the film will result from the failure to center the table. The most useful accessory in an X-ray room will be the X-ray table. With a table available, one will be able to take X-rays on patients who cannot stand or are unstable, without risking injury to the patient or the operator. (See Figure 1.6.)

Setting Up a New Radiographic Room

Office space is expensive, so one will not want to waste valuable space. The room should be 11 to 12 feet long in order to have the control booth aligned with the wall Bucky and tube. The room width should be 8 to 10 feet. If one budgets for 120 sq. feet, one should have a very comfortable X-ray room.

The darkroom will require plumbing and good ventilation and air conditioning. There should be negative air flow. It can be as small as 8 feet by 8 feet. Plan on having secondary containment for the fresh processing chemicals and the used fixer container. The chemical storage containers should have floating tops inside the container and airtight lids. The darkroom should have a deep sink and eyewash capabilities. Adequate cabinets for film storage are also important. The film should be stored vertically and never laid on its side. The film bin should be mounted under the countertop or attached to a wall.

The location of the X-ray room will impact the shielding requirements. The wall where the wall Bucky is will require at least 4 lb of lead per square foot or be an outside wall; 6 to 8 in. of concrete will usually meet local code for primary X-ray shielding. The wall of the control booth will also require 4 lb of lead and a leaded glass window. The other two walls and the door to the room should have 2 lb of lead. The lead does not need to extend higher than 7 feet.

Along with air conditioning in the office, proper electrical power is important. The minimum power should be 200 A into the office. The X-ray equipment will use 100 A of 240-V power; 120-V 30-A radiographic units are not recommended, including the 110-V high-frequency units. They lack power at the high ranges needed to X-ray large patients.

There should be a room where all extraneous light can be turned off to set up as the X-ray viewing room. Be sure and use only daylight replacement flourescent tubes in view boxes. A bright light will also be very useful for the occasional dark film or to see soft tissues.

1.2   Factors that Will Impact Image Quality: A Review of Physics Concepts

Technique Charts

The consistency of exposure, contrast, and density on the film will be controlled by the technique chart. The exposure time will be impacted by the focal spot selected and mA stations available on the control panel. Film quality will be only as good as the technique chart. If the X-ray machine controls the mAs (mA × time) in terms of time and mA station, recording the mAs on the technique chart is recommended.

Other useful information may include any tube angulation requirement of the view, film type, and filters and shielding needed for the view. Adjusting the factors for pathology, age, and body habitus, as well as equipment changes, is discussed later. All of these conversion factors are reflected in mAs.

The focal spot selection will impact the recorded detail. Whenever possible, the small focal spot should be used. This will provide the best possible geometric resolution. The small focal spot has less penumbra, or shadow effect. It also will have lower mA potential than the large spot. This will result in longer exposures, which may result in patient motion. For lumbar and full spine radiography, one should avoid exposure times greater than 0.5 seconds and use the large focal spot.

Types of Technique Charts

There are two basic types of technique charts: use a fixed mAs and vary the kVp, or use a fixed kVp and vary the mAs. Varying the kVp and using a fixed mAs will result in having no control of the contrast on the film. Small patients will be underpenetrated and large patients will have very low contrast on their films. The technical factors must be perfect or the film will be improperly exposed. The use of fixed mAs and variable kVp is not recommended.

The variable mAs and fixed kVp technique chart has numerous advantages. The use of the optimum kVp for the body part will provide the best possible contrast scale. It ensures that the body part will be properly penetrated. The fixed kVp chart will generally have the kVp set higher than when the mAs is fixed. This will reduce exposure to the patient. Last, fixed kVp provides more latitude in exposure factors and lower numbers of repeated films. The mAs will need to be wrong by more than 25% before it will affect image quality.

Getting Started Building a Technique Chart

Make sure the X-ray machine is calibrated properly and the film processor is cleaned and operating properly. If one has a step wedge and a friend with the same type of equipment, or two X-ray rooms, expose the step wedge in his room and then expose it in the X-ray room. Use exactly the same SID and technical factors for both exposures. Read a given step with an exposure between 1.20 and 2.20 optical density. Dividing the density of one film by the other film will give a conversion factor that can be used to convert the mAs from one machine to another.

There are also slide rule type technique conversion and formulation devices, such as the "Supertech." It comes with a penetrometer to establish the conversion factor for the unit. They also market a computer program that will print technique charts. This program works very well.

The following pages are techniques used by this author on a three-phase high-frequency generator using the Nolan Filter System and Kodak Lanex Regular Cassettes with Kodak TMG-1 or Clinic Select Green –1 film, equipment that can help start one's own technique charts. The positioning instructions provide the optimum kVp for each view.

Adjusting the Technique for Body Habitus and Pathology

This author's technique charts work for about 85% of the population. The charts are designed for relatively young patients of average build and musculature. Because the technical factors cause more than 50% of the number of repeated films, the use of technique charts is very important. It is also very important to know when to adjust the technical factors. Patients can be divided into three basic categories: easy to penetrate, normal, and hard to penetrate. The changes result from the relationship of X-rays as they pass through muscle, fat, or bone.

The Easy to Penetrate Patient: Reduce kVp by 4 to 6 kVp and leave mAs the same, or decrease the kVp by 10 kVp and double the mAs.

Post-menopausal female patients who do not take hormone therapy will generally suffer from osteoporosis. The loss of calcium in the bone will make the patient easier to penetrate and necessitate a reduction in kVp. Male patients over 60 years of age will also have some bone loss. Frail and atrophic patients will require the greatest reduction in kVp.

For the thoracic spine, patients with emphysema or active tuberculosis will require a reduction in kVp. Other disease processes such as aseptic necrosis, gout, fibrosarcoma, hemangiomas, Hodgkins disease, and many metastatic processes will require a reduction in kVp.

To a certain extent, the obese patient will be easier to penetrate than the normal habitus patient with the same measurement.

The Hard to Penetrate Patient: Increase kVp by 4 to 6 kVp and leave the mAs alone, or increase the mAs by 50 to 100% and leave the kVp alone.

The bodybuilder or someone with very high muscle mass cannot be X-rayed with the same technique as the normal patient. If the patient has very high muscle mass, a combination of increasing kVp by 6 to 10 kVp and increasing the mAs 25 to 40% may be required.

Additive disease processes will require a change in technical factors. If it is not a muscular process, leave the kVp the same and increase the mAs from 30 to 50%. Additive disease processes include acute kyphosis, chronic osteomyelitis, osteochondroma, osteoma, sclerosis, and Paget's disease.

For thoracic spine films, lung pathology such as atelectasis, pneumonia, pleural effusions, bronchiectasis, edema, and many malignancies will require an increase in the technique.

Collimation's Impact on the Technical Factors

Proper collimation and film size are factored into the technical factors of the technique chart. Based on the kVp and body part being imaged, one can estimate the amount of scatter radiation that will produce some of the density on the film. There are some basic rules about collimation. Collimation must be equal to or smaller than film size. Ideally, there should be three distinct borders on every film. At the same time, the film must demonstrate all of the anatomy of interest. If collimation is too tight, it will result in a repeated exposure. If the shutters are left wide open, there will be too much scatter radiation and the film will be dark.

Many general films are done on 14 in. × 17 in. films. Occasionally, one may want to do a coned down or highly collimated view to improve the image quality. The mAs will need to be increased to compensate for the reduced scatter radiation.

To convert from 14 in. × 17 in. to 10 in. × 12 in., multiply mAs by 1.20.
To convert from 14 in. × 17 in. to 8 in. × 10 in., multiply mAs by 1.4.

Film speed

Each film and screen system will have an assigned Relative Speed Value (RSV). Knowing and using the RSV, one can then adapt the technique from one speed system to another. If one mixes systems, one can get very inconsistent results. This author uses the Kodak Lanex Regular (400 RSV) system for all Bucky, spinal, and large extremity exams. For small extremity studies that are not taken Bucky, the Kodak Lanex Fine (80 RSV) system is used. The RSV is very similar to the ASA for photographic film. Very-high speed systems will be grainy and not suitable for fine detail. Detail systems will have a low RSV or ASA in photography.

Equipment Technique Adjustments

Single-phase equipment will require twice the mAs compared to three-phase or high-frequency generators. To convert from high frequency to single phase, double the mAs.

The grid ratio in the Bucky or film holder will impact the technical factors. Remember that the higher the ratio, the greater scatter control. In general, grids should always be used above 70 kVp. For extremities, body parts that measure less than 10 cm may be done Non-Bucky using extremity cassettes.

Conversion factors:

> Non-Bucky to 5:1 grid ratio: multiply mAs by 2
>
> Non-Bucky to 6:1 grid ratio: multiply mAs by 3.
>
> Non-Bucky to 8:1 grid ratio: multiply mAs by 4.
>
> Non-Bucky to 10:0 grid ratio: multiply mAs by 5.
>
> Non-Bucky to 12:1 grid ratio: multiply mAs by 6.

The conversion factors can be used to convert from one ratio to another by dividing the new ratio by the old ratio. As an example, to change from 6:1 to 12:1, divide 6 by 3. The factor would be to double the mAs.

Adjustment of Contrast

The 15% rule is used to adjust contrast while maintaining adequate density. It can also be used to reduce exposure times by increasing the kVp and lowering the mAs.

> To reduce mAs 25%, increase kVp 8% (lower contrast) (more shades of grey).
>
> To reduce mAs 50%, increase kVp by 15% (lower contrast) (more shades of grey).
>
> To double mAs, reduce kVp by 15% (increase contrast) (less shades of grey).

Technique Adjustment for Distance

$$\text{New mAs} = \text{Old mAs} \times (\text{Old distance})^2/(\text{New distance})^2$$

Geometric Properties that Affect Image Quality

One must endeavor to keep the patient as close to the film as possible. Object to film distance (OFD or OID) problems impact erect radiography much more than with recumbent radiography.

When the patient lies down, the body part is naturally as close to the film as possible. When the patient stands, the natural posture and the impact of shoulders will be graphically apparent. Precise positioning with minimal OFD will yield the best-quality images. As the body part moves away from the Bucky, its shadow or penumbra increases. This shadow effect makes sharp edges much less sharp and causes loss of detail.

The focal spot size will also greatly impact geometric detail. The large focal spot casts a larger shadow than the small focal spot. Images taken with the small focal spot with some OFD will be sharper than when the large focal spot is used. When the large focal spot and poor positioning with significant OFD is used, the image will be very blurry. The small focal spot has less heat dissipation and lower mA than the large focal spot. This will cause longer exposure times than when the large focal spot is used. If the patient cannot stand still or hold his/her breath, it is better to stop the motion by using the large focal spot. (This author typically tries to use exposure times of less than 0.5 seconds.)

The distance between the X-ray tube and the film will also impact detail. Increasing the source to image distance (SID) will reduce the effects of OFD. In using the part of the beam closer to the central ray, the photons have less divergence than the photons at the edges of the beam. The lateral cervical spine, chest, and A-P full spine are taken at 72 in. to reduce magnification and increase OFD.

Collimation Is Used to Control Scatter

Scatter radiation is the result of photons entering into action with matter or tissue. The larger the body part, the more scatter produced. If the beam is restricted to the area of interest, there will be less scatter radiation and better contrast. While the image is the same geometrically, the less off-focal photons will strike the film.

Collimation is the primary form of radiation protection for both the patient and the operator. The beam must be restricted to slightly less than film size so that one can see borders on two to three sides of the film. Often, the beam can be further restricted to just the area of interest. This will improve the image and protect the patient from needless radiation exposure. The positioning descriptions will help establish the area of clinical interest for proper collimation. Collimation that does not include the clinical objective will result in repeated images and more exposure to the patient. Collimation too tight or too small is nearly as bad as not collimating.

Compensating Filters Are Used to Adjust Exposure

Chiropractic leads the field of radiography in the use of filtration. Some body parts will have significant changes in overlying tissue. These parts need aluminum filters to remove some of the photons and equalize the exposure. The thoracic spine is a perfect example. The upper thoracic spine has just the air-filled lungs and chest tissue, while the lower thoracic spine has the heart and major vessels overlying the spine. If filters are not used, the upper spine is overexposed or the lower spine is underexposed. With the A-P full spine, exposure from the cervical spine to the pelvis must be equalized. Multiple filters are used to accomplish this.

The Beam Must Be Aligned to the Grid

Grid cut-off happens when there is an alignment problem with the grid. The grid will then stop the primary beam and produce linear artifacts on the film. Grid cut-off happens when:

    The beam is not perpendicular to the grid
    The grid is angled to the beam
    The wrong focal length grid is used for the SID
    The grid is backward to the beam

The most common problem is misalignment of the beam to the Bucky. If the tube is even slightly nonperpendicular, the edges or outside part of the film will be lighter than the middle part of the film. There will also be a loss of detail on the edges of the film. The same artifact will be seen if the grid is not focused to the SID being used.

1.3 Technique Charts and Technique Selection

Reading a Technique Chart

Each exam and view will require a different radiographic technique. Each body part thickness will also require different technical factors and perhaps added filters. The technique consists of:

1. mAs: the product of the mA times the exposure time. mAs determines the density of the film.
2. kVp: the peak kilovolts determines penetrating ability of the X-ray and the contrast scale of the image.
3. Focal spot size: decides the detail of the image. The focal spot selection also influences the mA selections available and heat loading of the tube. The small focal spot does not have as high an mA potential as the large focal spot. High-speed screens and film allow a greater use of small focal spots. The greater detail of the small focal spot can be undermined by motion due to patient movement. The indiscriminate use of the small focal spot can also result in shorter X-ray tube life due the lower heat dissipation of the small focal spot. All phantom images are done on the large focal spot.
4. (Optional) Power: the MP300 and MP500 allow the selection of low, medium, or full power. This is another way of allowing the adjustment of mA settings. This allows the operator to select a longer exposure time. Remember that 10 mAs is the same if the factors are 100 mA and 0.10 s or 200 mA and 0.05 s. This is the Reciprocity Law of X-ray.
5. Spot or point filters: added to equalize density.
6. Other information: such as cassette type, FFD, and even cassette size. The technique chart is made to standardize the variables of radiography.

Types of Technique Charts

There are two types of technique charts: (1) fixed kVp and variable mAs and (2) fixed mAs and variable kVp.

Fixed kVp technique charts are preferred for a number of reasons.

1. Because kVp controls contrast, these charts provide the optimum contrast of the image.
2. They assure that the body part is properly penetrated.
3. The kVp controls the level of scatter radiation; therefore, using the optimum kVp will produce consistent levels of scatter radiation.
4. Fixed kVp techniques also aid in the control of radiation exposure. Higher-energy photons produced with optimum kVp tend to pass through the body without interacting with the atoms of the body. Consequently, the ionizing effects are lower than when low kVp is used. The use of the highest kVp that will provide satisfactory contrast should be used to keep the exposure to the patient as low as possible.

Fixed mAs and variable kVp technique charts have a fixed mAs and variable kVp. Very small patients will not be adequately penetrated. This type of chart can produce good-quality images if the patient habitus, collimation, and other variables are always the same. This type of chart has less latitude than the fixed kVp chart. Latitude is the margin for error in the technique or patient positioning.

Technical Factors and Their Impact on Image Quality

Each body part or region has an ideal kVp range to achieve optimum contrast. The type of tissue being studied also decides the kVp range that will achieve the contrast desired. Chest X-rays, where soft tissue and lung detail is essential, require high kVp (above 90 kVp). This is a long gray scale or low contrast study. Rib, T-spine, or sternum studies use lower kVp (70–80 kVp) and high contrast. The lower kVp produces shorter gray scale or higher contrast image. The technique charts should reflect the optimum kVp for the type of screen film combinations used. Rare-earth screens lose speed at very low kVp (below 60 kVp). This author does not use the range below 60 kVp on patients.

Optimum kVp for Common Body Parts

Body Part	Optimum kVp
Small extremities	55–60
Large extremities	65–70
Skull	80
Abdomen	70
Chest	110–125
Spine	70–80
Pelvis	70
Shoulder	70
Ribs	70

Impact of Patient Body Habitus and Pathology on Technical Factors

Most technique charts are based on the average degree of muscularity and body fat. The correctly generated technique chart will work 85% of the time. The type of tissues being X-rayed will affect the final technical factors used. A patient with higher muscle development or increased fatty tissues will require a change in the technique from the one on the technique chart. Body fat is very harmful for erect radiography because, typically, it drops down into areas of clinical significance. Very obese patients may require recumbent radiography.

When evaluating a film with technique errors, first look to see if adequate penetration exists. If penetrated, adjustments in density or mAs will need to be made. If not penetrated, kVp should be increased. Remember that mAs must be increased by more than 25% to make any visible change in the image. There will be times that the experienced radiographer will adjust both.

Increased Body Fat. Leave kVp same and increase mAs by 40 to 80%, or decrease kVp by 6 to 10 kVp and double mAs.

Increased Muscularity. Increase kVp by 6 to 10 kVp and mAs by 20 to 40%.

Certain pathological conditions also will affect the technical factors. Osteoporosis and osteopenia will require a reduction in kVp by 6 to 10 kVp in the thoracic and lumbar examinations.

Equipment and Its Impact on Technical Factors

Impact of Technique Changes Depends on the Speed of the Screen Film Combination

Each screen and film combination will have an RSV. Knowing the RSV will allow one to adjust the technical factors from one combination to another. Technique charts used by the author are based on a 400 speed system (Kodak Lanex Regular) for spines and Bucky studies, and 80 speed (Kodak Lanex Fine) for Non-Bucky extremities.

> To change from 400 speed to 200 speed, double the mAs.
> To change from 400 speed to 100 speed, increase the mAs 4 times.
> To change from 400 speed to 80 speed, increase mAs 5 times.
> To change from 80 speed to 400 speed, divide mAs by 5.

High-frequency or three-phase techniques can be changed to single-phase factors by doubling the mAs.

Impact of Collimation on the Technique

Proper collimation should be factored into technique charts. Collimation is one of the main factors in controlling radiation exposure and scatter radiation. The collimation should never be larger than the film size. Ideally, three borders of collimation should be seen on most films. If the collimation is incorrect, the film may be dark or lose detail because of excessive scatter radiation. Occasionally, one will need to do spot or coned down views. Because of the tight collimation, the full-size technique will result in a light or underexposed film.

> To convert from 14×17 to 10×12, multiply the mAs by 1.25.
> To convert from 14×17 to 8×10, multiply the mAs by 1.40.

The Control of Contrast Using Technical Factors

The operator can control contrast by the selection of mAs and kVp. Virtually any study can be done with a variety of mAs and kVp combinations. A small kVp change can result in a major change in the image. Small changes in mAs have a lesser impact. To see a change in density because of changing mAs, one needs to change it by at least 20%. (A change of 4 kVp is seen on the image in our kVp ranges.)

Basic Rules For Adjusting Contrast

1. To reduce mAs 25%, increase kVp 8%.

2. To reduce mAs 50%, increase kVp 15%.

3. To increase mAs 100%, reduce kVp 15%.

4. For the 60 to 90 kVp range, a change of 10 kVp is equal to 15%.

Disadvantages of High mAs and Low kVp Techniques

1. Focal spot blooming due to an overload of photons for the focal spot cup can generate off-focal radiation. This results in a loss of detail.

2. The images have a short scale of contrast, resulting in a loss of latitude. The technique must be perfect because of the high and sharp contrast between structures.

3. Beside blooming, perceived detail can be lost because of a lack of shades of gray. The techniques make a film of good density, but low on contrast.
4. The actual technique results in more heat units on the X-ray tube that can shorten tube life.
5. Dense body parts stand out and less soft tissue is seen.
6. High mAs low kVp techniques result in higher patient exposure.
7. If the body part is not penetrated, detail of the inner structures will be lost.

Object To Film Distance (OFD) and Focal to Distance (FFD): Impact on Image Quality

The impact of object to film distance (OFD) on image quality depends on the focal size and the focal film distance. In some studies in radiography, OFD is increased to produce a better film. This is true in mammography but it requires special X-ray equipment with very small focal spots (<0.3 mm). OFD will be further discussed in material covering detail.

In general radiography, OFD is minimized to achieve optimum image quality. This is particularly true for the equipment used by this author with 1.0 and 2.0 mm focal spot sizes. The greater the OFD, the greater magnification of the image is seen at 40 in. focal film distance (FFD).

1. If the object of interest is far from the film, the FFD is increased to reduce the penumbra present with even a small focal spot. (This is why this author takes the lateral C-spine at 72 in. FFD.)
2. Greater image clarity is seen in the anatomy closest to the film in short focal distances. In rib X-rays, the anterior ribs are seen better on the P-A views. Patella views are done P-A for the same reason.
3. Chest X-rays are done at 72 in. FFD to reduce magnification so as to see the heart and other pulmonary structure in their true size.
4. Excessive OFD will result in a light film because the air gap between the patient and the film will filter some of the scatter radiation needed to produce the required density on the film.
5. The radiation exposure to the patient is reduced when longer FFDs are used. The soft undesirable photons do not reach the patient. Therefore, it is ideal to use the shortest OFD and the longest possible FFD to reduce radiation exposure to the patient.

1.4 Working in a Darkroom with an Automatic Processor

The darkroom (see Figure 1.7) can be rather intimidating when one first uses it. After becoming familiar with the location of the film, I.D. camera, cassette latch, and feed tray, it will be easier and more enjoyable. The film-processing chemicals and the used fixer are usually stored in the darkroom. To keep the fumes to a minimum, the lids to the tanks are closed. The darkroom is also well ventilated, and the exhaust from the processor dryer is vented out of the darkroom. The darkroom should be as safe and as pleasant as possible.

The Sequence

1. Place exposed cassettes on counter, yellow side up, with I.D. blocker toward the wall (Figure 1.8).
2. Put the flash card in the I.D. camera under the clip with the printing facing up.
3. Press the button on the processor to take processor off the standby mode.
4. Close and lock the darkroom door.
5. Open cassette enough to get the film out of the cassette (Figure 1.9).

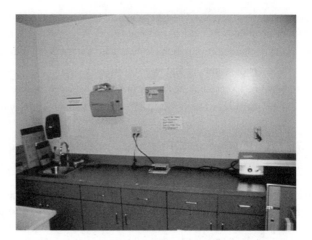

FIGURE 1.7
Darkroom work surface.

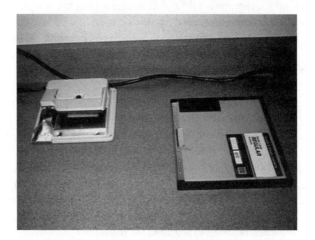

FIGURE 1.8
Cassette, back side up.

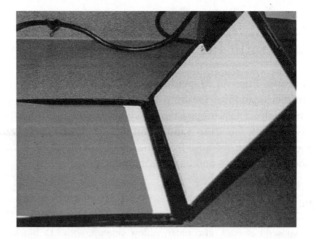

FIGURE 1.9
Cassette opened.

6. Grasp film by the edges with clean and dry hands and slide it over the flash card.

7. Align the edge of the film with the edge of the clip that holds the card in the camera.

8. Push down on the bar on top of the camera (Figure 1.10) until a light flash is observeed in the camera window.

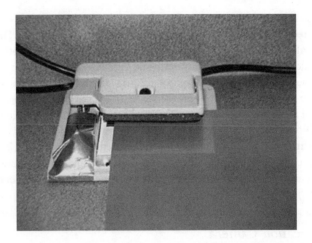

FIGURE 1.10
I.D. camera.

9.   Place film on the feed tray lengthwise next to the left rail and slightly push the film into the processor. The light over the processor will go out when the processor has accepted the film.

10. Locate the film bin and slowly open the bin. Locate the fresh film size. Remove the lid from the box and take a sheet of fresh film from the box. Put the lid back on the box. While the bin is open, an alarm will sound as a reminder that the bin is open.

11. Place the fresh film in the cassette and latch close the cassette.

12. When the exposed film is fully in the processor, a beep will be heard and the safelight over the processor will come back on. It will be safe to feed the next film into the processor or unlock the door and leave the darkroom.

Note: When processing multiple films, one can wait until all of the exposed film is fed into the processor before reloading the cassettes. Initially, this will be easier than reloading each cassette as one processes the film.

The Cassette

This author uses the Kodak X-Omatic cassettes. The border on the outside of the cassette signifies the type of screen inside the cassette: gray-bordered cassettes with high-detail Lanex fine screens for extremities and black-bordered cassettes for Lanex regular screens (see Figure 1.11). This type

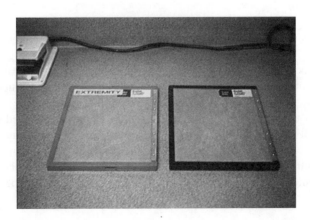

FIGURE 1.11
Cassette types.

of cassette is unique in its design. The cassette — front and back — when opened has a slight bow. The screens on the front side have foam rubber behind them. The bow and the foam rubber combine to allow excellent screen-to-film contact. When the cassette is closed, all of the air is forced out and good contact is achieved. The cassettes are also very easy to open.

When the cassette is turned yellow side up, there is a stainless steel latch. Lifting the latch will open the cassette. Do not open the cassette all the way. Open it just enough to remove the film; this will add life to the cassette. Eventually, the plastic hinge side will break; then, the cassette is facing yellow side up, and one also sees a black window. This is an area of the cassette where patient information (or I.D. identification) is printed on the film. Kodak makes an I.D. camera that will automatically open this window and flash the information on the film, along with the time and date. (This particular camera costs over $1000 and is beyond the needs of the office.) The information is printed on the film in the darkroom using the manual I.D. camera.

The Identification Camera

The identification (I.D.) camera is used to print the patient information on the film (see Figure 1.12). The flash card is placed in the camera with the typed or printed information face-up. A spring steel clip will hold the flash card in place. The exposed film is placed on top of the flash card with the left side of the film next to the clip that holds the card in place. (One may need to use a finger to feel the film next to the card.) The bar or handle on top of the camera in pushed down. This will activate a light that will produce a contact print of the information on the film. When activated, one observes a flash of red light through a window on the top of the camera. In some situations, the camera is mounted in/on the wall, but the operation principles are the same.

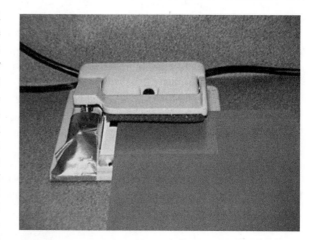

FIGURE 1.12
Film in I.D. camera.

The Processor

Once the patient information has been printed on the film, it is ready to be fed into the processor (Figure 1.13). This should be done as soon as possible to avoid fogging of the film by the safelights.

If the processor is on standby, it will not accept the film. A button to the left of the feed tray will take the processor off of standby. The button should be pressed upon entry into the darkroom to process the film because it is easier to locate with more light.

The film is fed lengthwise into the processor along the left feed tray rail (see Figure 1.14). Feeding small films down the middle of the tray can result in a jammed processor. As soon as the film enters the processor, the safelight over the feed tray will go out. It will come back on after the film is fully inside the processor. Never try to pull a film out once the entrance rollers have taken the film; this will get developer on the rollers and feed tray. The developer will put artifacts on the films.

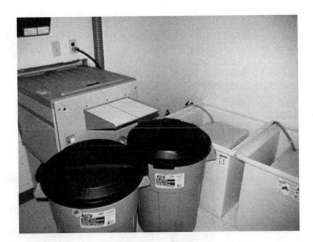

FIGURE 1.13
Film processor.

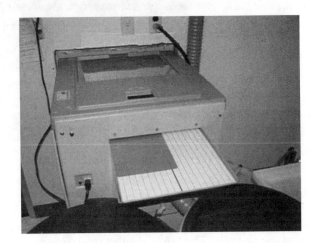

FIGURE 1.14
Feeding film into processor.

Processor jamming or malfunctions are generally rare but may happen at any time. If one should hear any banging or uncommon noises coming from the processor, do not feed more films into it until the noise is investigated by the radiographer. When the processor top is removed to investigate the noise, eye protection and gloves should be worn. In the event of getting chemicals in one's eyes, use the eyewash for 15 minutes and then seek medical care.

Processing Chemicals and Hazardous Waste

Avoid contact with the processing chemicals. The developer contains hydroquinone, which is considered a hazardous material. The fixer in the processor contains silver, making it a hazardous waste; it cannot be disposed of down any drain. The barrels in front of the feed tray contain the used fixer. The used fixer is removed and disposed of by a hazardous waste removal company.

The fresh chemicals and waste are within secondary containment. This is designed to capture the chemical if the primary container leaks. The fresh developer and fixer are not considered hazardous waste and can be dumped down a drain with water to dilute the chemicals. Always wear eye protection and gloves when handling processing chemicals. Avoid contact with clothing and skin.

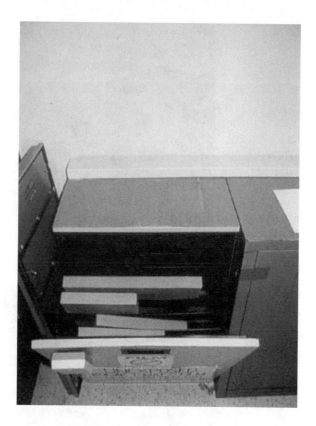

FIGURE 1.15
Film bin.

The Film Bin

The fresh film is stored in the film bin (Figure 1.15). The bin opens by pulling the handle on the front toward the operator. The bin is divided into sections so that each film size can be stored separately from the others. The smallest film is toward the front; this provides better balance for the bin when a counter is not installed over the bin. Do not remove the box from the bin. Remove the top and get the unexposed film. Immediately place the unexposed film in the cassette and close the cassette. Always replace the top on the box in the film bin. Close the bin in which the cassette has been reloaded.

The Film

The film has emulsion on both sides so one does not need to be concerned about how it goes in the cassette. The box has a metallic paper wrapper inside. There is a piece of white cardboard on each side of the film to protect the film. Do not remove the cardboard; it is thicker than film, so one should be able to distinguish it from the film. Always make sure that hands are clean and dry when handling the film. Use a light grip on the edges of the film to avoid bending the film base; which would cause a crinkle artifact on the film.

Film should always be stored in a cool, dry place. The film stock should be rotated. Use the oldest box when replacing the film in the film bin. If the X-ray facility is in an office, do not turn off the air conditioning on weekends, as heat will fog the film very quickly. The film will also fog when it gets old and out of date. Be careful when purchasing film; fresh film will have a shelf life of at least 12 months.

Conclusion

Working in the darkroom requires proper care of the equipment located therein. The safelight needs to be monitored to ensure that the filtration is correct. The correct wattage bulb must be installed in the safelight. The darkroom should be checked for light leaks and any leaks should be repaired.

The countertop needs to be clean and free of dust or liquids that could produce artifacts on the film. The processor should be in good working order and totally warmed up before films are processed. The water must be turned on to provide adequate washing of the film and cooling of the developer. Always feed the film into the processor next to one of the feed tray rails. (This author always uses the left rail as it is closest to the film transport drive.) Small films such as 8 in. × 10 in. films can jam the processor if fed crooked or down the middle of the tray.

The fresh chemical tanks should be monitored and not allowed to run dry. The lids on the tanks should always remain on the tanks to avoid fumes and oxidation of the chemicals. Remember that fresh chemicals are not hazardous waste and can be dumped down the drain when diluted with water. When working with chemicals, eye protection and gloves should be used. Avoid contact of chemicals with clothing.

The used fixer is a hazardous waste and should never be dumped down a drain. It contains silver, which is toxic to aquatic life. Follow local hazardous waste regulations. Generally, containers holding used fixer must be labeled as hazardous waste and put in secondary containment.

The film must be stored in a cool, dry space. It should be handled only by the edges and in a properly safelighted darkroom. Hands should be clean and dry when handling film or touching the screens in the cassette. The film bin is opened only when the door to the darkroom is locked and the safelight is on. Avoid taking the film box out of the film bin. Take the top off, retrieve a fresh sheet of film, and replace the top. Close the bin when finished with the bin.

The cassettes should be cleaned periodically. When loading and unloading, avoid opening them all the way. Just open them far enough to remove or replace the film. This will add years to the life of the hinges of the cassette.

1.5   Film Processing and the Environment

The improper handling of film-processing chemicals can be hazardous for both the operator and the environment. Larger offices and medical imaging departments must deal with the Office of Occupational Health and Safety regulations, which have "Worker's Right to Know" requirements. It is equally important for the operator and office staff to know what they are dealing with when at work. Upon request, the manufacturer or supplier of film-processing chemicals will provide a document known as the Material Safety Data Sheet (MSDS); it lists the chemical composition of the product and hazards associated with its use. Many counties require the Hazardous Waste Diamond Code System established by the National Fire Prevention Association. Working-strength developer and fixer have a slight health hazard (Blue) One Code. Fire (Red), Reactivity (Yellow), and Specific Hazard (White) Codes are all zero.

Most state and local governments have hazardous chemical and waste regulations that one must follow if films are processed in the office. The company that provides film-processing supplies will help meet these requirements. The actual manufacturer of the chemicals will also be of great assistance. If the operator has a copy of the MSDS, it will be easier to meet the hazardous materials standards.

The Darkroom

Operator safety is as important as the environment. Facilities to wash hands and eyewash facilities should be available. Eye protection and rubber gloves must be used when handling the processing chemicals. Fresh chemicals should be stored in air-tight containers with floating tops to minimize oxidation in the tanks. Keeping the lids on the tanks when not adding fresh chemicals will reduce the fumes in the darkroom. Ventilation is the key factor for operator protection. The fumes from the chemicals will damage the processor — so imagine what they can do to the operator without good ventilation. There should be eight to ten air changes per hour. The exhaust from the processor should be directed out of a separate exhaust.

The darkroom should be painted a light pastel color. Flat or semigloss paint should be used. Never use high-gloss paint, as it will reflect light leaks. Light colors will reflect some of the light from the safelight to better illuminate the work area of the darkroom. One or more safelights can be installed. The safelight should be a filter that is consistent with the type of film being used. The safelight should be 4 feet above the work surface.

Developer

The developer contains some fairly hazardous chemicals. If mixing one's own chemicals, one will be exposed to much higher chemical concentrations. Today, most offices and even major medical institutions have ready-mixed chemicals delivered in working strength. This significantly reduces exposure because working-strength processing chemicals are about 85 to 90% water.

The developer has a slight odor and is yellow in color. It turns brown as it ages and becomes exhausted. It is the first chemical that the film is exposed to during processing. It is also easily contaminated if even minute amounts of fixer are put into the developer tank.

The principal ingredients of developer are:

Ingredient	Concentration	Action
Water	85–90%	Solvent
Potassium sulfite	5–10%	Preservative
Hydroquinone	2%	Develops exposed silver bromide
Potassium acetate	1–5%	
Glutaraldehyde BIS (sodium bisulfite)	1–5%	Hardener
Potassium hydroxide	1–5%	Accelerator

The most hazardous chemicals in the developer are hydroquinone, potassium hydroxide, and glutaraldehyde. They can cause skin and eye irritation, and some people will be allergic to the chemicals. Developer will permanently stain and ruin clothing. Gloves and eye protection with side shields should be used when handling the developer. Hydroquinone can be absorbed through the skin. Wash thoroughly after any contact with developer. An eyewash bath should be available.

The used developer can retain some silver if the processor is not operating properly. Many counties require testing the developer for silver before disposal. They may require an LD50 test to prove that it can be dumped down the drain. The test involves pouring used developer into a container with live minnows. If the minnows die, the chemical is deemed a hazardous material. This test is very expensive; but if Kodak chemicals are used, they can provide a copy of the test. Both fresh and used developer can be safely disposed of in the normal sewer system. As with all chemicals, dilute with water when disposing of the developer. The tanks that hold fresh developer should be air-tight and have a floating inner lid to reduce oxidation of the developer and minimize fumes in the storage area. This oxidation or reduction reaction starts as soon as the developer is mixed.

Oxidized developer will turn dark brown. It will also smell like ammonia.

Fixer

The fixer has a rather offensive smell, similar to vinegar or acetic acid. It is a clear liquid. Until film comes into contact with the fixer, it is relatively harmless and can be disposed of through the sewer system. It is corrosive to metal. The fixer tank in the processor will need to be replaced periodically. The function of the fixer is to stop development and remove the unexposed silver bromide from the film emulsion. The remaining emulsion is then hardened.

The principal ingredients of the fixer are:

Component	Weight %	Function
Water	80–85%	Solvent
Ammonium thiosulfate	10–15%	Removes unexposed silver bromide from film
Sodium thiosulfate	1–5%	Removes unexposed silver bromide from film
Acetic acid	1–5%	Stops development, preservative
Ammonium sulfite	<1%	Preservative
Gluconic acid	<1%	

The hazards of handling fresh fixer are due to its acidic nature. The smell and fumes can be irritating to the respiratory system and eyes. It will also irritate the skin. Both skin and eye protection should be used when working with or handling fresh fixer. Tanks that hold the fresh fixer should be air tight to keep the fumes to a minimum.

Used fixer is a hazardous material due to the silver content. It must be disposed of by licensed hazardous waste companies. They are able to remove and recycle the silver. Most states will require the shipment to be manifested as other toxic substances. Keep the used fixer in secondary containment. A plastic garbage can with a lid works very well as secondary containment. If the container leaks, the waste fixer will be captured in the plastic waste can. Check the hazardous waste container for possible leaks or overflow on a weekly basis. It can be very expensive to remove the silver from floors and carpets.

Wash Water

The last solution that the film goes through during processing is water. The wash water removes any residual fixer from the film before it goes into the dryer. There should be a continuous flow of cool fresh water into the wash tank when films are being processed. If there is not a continuous water flow, the silver bromide in the residual fixer in the wash water will require hazardous waste treatment. In hospitals, the wash water from motion picture film processors is treated before discharge because of the perforations on the 135 mm film. The perforations will carry too much fixer into the wash water.

Conclusion

By being familiar with the chemical properties and characteristics of these chemicals, when a processor has a leak, one will be able to safely contain and clean up the leak. Immediately kill the electrical power to the processor.

If the leak is yellow or brown, it will usually be developer. A clear liquid that is odorless will usually be wash water. This is probably the most common leak. Algea like to grow in the wash tank. It can clog the wash tank overflow. In either of the above situations, simply mop the liquid, as it does not require hazardous waste treatment.

If the spill smells like vinegar or acetic acid and is clear, it is probably fixer and requires hazardous materials handling. The spilled fixer and all materials used to clean up the spill will be contaminated. They will need to be disposed of by a hazardous waste facility. Fixer spills are rare. One will need to have a contingency plan to handle a fixer spill in a darkroom. Spill containment kits are not very expensive. The Contingency Plan for Palmer College of Chiropractic–West is included.

Palmer College of Chiropractic-West Contingency Plan X-ray Department Processor Spill Procedures

Policy

The release of any liquids from the automatic processor shall be immediately evaluated for the potential of a hazardous waste release. The color and odor of the spill will suggest the nature of the spill. If the spill is fixer from the processor, it is a hazardous waste spill.

Chemical Storage Policy

Fresh fixer and developer are stored in tanks with secondary containment. Air-tight lids shall always be installed to minimize fumes and oxidation of the chemicals. Used fixer is automatically dumped into ORM-E containers that are in secondary containment. Used fixer is removed from Palmer College by an approved hazardous waste hauler, California Radiographics.

Processor Spill Procedures

1. In case of a liquid spill from the automatic film processor, the processor shall be immediately turned off and unplugged from the power. The water shall be turned off.

2. The cover to the processor will be removed and a determination as to the source of the leak shall be made. The color and odor of the spill will help in this process.

    a. If the color is brown or not clear, it is a spill from the developer tank or clogged overflow drain.

    b. If the spill is clear and odorless, it is water from the wash tank. This is the result of algae buildup in the drain. This is the most common source of a processor spill.

    c. A clear liquid spill with the smell of acetic acid or ammonia is a fixer spill. A tank rupture or leak in the plastic tubing going to the hazardous waste storage bottle must be suspected. This is a hazardous waste spill.

3. Once the source of the spill is decided, corrective action shall be taken to correct the problem. If it is a hazardous waste spill, notify the appropriate personnel. A spill containment kit stored under the main cabinet in the darkroom shall be obtained and the department shall follow the direction of supervisor in charge. The Spill Containment Kits are stored in the darkroom at all clinics.

4. Processor service provider shall be notified if repairs are needed on the processor before turning on power or the water.

5. The Incident Report Form shall be completed for any chemical spill. If the spill is used fixer, the orange Palmer College Emergency Incident Report shall be started.

Developer Tank Leak (brown or yellow colored leak)

1. Developer should always be handled with gloves and eye protection in place. Developer contains some hazardous chemicals. Contact with the skin and clothing must be avoided. Refer to the Material Safety

Data Sheet for more details. It is not a hazardous waste when diluted with water and can be cleaned up using normal housekeeping methods. Liquid from the cleanup does need to be diluted and can be dumped down a drain with fresh water.

2. It will stain any clothing contaminated. The spill should be completely cleaned up and surfaces of the processor dry before normal service is resumed.

3. In some processors, an overflow from the wash tank can contaminate the fixer and developer and result in this type of spill. If the developer is milky in appearance, it is probably contaminated by some fixer. This will require a complete chemical change and new developer filter. The service company must be notified. In this case, the developer in the processor must be considered hazardous waste. Processor quality control should be done before cases are processed to assure that the developer is not contaminated.

Wash Water Leak (clear and odorless liquid)

1. Wash water can be cleaned up using typical housekeeping methods. No significant hazards or precautions need to be taken.

2. Monthly cleaning of the processor and draining of the wash tank at shutdown will help control algae. Algae is the primary cause of wash water spills as it will clog the drain.

3. All components of the processor must be dry before power can be turned on and operation resumed.

4. Processor quality control must be done before resuming operations.

Fixer Spill (clear liquid with the smell of vinegar or acetic acid)

1. If the leak is coming from the tank or lines going to silver recovery, it is a hazardous waste spill. If the tank and line to recovery are intact, it can be from the replenisher pump or line coming from the fresh chemical tank. If the pump is the source of the leak, it is not a hazardous waste spill and the same protocol as for developer spills can be used.

2. The area of the spill needs to be contained as quickly as possible with a spill kit. The use of booms are encouraged. Liquids can be vacuumed using a wet/dry vacuum and then poured into the hazardous waste drums.

3. Booms or any other material used to clean up the spill shall be placed into a plastic pail and labeled as hazardous waste.

4. The disposal of the waste shall be in accordance with Title 22 requirements for hazardous waste disposal. A manifest shall be completed and disposal shall be in a hazardous waste facility.

5. Any release of hazardous waste must be reported to the appropriate county agencies.

Manual and Automatic Processing

Manual Processing

There are two basic methods of processing radiographic film. Prior to the 1960s, the most common way to process X-ray films was by manual processing. The entire process from removing the film from the cassette to having a film ready to be interpreted would take about 1 hour. Much of this time was devoted to film drying. Today's automatic processors can completely process a film in 30 seconds using special film and chemicals. Most processors used today process the film in 90 to 140 seconds for general radiographic film. The developer temperature is commonly from 91 to 95°F.

Manual processing is sometimes referred to as the Time and Temperature Method of processing. The developer and fixer tanks were immersed in a large container of water. The typical manual processing developer or fixer tank would hold about 5 gallons. The temperature of the chemicals was controlled by the temperature of the wash water. The water temperature was controlled by a large mixing valve. The optimum developer temperature was 68°F. The chemicals had to be stirred each morning and the level checked. The film was clipped on a special metal hanger after it was removed from the cassette. With the film in the developer tank, the hanger was tapped against the sides of the tank or dipped in and out of the tank to provide agitation of the developer. At 68°F, the timer was set for 5 minutes to have complete development of the film.

With great care, the film was removed from the developer tank. The object was to avoid having the developer on the film drain back into the developer tank. The used developer was drained into the wash water. The film would either be placed into a stop bath tank, which stopped development, or into continuous running water for at least 30 seconds.

The film was then placed in the fixer tank for the amount of time recommended by the film manufacturer. The film had to be agitated for the first minute of fixation. The typical fix tank time was from 5 to 10 minutes. The film was then placed in the wash water for 5 to 30 minutes. The water flow going into the wash tank was changed about eight times per hour. The films had to be carefully spaced in the tank to ensure that the water cleaned all of the film and ran over the top of the film holder.

If possible, a tank containing a wetting agent was the next stop for the film before it went into the dryer. The wetting agent would minimize the water spots on the film much like additives used today for automatic dishwashers. As much of the liquid was allowed to drain back into the tanks before the film was hung on racks to air dry or placed in the dryer. Some of the film was prone to cracking if left in the dryer too long. When dry, the film was removed from the hangers and the edges clipped.

The person who manually processed films wore a long rubber apron and gloves to avoid skin contact with the chemicals. After each process, fresh chemicals were added to the tanks to replenish the chemicals.

There are some people who continue to manually process films today. Unfortunately, many of the most modern films cannot be manually processed. The hazards of working with film processing chemicals is significantly higher with manual processing.

Introduction to Automatic Processing

The cost of automatic processors has dropped over the years. A reasonably good desktop 90-second processor can be purchased for about $2000. The original Paku processor used in 1943 cost $43,000 and would fill an 8 × 10 ft room. In current dollars, the cost would be $120,000. It took 45 minutes to process the film. Eastman Kodak developed an offset roller film transport system with their X-OMAT processor that made them more reliable; this system is the foundation of all automatic processors sold today. The film travels through the processor tanks in a serpentine path, which provides superior agitation and uniform development.

The operator must still be careful in the darkroom. The film used for automatic processing has a thinner layer of emulsion on the film to speed the development. It needs to be handled with care. The film should be handled by its edges with very clean and dry hands.

The film should always be placed lengthwise into the processor next to the rail of the feed tray. Small films are prone to jam in the processor if not fed lengthwise. The replenishment of the chemicals is also impacted by the way the film is placed in the processor.

Only one film can be placed in the processor at a time. The processor will make an audible tone when it is safe to place the next film into the processor. This time will depend on the size of the processor tanks as well as the total processing time. A desktop unit will run slower than a larger processor because of the smaller tanks. Development depends on the temperature of the developer and the amount of time the film is immersed in the developer. Processors are rated in terms of the number of 14 in. × 17 in. films that can be processed in 1 hour.

It is equally important that one does not turn on any white lights or open the darkroom door until the film is completely in the processor and the audible tone has sounded. Chapter 2 will cover working in the darkroom and processing films with automatic processing.

The following sections are examples of Material Safety Data Sheets (MSDSs) for markers and processing solutions.

1.6 Sample MSDS for Working-Strength Developer

Material Safety Data Sheet

200000418/F/USA - C-0133.500D

Approval Date: 2/16/1994

Print Date: 2/19/1994

Page 1

---

1. Chemical Product and Company Identification

Product Name: Kodak RP X-OMAT Developer Replenisher Working Solution

Catalog Number (s)   124 9259 - To Make   10 gallons (U.S.)
                     171 6828 — To Make 20 gallons (U.S.)
                     131 8989 — To Make 200 gallons (U.S.) — Part A
                     817 0748 — To Make 200 gallons (U.S.) — Part A
                     162 0509 — To Make 200 gallons (U.S.) — Part B & C

Manufacturer/Supplier: EASTMAN KODAK COMPANY, ROCHESTER, NY 14650

For Emergency Health, Safety & Environmental Information, call: 716-722-5151

For Other Information, call the Marketing and Distribution Center in your area.

Synonym(s): KAN 441665, C-0133.500, Contains: PCD 5468 - Part A, PCD 5228 — Part B, PCD 5250 — Part C

---

2. Composition/Information on Ingredients

Weight %	Component	(CAS Registry No.)
85–90	Water	(007732-18-5)
5–10	Potassium sulfite	(010117-38-1)
2	Hydroquinone	(000123-31-9)
1–5	Potassium acetate	(000127-08-02)
1–5	Glutaraldehyde bis (sodium bisulfite)	(007420-89-5)
1–5	Potassium hydroxide	(001310-58-3)

---

3. Hazard Identification

[WARNING] CONTAINS: Hydroquinone (000123-31-9), potassium hydroxide (001310-58-3)

CAUSES SKIN AND EYE IRRITATION

MAY CAUSE ALLERGIC SKIN REACTION

HMIS Hazard Ratings:

Health — 2   Flammability — 0   Reactivity — 0   Personnel Protection — C

NFPA Hazard Rating:

Health — 1,   Flammability — 0,   Reactivity (Stability) — 0,

Note: HMIS and NFPA ratings involve data and interpretations that may vary from company to company. They are intended only for rapid, general identification of the magnitude of a specific hazard. To adequately deal with the safe handling of this material, all information contained in this MSDS must be considered.

---

4. First-Aid Measures

Inhalation: Move to fresh air. Treat symptomatically. Get medical attention if symptoms occur.

Eyes: Immediately flush with plenty of water for at least 15 minutes. Get medical attention.

Skin: Immediately flush with plenty of water and wash with a non-alkaline (acid) type skin cleaner. If skin irritation or an allergic reaction develops, get medical attention. Remove contaminated clothing and shoes. Wash contaminated clothing before reuse. Destroy or thoroughly clean contaminated shoes.

Ingestion: Drink 1–2 glasses of water. Seek medical attention.

5. Fire-Fighting Measures

Extinguishing Media: Use appropriate agent for adjacent fire.

Special Fire-Fighting Procedures: Wear self-contained breathing apparatus and protective clothing. Fire or excessive heat may produce hazardous decomposition products.

Hazardous Combustion Products: None (noncombustible), (see also Hazardous Decomposition Products section).

Unusual Fire and Explosion Hazards: None

6. Accidental Release Measures

Flush to sewer with large amounts of water. Otherwise, absorb spill with vermiculite or other inert material, then place in a container for chemical waste. Clean surface thoroughly to remove residual contamination.

7. Handling and Storage

Personal Precautionary Measures: Avoid contact with eyes, skin, and clothing. Use with adequate ventilation. Wash thoroughly after handling. The routine use of a non-alkaline (acid) type hand cleaner and regular cleaning of working surfaces, gloves, etc. will help minimize the possibility of a skin reaction.

Prevention of Fire and Explosion: No special precautionary measures should be needed under anticipated conditions of use.

Storage: Keep container closed. Keep away from incompatible substances (see Incompatibility section).

8. Exposure Controls/Personal Protection

Exposure limits:
  ACGIH Threshold Limit Value (TLV):
    Hydroquinone: 2 mg/m^3 TWA
    Potassium hydroxide: 2 mg/m^3 ceiling
  OSHA (USA) Permissible Exposure Limit (PEL)
    Hydroquinone: 2 mg/m^3 TWA
    Potassium hydroxide: 2 mg/m^3 ceiling

Ventilation: Good general ventilation (typically 10 air changes per hour) should be used. Ventilation rates should be matched to conditions. Use process enclosures, local exhaust ventilation, or other engineering controls to maintain airborne levels below exposure limits.

Respiratory Protection: None should be needed.

Eye Protection: Wear safety glasses with side shields (or goggles).

Skin Protection: Wear impervious gloves and protective clothing appropriate for the risk of exposure.

Recommended Decontamination Facilities: Eye bath, washing facilities, safety shower.

9. Physical and Chemical Properties

Physical Form: Liquid

Color: Yellow

Odor: Slight

Specific gravity: (water = 1) 1.086

Vapor pressure at 20°C (68°F): 24 mbar (18 mmHg)

Vapor density (air = 1): 0.6

Volatile fraction by weight: 85–90%

Boiling point: >100°C (>212°F)

Solubility in water: Complete

pH: 10.3

Flashpoint: None

10.   Stability and Reactivity

Stability: Stable

Incompatibility: Strong acids

Hazardous Decomposition Products: Carbon dioxide, carbon monoxide, sulfur dioxide

Hazardous Polymerization: Will not occur

11.   Toxicological Information

Effects of exposure:
   Inhalation: Expected to be low hazard for recommended handling.
   Eyes: Causes Irritation
   Skin: Causes irritation. May cause allergic reaction.
   Ingestion: Expected to be low ingestion hazard. May cause irritation of the gastrointestinal tract.

12.   Ecological Information

Introduction: This environmental effects summary is written to assist in addressing emergencies created by an accidental spill which might occur during the shipment of this material, and, in general it is not meant to address discharges to sanitary sewers or publically owned treatment works.

Summary: Data for the major components of this material have been used to estimate the environmental impact of this material. This material has not been tested. This material is a moderately alkaline aqueous solution, and this property may cause adverse environmental effects.

It is expected to have the following properties: A low biochemical oxygen demand and little potential to cause oxygen depletion in aqueous systems, a high potential to affect some aquatic organisms, a moderate potential to affect secondary waste treatment microbial metabolism, a low potential to affect germination and/or early plant growth, a low potential to persist in the environment, a low potential for bioconcentrate. After a large amount of water, followed by secondary waste treatment, this material is not expected to cause adverse environmental effects.

13.   Disposal Considerations

Discharge, treatment, or disposal may be subject to national, state, or local laws. Flush to sewer with large amounts of water.

14.   Transport Information

For transportation information regarding this product, please phone the Eastman Kodak Distribution Center nearest you.

15.   Regulatory Information

Material(s) known to the State of California to cause cancer: None

Material(s) know to the State of California to cause adverse reproductive effects: None

Carcinogenicity Classification (components at 0.1% or more):

   International Agency for Research on Cancer (IARC): None

   American Conference of Governmental Industrial Hygienists (ACGIH): None

National Toxicology Program (NTP): None

Occupational Safety and Health Administration (OSHA): None

Chemical(s) subject to the reporting requirements of Section 313 or Title III of the Superfund Amendments and Reauthorization Act (SARA) of 1986 and 40CFR Part 372: Hydroquinone

16.   Other Information

U.S./Canadian Label Statements

Contains: Hydroquinone (000123-31-9), potassium hydroxide (001310-58-3)

WARNING

CAUSES SKIN AND EYE IRRITATION

MAY CAUSE ALLERGIC SKIN REACTION

Avoid contact with eyes, skin, and clothing.

Wash thoroughly after handling.

First Aid: In case of eye contact, immediately flush eyes with plenty of water for at least 15 minutes. In case of skin contact, wash skin with soap and plenty of water. Get medical attention. Remove contaminated clothing and shoes. Wash before reuse. Destroy or thoroughly clean shoes.

Keep out of reach of children.

Additional precautions for containers greater than 1 gallon of liquid or 5 pounds of solids:

Since empties containers retain product residue, follow label warnings even after container is emptied.

The information contained herein is furnished without warranty of any kind. Users should consider these data only as a supplement to other information gathered by them and must make independent determinations of the suitability and completeness of information from all sources to assure proper use and disposal of these materials and the health and safety of employees and customers and the protection of the environment.

Note: This is an example of a MSDS sheet for developer. For definitive information or current data, contact the manufacturer of the developer that your facility purchases.

1.7   Sample MSDS for Working-Strength Fixer

Material Safety Data Sheet

200000601/F/USA - C-0026.000J

Approval Date: 2/16/1994

Print Date: 2/19/1994

Page 1

1.   Chemical Product and Company Identification

Product Name: Kodak RP X-OMAT Fixer and Replenisher Working Solution

Catalog Number(s)   180 5076 — To Make   4 gallons (U.S.) — Part A
180 5118 — To Make   20 gallons (U.S.) — Part A
180 5134 — To Make 200 gallons (U.S.) — Part A
804 4083 — To Make 200 gallons (U.S.) — Part A
820 6112 — To Make 200 gallons (U.S.) — Part B

Manufacturer/Supplier: EASTMAN KODAK COMPANY, ROCHESTER, NY 14650

For Emergency Health, Safety & Environmental Information, call : 716-722-5151

For Other Information, call the Marketing and Distribution Center in your area.

Synonym(s): Part A : KAN 448590; PCD 5538: D-0026.000, Working solution: KAN 965743; contains: PCD 5538 — Part A, PCD 5597 — Part B

2. Composition/Information on Ingredients

Weight %	Component	(CAS Registry No.)
80–85	Water	(007732-18-5)
10–15	Ammonium thiosulfate	(007783-18-8)
1–5	Sodium thiosulfate	(007772-98-7)
1–5	Acetic acid	(000064-19-7)
<1	Ammonium sulfite	(010196-04-0)

3. Hazard Identification

LOW HAZARD FOR RECOMMENDED HANDLING

4. First Aid Measures

Inhalation: If symptomatic, move to fresh air. Get medical attention if symptoms occur.

Eyes: Immediately flush with plenty of water for at least 15 minutes. Get medical attention.

Skin: Immediately flush with plenty of water and wash with a skin cleaner. Get medical attention if symptoms occur.

Ingestion: Drink 1–2 glasses of water. Seek medical attention.

5. Fire-Fighting Measures

Extinguishing Media: Use appropriate agent for adjacent fire.

Special Fire-Fighting Procedures: Wear self-contained breathing apparatus and protective clothing. Fire or excessive heat may produce hazardous decomposition products.

Hazardous Combustion Products: None (noncombustible), (see also Hazardous Decomposition Products section).

Unusual Fire and Explosion Hazards: None

6. Accidental Release Measures

Flush to sewer with large amounts of water.

7. Handling and Storage

Personal Precautionary Measures: Use with adequate ventilation. Wash thoroughly after handling.

Prevention of Fire and Explosion: No special precautionary measures should be needed under anticipated conditions of use.

Storage: Keep container closed. Keep away from incompatible substances (see Incompatibility section).

8. Exposure Controls/Personal Protection

Exposure limits:
  ACGIH Threshold Limit Value (TLV):
    Sodium bisulfite: 5 mg/m3 TWA
    Acetic acid: 10 ppm TWA, 15 ppm STEL

OSHA (USA) Permissible Exposure Limit (PEL)

Sodium bisulfite: 5 mg/m3 TWA

Acetic acid : 10 ppm

Ventilation: Good general ventilation (typically 10 air changes per hour) should be used. Ventilation rates should be matched to conditions. Use process enclosures, local exhaust ventilation, or other engineering controls to maintain airborne levels below exposure limits.

Respiratory Protection: None should be needed.

Eye Protection: Wear safety glasses with side shields (or goggles).

Skin Protection: Wear impervious gloves and protective clothing appropriate for the risk of exposure.

Recommended Decontamination Facilities: Eye bath, washing facilities, safety shower.

9.   Physical and Chemical Properties

Physical Form: Liquid

Color: Colorless

Odor: Slight ammonia or vinegar

Specific gravity: (water = 1) not available

Vapor pressure at 20°C (68°F): 24 mbar (18 mmHg)

Vapor density (air = 1): 0.6

Volatile fraction by weight: 81%

Boiling point: >100°C (>212°F)

Solubility in water: Complete

pH: 4.1

Flashpoint: None

10.   Chemical Product and Company Identification

Stability and Reactivity

Stability: Stable

Incompatibility: Strong acids

Hazardous Decomposition Products: Ammonia, sulfur dioxide, nitrogen oxides (NOx)

Hazardous Polymerization: Will not occur

11.   Toxicological Information

Effects of Exposure:

Inhalation: Expected to be low hazard for recommended handling.

Eyes: No specific hazard. May cause transient irritation.

Skin: Low hazard for recommended handling.

Ingestion: Expected to be low ingestion hazard.

12.   Ecological Information

Introduction: This environmental effects summary is written to assist in addressing emergencies created by an accidental spill which might occur during the shipment of this material and, in general, it is not meant to address discharges to sanitary sewers or publically owned treatment works.

Summary: Data for the major components of this material have been used to estimate the environmental impact of this material. This material has not been tested. This material is a moderately alkaline aqueous solution, and this property may cause adverse environmental effects.

It is expected to have the following properties: A low biochemical oxygen demand and little potential to cause oxygen depletion in aqueous systems, a high potential to affect some aquatic organisms, a moderate potential to affect secondary waste treatment microbial metabolism, a low potential to affect germination and/or early plant growth, a low potential to persist in the environment, a low potential for bioconcentrate. After a large amount of water, followed by secondary waste treatment, this material is not expected to cause adverse environmental effects.

13. Disposal Considerations

Discharge, treatment, or disposal may be subject to national, state, or local laws. Flush to sewer with large amounts of water.

14. Transport Information

For transportation information regarding this product, please phone the Eastman Kodak Distribution Center nearest you.

15. Regulatory Information

Material(s) known to the State of California to cause cancer: None

Material(s) know to the State of California to cause adverse reproductive effects: None

Carcinogenicity Classification (components at 0.1% or more):

International Agency for Research on Cancer (IARC): None

American Conference of Governmental Industrial Hygienists (ACGIH): None

National Toxicology Program (NTP): None

Occupational Safety and Health Administration (OSHA): None

Chemical(s) subject to the reporting requirements of Section 313 or Title III of the Superfund Amendments and Reauthorization Act (SARA) of 1986 and 40CFR Part 372: None

16. Other Information

U.S./Canadian Label Statements

LOW HAZARD FOR RECOMMENDED HANDLING

Keep out of reach of children.

Additional precautions for containers greater than 1 gallon of liquid or 5 pounds of solids:

IN CASE OF SPILL: Absorb spill with inert material, then place in a chemical waste container. Flush residual spill or area with water. For large spills, dikes for later disposal. Prevent runoff from entering drains, sewers, and streams.

The information contained herein is furnished without warranty of any kind. Users should consider these data only as a supplement to other information gathered by them and must make independent determinations of the suitability and completeness of information from all sources to assure proper use and disposal of these materials and the health and safety of employees and customers and the protection of the environment.

Note: This is an example of a MSDS sheet for developer. For definitive information or current data, contact the manufacturer of the developer that your facility purchases.

Chapter 2

Radiation Safety in Chiropractic Radiography

The Radiographic Room

Radiation safety starts with the design of the radiographic room. There are state and federal standards for the shielding of the room that must be met. It is important that the radiation, both primary and scatter, be limited to the radiographic room. The dressing area, office, and adjoining spaces should be radiation-free. Shielding needs to extend up 7 feet in the walls of the room. The door to the room may need to be lead lined. Consult a radiation physicist to perform the shielding calculations for the X-ray room. Retain the report as part of office permanent records.

When designing the room, allow for a control booth that is large enough for the operator, the control panel, technique charts, and enough cassettes to complete the study. A leaded glass window for observing the patient while remaining fully shielded is very important for operator safety. Being able to monitor the patient just before and during exposure is important in reducing errors.

The rooms should be large enough to perform all of the studies that may be needed by the patient. It is advisable to own a radiographic table for taking extremity and recumbent views. The size of a table and the ability to get 6 feet from the wall Bucky film holder should be considered when allotting space for X-ray. There should also be space in the room to store radiographic positioning sponges, compensating filters, lead blockers, and gonad protection.

Make sure that the film storage and darkroom will not be subjected to scatter or primary radiation. The author does not recommend that the darkroom be attached to the X-ray room. Both the operator and the patients will be exposed to the processing chemical fumes. The darkroom should be close enough to reduce any possibility of injury while carrying cassettes to the darkroom. If the X-ray control room is too small to hold the unexposed cassettes, storage space should be provided in the darkroom. Air conditioned space must be available to store the unexposed and fresh film.

It is nice for the patient's modesty to have the dressing area adjacent to the radiographic room. If it opens into the room, one will be limited to only one patient at a time changing into the gown.

Film and Screen Combination and Equipment Type

The relative speed value (RSV) of the screen and film combination will have a dramatic impact on radiation exposure. As with photographic film, the higher the RSV, the lower the exposure needed to produce a good radiograph. For Bucky work, rare-earth screens are now the community standard. The typical RSV for these systems is from 400 to 800. Older calcium tungstate screens ranged from 100 for par speed to 200 for high speed or high speed plus. The 400 speed system will require 25% of the exposure that a 100 speed system needs to produce the same density on the film. System speeds range up to about 1600. The very high speed systems will typically produce a lot of noise or a grainy image that will potentially impact resolution; these are not recommended for general radiography. Extremity radiography should not be done on 400 speed or higher imaging systems. The kVp must be reduced so low and the resolution becomes so poor that fine detail is lost. Special fine detail cassettes should be used for Non-Bucky extremity studies.

To achieve the desired image quality and low radiation exposure, the film should match the screens. One does not necessarily need to use the same manufacturer, but make sure that the light spectrum or sensitivity of the film matches the spectrum produced by the screens. Green-sensitive film is used with green light-producing screens. The older calcium tungstate screens produced a blue/green light.

The type of radiographic generator will have a significant impact on radiation exposure. The more efficient the beam generation, the lower the exposure needed to produce the same film. Single-phase units need twice as much exposure compared to three-phase or high-frequency generators. The typical patient exposure is reduced by over 35% when high-frequency or three-phase generators are used. Exposure times are faster, so the small focal spots can be used to improve detail.

Proper installation is very important. Improperly installed wall grids result in grid cut-off. The grid must be perfectly perpendicular to the beam. Misalignment by more than 2° will produce grid cut-off. The grid ratio should be high enough to provide proper cleanup of the film. The minimum grid ratio should be 10:1 for good spinal radiography. The collimator must also be accurately calibrated in terms of source to film distance and restriction. Federal law requires accuracy to within 2%. At 40 in. SID, the tolerance is about 0.8 in. The author prefers to have the shutters adjusted tight within these tolerances; that way, when collimated slightly less than film size, one seee a border on the film.

Accessories such as calipers, the Nolan filtration system, lead blockers, lead aprons, and radiographic sponges are some of the key tools for proper radiation safety. The proper use of these items will demonstrate a commitment to keep the exposure for the patient as low as reasonably achievable (referred to as the ALARA standard). The use of compensating filters will reduce the exposure to parts of the patient's anatomy that are less dense. It will improve image quality as well as lower the dose for the patient. Lead blockers are used to eliminate any film fogging from scatter radiation on extremity views. This will reduce the number of retakes. Lead aprons are used by the patient for gonadal protection and by the operator if there is a need to be in the room during an exposure.

Operator Radiation Safety

If the control booth of the radiographic room is properly shielded and a leaded window large enough to monitor the patient is provided, plain film radiography should never present any health hazard to the operator. The operator should always stand completely within the control booth, and avoid peeking around the edge of the primary barrier during the exposure.

The primary radiation exposure to radiologic technologists and radiologists in medical radiography is during fluoroscopic studies and portable radiography. Even in these instances, they can remain safe if they stay as far away from the radiation sources as possible. Since fluoroscopy is generally not used in chiropractic, this source of exposure is not a significant factor for the chiropractor.

The only potential hazard would be when holding patients or doing stress views that would require them to be in the room during the exposure. The holding of patients should be avoided except in emergency situations, which are unlikely in chiropractic. A family member should be used to hold a patient if it is necessary. They should be given a coat-type lead apron and leaded gloves of 0.5 mm lead. They should stand as far away from the primary beam as possible. The coat-type lead apron and leaded gloves should be used by the operator when stress views of an extremity are necessary.

If one is concerned about exposure potential, film badges for exposure monitoring are available. They typically cost only a few dollars per month and can be used to track lifetime exposure. In 3 years of chiropractic radiography, this author has not received any exposure. As long as fluoroscopy is not used and the X-ray room is shielded, one can expect no significant radiation exposure. This is important to doctors who are planning a family or may be pregnant. A pregnant radiographer is legally allowed 500 millirems during pregnancy.

Patient Radiation Safety

The safety of the patient depends on the quality of the radiographic system and the training and work practices of the operator. The proper use of calipers to obtain accurate measurements of the patient is the first step. Accurate measurements are used with the technique charts to achieve optimum exposure. Exposure errors with the film being too light or underexposed and the film being too dark or overexposed account for over half of the repeated films. Accurate technique charts and measurements would significantly reduce this trend. The operator should also know when to adjust the technical factors due to body habitus or pathologic factors. Each repeated film will add unnecessary exposure to ionizing radiation to the patient. Radiation exposure is culumative, as are its effects on the tissues.

The placement of the patient in relation to the beam can significantly reduce radiation exposure. Sometimes, the actual positioning can be modified from A-P view to P-A view to reduce exposure. Not placing the patient's lower extremities under the table used for upper extremity views will significantly reduce exposure to the blood-producing organs of the body.

Each region of the body has an optimum kilovoltage to properly penetrate the bone and tissues. For this reason, fixed kilovoltage technique charts should be used in general radiography. Because optimum penetration is so important, the highest possible kilovoltage (kVp) and lowest possible mAs should be used to keep the exposure to the patient as low as possible. The better penetrating beam will have a lower ionizing effect on the tissues. This will also provide proper contrast on the films and greater latitude in exposure.

The second major factor for patient radiation exposure is collimation of the beam. The area of exposure should never be larger than the film being used. The best was to prove this is to always collimate slightly smaller than film size. If the anatomy of clinical interest is smaller than film size, collimate to the anatomy. Restrict the beam to skin side to side on views of extremities and the cervical spine. In order to correctly collimate, one must know the essential anatomy for each view. Collimating so tight that the area of clinical interest is missed will result in a retake and more unnecessary exposure to the patient.

Some form of gonad protection should be used for all radiographic procedures except when it will obscure clinically necessary anatomy. A leaded half-apron is very useful for gonad protection for cervical spine and thoracic spine studies. Putting it on the patient demonstrates a conscious concern for the safety of the patient that the patient will appreciate. The apron should contain 0.5 mm lead for effective gonadal protection. The Nolan filtration system provides a lead bell for male patients and a heart-shaped filter for female patients. The Nolan system also provides a shadow-type gonadal shield for lateral and oblique lumbar spine views. Other companies manufacture different types of shadow shields that mount to the collimator and different contact shields that the patient can wear during radiography. Studies have demonstrated that contact shielding will provide the best possible protection.

Male patients are easier to shield. The Nolan filtration system provides a bell-shaped shield that is attached to a belt. If the bell is properly placed on the patient, it will provide good protection from the primary radiation for A-P views. The only exposure the patient will receive is secondary from the body. The collimator-mounted, shadow-type gonad shield works well on lumbar posterior or anterior oblique and lateral views of the lumbar spine. For male patients, it should be about 2 to 3 in. below the ASIS.

Female patients present a more difficult shielding problem. The exact location of the patient's ovaries is not known. The ovaries are usually located below the ASIS; and if a lead shield is used, it would cover the sacrum and sacroiliac joints. The irradiation of the ovum is dangerous at any time, and all possible steps should be taken to keep the exposure to a minimum. A heart-shaped filter can be used to reduce the exposure, or one can take the film P-A. Changes in positioning can be very useful for lumbar spinal views and serial scoliosis studies of the female patient of child-bearing age. By taking the film P-A, the pelvic bones will absorb most of the radiation and reduce the exposure to the ovaries by over 50%. For other lumbar spine views, the shadow-type gonad shield is used but placed at the level of the ASIS. The P-A full spine will also reduce exposure to the breast tissues for serial studies. The author does not recommend P-A views for the initial film because the divergent rays will degrade the cervical spine. Paraspinal shadow-type shields are used for the full spine to reduce breast and lung exposure.

There is what is called the Five Centimeter Rule, which states that with a properly functional collimator, anatomy more than 5 cm away from the beam will not receive significant primary radiation exposure. What exposure that anatomy will receive will be from scatter radiation within the patient's body. The use of the lead apron will provide no added protection other than to reassure the patient. However, reassurance is very important and helps build a stronger patient–doctor relationship.

The greatest concern in terms of radiation is the potential risk of exposure to a pregnant patient. The most dangerous time to expose a pregnant patient is when the embryo is in the earliest stages of development. This is also the time when the patient may not know that she is pregnant. For patients of child-bearing age (10 to 50 years), one can use the Ten Day Rule. The Ten Day Rule states that the safest time to radiograph a female of child-bearing age is within 10 days of the onset of menses. This may not be convenient for the acute patient. The use of birth-control measures and lifestyle can also be used. Under all circumstances, the patient should be asked if there is any potential of being pregnant and when was the start of their last menses. There should also be a sign in the dressing room in the languages of the patients that directs them to let the doctor/operator know if they may be pregnant.

Radiography of the Pregnant Patient

A pregnant patient should not be radiographed unless her symptoms are of such significance that proper care would be jeopardized without such radiographs. If films are needed, consultation with an orthopedist, radiologist, or obstetrician should be sought. The area of clinical interest will be one of the key factors when taking radiographs of a pregnant patient. The lumbar spine or pelvic region would provide the greatest potential harm and concern. The exposure to general radiography should not be a concern for any decision to terminate a pregnancy. The cervical spine and extremities are generally far enough away from the fetus that they add little risk to its development when a lead apron is used. Even the thoracic spine study consisting of A-P and lateral views will add only about 0.5 millirems to the fetal radiation exposure. Any exposure is going to add to the anxiety of the patient and should be avoided if possible.

Quality Assurance and Quality Control

The greatest potential for across-the-board radiation safety is to have functional quality assurance and quality control processes. The monitoring of machine radiation output and analysis of repeated films can help reduce the exposure to the patient. One should be able to tell the patient what the

TABLE 2.1
Potential Methods for Reduction of Patient Exposure

Method	Impact on Image Quality	Actions to Account for Impact
High kVp/low mAs techniques	Reduces contrast	Use optimum kVp for body part and view Use technique charts
Filtration	May reduce contrast	Use filters to equalize exposure Make sure that tube's half value layer is correct
Collimation	Increases contrast	Collimate to slightly less than film size or to area of clinical interest
Compression	Increases contrast	Obese patients may need to be imaged in prone or recumbent position
High-speed screens	Decreases detail	Use highest speed system that provides optimum detail
High-speed film	Decreases detail and increases mottle	Match film to screen system
Grid removal	Decreases contrast	Avoid, if possible, severe impact on quality. Use non-Bucky holder when indicated
Quality assurance that reduces repeats	Improved and consistent exposure	Includes processor quality control, preventive maintenance
Selection of procedures and views	Use body to reduce exposure to gonads	P-A lumbo-pelvic and anterior oblique use the bone to shield ovaries
Gonad shielding	Lead apron used for most views for patient assurance	Gonad shielding used when it will not interfere or cover area of clinical interest
Monitoring and communication with patient	Avoid retakes Ten Day Rule to avoid exposure of pregnant patient	Breathing instruction, gowning, and positioning direction avoids retakes

average-size patient would receive in radiation exposure for each examination that is routinely performed.

Having preventive and corrective service performed on X-ray and film processing equipment will keep the equipment operating at peak efficiency. One will be able to establish reliable technique charts and accurately collimate the film. One should also ensure that hazardous waste is properly handled; and in many cases, reduce waste. Quality assurance and quality control programs will be covered in detail later in this book (see Chapters 19 through 23).

The chart in Table 2.1 covers the basic principles of patient radiation protection. The remainder of the chapter is a sample radiation safety plan similar to ones used in medical radiology departments.

2.1   Sample Radiation Plan

Palmer College of Chiropractic–West is committed to ensuring that the level of ionizing radiation exposure to the staff, students and patients is as low as reasonably achievable. This is commonly known as ALARA.

The use of radiography in the field of chiropractic is the primary potential source of ionizing radiation exposure. The proper use of radiographic services is the key to keeping the exposure at achievable levels. The program is divided into three primary sections.

1.   The Radiographic Quality Assurance Program is used to monitor the performance of the radiographic equipment. This plan monitors and controls the variables of radiography to ensure that all equipment is in safe and proper working condition for both the operator and patient. This program also monitors radiation exposure to the patient.

2. Radiation monitoring via personnel monitoring for full-time X-ray personnel and area monitors is used to ensure that the occupational exposure to controlled and uncontrolled personnel is within regulatory limits as defined in Federal Codes 10 CFR-19 and 20 and the California Radiation Control Regulations (CCR), Title 17.

3. Policies and procedures are developed to establish standards of operation of radiographic equipment. The principles of radiation control as defined in state regulations and professional standards are the guidelines for these policies and procedures.

The Radiographic Quality Assurance Plan

The Radiographic Quality Assurance Plan is designed to provide the necessary monitoring of operational effectiveness of the radiographic systems used in the clinics. The monitoring and quality control of the variables of conventional radiography are key elements of the program to keep the radiation exposure to patients and staff as low as reasonably achievable.

The accuracy of equipment calibration — including collimator, kVp, and mAs — is monitored on a routine basis. The radiographic equipment receives preventive and corrective maintenance as recommended by the manufacturer.

The condition of the accessories — including grids, gonadal shields, and cassettes — is monitored. The cassettes and screens are cleaned monthly.

Patients are not exposed until the film processor is monitored and within operational standards. The processing equipment receives regular cleaning and preventive maintenance.

The repeat film rate for the clinics is monitored quarterly. The results of this monitoring are reported to the Chief of Clinics and the Chief of each clinic by the radiographer.

Radiation Exposure Monitoring

The area surrounding the radiographic equipment is considered a controlled area. Area control monitors are used to monitor the levels of exposure in these areas. The areas selected for monitoring within the X-ray department are those areas that may be occupied by staff or public during the performance of radiographic procedures. The monitoring is located as follows.

1. Tasman (Main Campus) Clinic
    a. Darkroom
    b. Control booth for Radiographic Room One
    c. Control booth for Radiographic Room Two
    d. Patient waiting/dressing room
    e. Radiologist office
2. Benton Clinic
    a. Radiology resident office
    b. Control room for radiographic room
3. Outreach Clinic
    a. Operator booth
    b. Corridor
    c. Darkroom

The film badges (or dosimeters) are changed on a monthly basis. The reports are monitored by the Radiographer of Palmer College. The Radiographer and Radiologists and Radiology Resident are the only personnel monitored; they are thus considered controlled personnel. The maximum legal exposure limit for these workers is 5 rem (0.05 Sievert) per year. The quarterly exposure limits have been eliminated with the current 10 CFR-20 regulations. ALARA requires that a limit be set below the legal limit. Most radiologic facilities set the limit at 10% of the legal limit (500 mrem or 0.005 Sv per year). This 10% below the limit is also the limit where film badges or personnel monitoring is required; 500 mrem is also the legal limit for exposure of declared-pregnant controlled personnel during the gestational period.

The radiation exposure limits for the remaining staff and students of Palmer College is 0.1 rem (1 mSv), as established by 10 CFR-20. The areas control monitoring film badges that are changed monthly. These control monitors are in fixed locations and monitor the total exposure in a specific area.

The dose in any unrestricted radiation control area may not exceed 0.002 rem or 0.02 mSv. The area control monitors in the dressing or waiting areas are used to ensure compliance with these limits. The exposure potential to staff is significantly reduced by the use of modern high-frequency and nonceiling-mounted radiographic equipment. The lack of fluoroscopic and portable radiographic equipment has the greatest impact on the low exposure potential. The X-ray exposure cannot be initiated outside the operator area or control booth. This implies that the monitoring of the control booth will detect any exposure to any staff during the month.

Radiation Safety Policies for the Staff

1. Radiographic equipment can be operated only by qualified and competent personnel. Students must have successfully completed the course on Radiologic Physics and started PB-322 Radiographic Positioning before they are allowed to produce a radiograph of a phantom. This image is under the direct supervision of the Radiographer. No exposures can be made by untrained personnel.

2. Before the use of X-ray on patients, the student must complete a series of ten sets of radiographs of phantoms meeting the same clinical quality standards used for patient studies and pass a clinical competency test. The performance of radiography on patients is then under the direct supervision of a Resident Radiographer. A more senior and experienced intern provides peer assistance during all human or patient radiographs.

3. No X-ray personnel may hold a patient during the radiographic exposure.

4. The door to the X-ray room must be closed during any radiographic exposure.

5. The operator will assure that only essential personnel remain in the room and they are behind the shielded barrier before initiating a radiographic exposure.

6. Staff will knock on the door of a closed radiographic room and gain entry by the operator opening the door. The doors to radiographic rooms will remain open when exposures are not being made. The doors will never be locked when the room is occupied.

7. The primary X-ray beam should never be directed at the control area.

8. Personnel will exercise care and caution when working in radiology to avoid the potential of unnecessary X-ray exposures.

9. The operator must stand completely behind the barrier in the control area when making a radiographic exposure.

Radiation Safety Policies for Patients

1. Radiographic procedures shall be done only by personnel adequately instructed in the safe operation of the equipment and deemed competent in the safe use of radiographic equipment.

2. No radiographic machine shall be operated if it does not meet the current safety, shielding, and performance standards as established by the California Radiation Control Regulation, Title 17.

3.	Radiographic studies of female patients of child-bearing age are performed following the Ten Day Rule. The safest time to X-ray females of child-bearing age is within 10 days of the onset of menses. Unless there are strong clinical reasons to radiograph the patient outside this window, the studies will be scheduled according to this rule.

4.	The radiographic field shall be restricted to the area of clinical interest and/or film size, whichever is smaller. There shall be evidence of collimation or beam restriction on all radiographs on three borders of the film. Collimation shall not be so restricted as to not visualize the area of clinical interest or result in a repeated exposure.

5.	Gonadal shielding shall be used for all X-ray studies of patients that have not passed the reproductive age in which the gonads are in the direct beam or scatter exposure, except cases in which this would interfere with the diagnostic procedure. The use of gonadal shielding is not a substitute for proper collimation. Gonadal shielding shall be the equivalent of 0.5 mm lead. Gonadal shields and aprons shall be tested semi-annually.

6.	The technical factors used to produce the radiograph shall be in accordance with the technique charts provided and based upon the proper measurement of the patient with calipers.

7.	Point and compensating filters shall be used to reduce the exposure in areas that are prone to be overexposed and as a means to reduce the total exposure for the patient.

8.	The Radiographic Quality Assurance Standards shall be followed when patients are being exposed to X-rays. The principles of proper sequencing of the steps needed to be performed to correctly produce a radiograph shall be adhered to by interns. The watching of the patient to avoid motion artifacts or repeated films is a key element of these standards.

9.	The Radiographer or Resident assigned to X-ray shall closely monitor and supervise the performance of each radiographic procedure done by the interns. The intern performing the radiographic study may be helped by a more senior intern assigned as the "Intern of the Day." Credit for the I.O.D. assignment shall be withheld if the intern makes significant errors resulting in additional exposures to the patient. The radiographer or resident shall take charge of the study when he/she feels that the interns are not capable of safely performing the study. This action shall be discussed with the interns at the conclusion of the study and corrective measures shall be recommended.

10.	Radiographic procedures must be authorized by a clinician and have clinical reasons for their performance. The clinical history of the patient shall be monitored by radiology staff. The clinical benefit of the radiographic study must outweigh the risks of exposure to ionizing radiation.

11.	Radiographic screening or educational studies authorized by the clinician shall be restricted to the minimum number of films and level of X-ray exposure.

## 2.2	The Use of Compensating Filters and Gonadal Protection

Compensating Filters

Aluminum compensating filters are used to compensate or reduce the exposure to areas of the body that are less dense yet in the field of view. There are two principal types of filters used with the Nolan filter system. Cervicothoracic filters are used to reduce the exposure to the upper thoracic spine. It is commonly called the thyroid filter for this reason. There are two of these filters. The larger version is for 40-in. SID films and the smaller for 72-in. SID films. The other type of filter is the point filter. These filters are unique to the Nolan filter system. There are four filters of different thicknesses. They are used to fine-tune the exposures and can be used singularly or in combination.

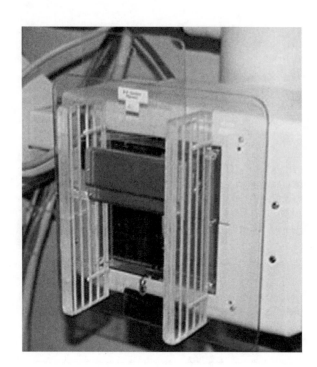

FIGURE 2.1
40 in. Cervicothoracic filter.

40 in. Cervicothoracic Filter

Use

A-P thoracic spine

Placement

Down from top until light is seen at top. Pulled up to close off the light. Thickest part is placed up toward the cervical spine. (See Figure 2.1.)

72 in. Cervicothoracic Filter

Use

A-P full spine

Placement

Down from top until light is seen at top. Pulled up to close off the light. Thickest part is placed up toward the cervical spine. (See Figure 2.2.)

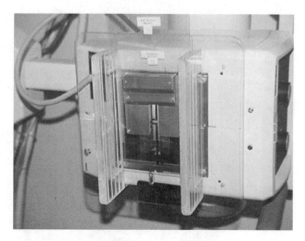

FIGURE 2.2
72 in. Thyroid filter and para-spinal shield.

Point Filters

Use

Lateral thoracic spine

Placement

From below the axilla down or from the horizontal central ray down. The area of the shoulders is the thicker part of the lateral thoracic spine. Number of filters determined from technique chart.

Use

Lateral lumbar spine on female patients

Placement

From the horizontal central ray up. The filter is used to compensate for the narrow waist and broader hips of female patients. Number determined by taking lateral measurement at umbilicus and at trochanter. The product of trochanter minus umbilical measurement minus 5 will be the needed filtration. (See Figure 2.3.)

Use

A-P full spine

Placement

From xiphoid tip up or horizontal central ray up. Used with the thyroid filter to reduce exposure to the cervical and thoracic spine. (See Figure 2.4.)

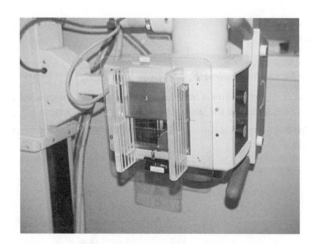

FIGURE 2.3
Gonad shield and point filters.

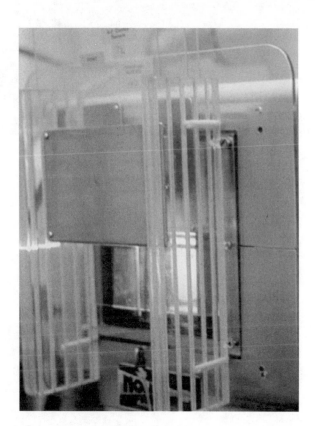

FIGURE 2.4
Point filter.

Gonadal Protection

Three basic forms of gonadal protection are used. Half or full lead aprons can be very effective because they cover more than just the gonads. Contact shields include the bell for males and a heart-shaped filter for females. These shields are attached to the patient using a belt. The other shield is called a shadow shield. It is installed in the filter holder on the collimator. The shadow gonad shield is shaped like a quarter of a pie and is used on lateral and oblique lumbar views. The para-spinal blocker is also a radiation protection device that reduces exposure to the breast and lung tissues.

Gonadal and Radiation Protection Shielding

1. The *Half Lead Apron* is used for all cervical spine, thoracic spine, and shoulder views. It can be draped over the abdomen for lower extremity views. (See Figure 2.5.)

2. The *full or coat lead apron* is used for upper and lower extremity views other than the shoulder region. (See Figure 2.6.)

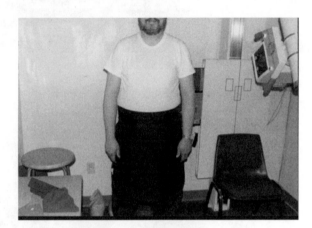

FIGURE 2.5
Half lead apron.

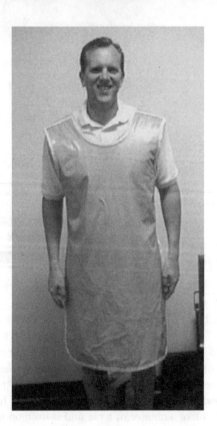

FIGURE 2.6
Coat lead apron.

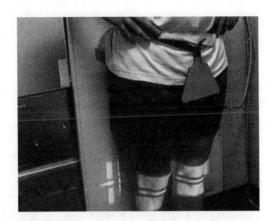

FIGURE 2.7
Bell gonad shield.

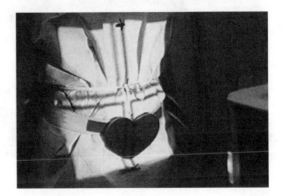

FIGURE 2.8
Heart-shaped filter.

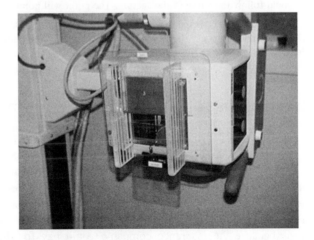

FIGURE 2.9
Lateral gonadal shield.

3. The bell (Figure 2.7) is placed below the most inferior aspect of the symphysis pubis of male patients for A-P full spine, A-P lumbopelvic, A-P pelvis and hips, sacrum and coccyx views, and upright knee views.

4. The heart-shaped filter (Figure 2.8) is used for the A-P full spine and A-P lumbopelvic views on female patients. The female lumbopelvic view is generally done P-A to reduce exposure and no shield is needed.

5. The shadow lateral gonadal shield (Figure 2.9) is used for lateral views of the lumbar spine, sacrum, and coccyx. It is used for oblique views of the lumbar spine and sacroiliac joints. For male patients, it

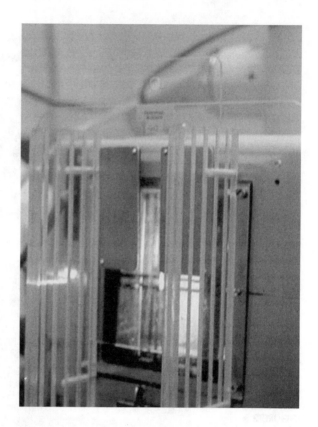

FIGURE 2.10
Para-spinal blocker.

is placed about 2 to 3 in. below the ASIS. For female patients, it goes just below the ASIS. The curved side should follow the curve of the sacrum. The point will point to the pubic region.

6. The para-spinal blocker (Figure 2.10) is used for the A-P full spine. At Palmer, it goes down to the level of the xiphoid process. If not interested in seeing the abdominal structures, it can be placed down to the level of the iliac crest.

2.3   Indications for Radiography and Imaging Studies

It is highly unlikely that every patient that comes to the office will need radiographs. If the patient had films taken recently at a hospital or outpatient imaging center, one should obtain those films from that facility. With the high cost of health care, and as managed care makes greater inroads into chiropractic, one may be faced with justification for the studies that one orders. Under capitated care, unnecessary studies will cost money. The days of the "shotgun approach" to the delivery of health care are thankfully gone. The medical industry once used multiple, expensive tests to make the diagnosis because the insurance company would pay for them. It was easier to have the radiologist make the diagnosis or rule out a disease process. There was a cartoon showing two medical doctors discussing the purchase of a huge cabin cruiser. The caption was, "To think I fought Medicare for years!!!" When health care began using significant resources, the system was forced to change.

If planning to operate an office on a fee-for-service method, one should be able to explain why the patient should pay for the X-ray exam and what benefit it will have for the patient. Remember that one of the reasons why chiropractic is so successful is because of its cost effectiveness. The chiropractor is able to treat and relieve pain for much less cost than medical or surgical intervention. This includes both treatment and reduced loss of work time. If all patients have extra radiographic studies — justified or not justified — that erodes the cost effectiveness.

While the use of modern radiographic equipment and film will reduce the radiation exposure for the patient, it does not eliminate it. There are always inherent risks for the patient when exposed to ionizing radiation. It is very important to consider the potential risks and benefits for the patient before films are taken. The likelihood that the exam will be of benefit in establishing or refuting a diagnosis is another important consideration. In this age of frequent legal action, one must also consider the risk of liability if the examination is requested or not requested.

Baysean Analysis or Physical Examination and Complete History

The best tool for determining if a patient needs X-ray tests will always be a complete clinical history and a complete physical examination. The X-ray examination should be indicated based on finding from the history and physical examination of the patient. This type of decision-making process is called Bayesian analysis. Ask yourself the following questions:

1. Will X-rays affect my diagnostic certainty about the differential diagnosis I am considering? If so, how much?
2. Will the information expected to be provided by the X-rays change my diagnostic thinking enough so that it will significantly affect my choice of treatment?

Bayes Theorem

Another important consideration is the sensitivity and specificity of the diagnostic examination; the diagnostic accuracy of the examination must be considered. Would an MRI or CT scan yield more information than a limited lumbar spine X-ray view? If the study is not to be read by a radiologist, one should also consider if one has the ability to see the disease process on films. One's impression based on clinical finding, physical examination, clinical experience, and intuition will impact the decision. Based on one's own experience, how probable is it that the disease exists? Based on these same processes, how convinced is one that the disease process can be excluded? If one is convinced that a disease process exists, the action level is the point at which treatment is instituted. Again, the ability to evaluate the patient's symptoms, as gathered by the physical examination and clinical history, X-ray tests are used when one does not know what is causing the problem and one cannot determine how to treat the patient (take action), or one is uncertain if a disease process exists (exclude the disease process).

The Bayes Theorem can be summarized as follows: "It essentially means that if a test gives either a positive or negative result, then the chance of the patient having or not having the disease in question depends not only on the sensitivity or specificity of the test, but also on the pretest probability of the presence of the disease."

Once the doctor has arrived at a pretest probability of a certain condition, he/she must then consider if the probability is below exclusion or above the action level. If below the exclusion level, the doctor is convinced that the disease process in question is not present and no further tests are needed at that time. If above the action level, the doctor is certain enough that the condition or disease is present, and that he/she initiates a trial treatment plan and no further or additional tests are needed at this time. It is when the patient lies *between* the exclusion and action levels that a diagnostic test with a reasonable degree of sensitivity and specificity for the detection of that condition should be performed to move probability to one of the diagnostic levels.

The Palmer College–West Clinic Indications for Radiography

The following indications for the use of radiography are used by the clinics of Palmer College of Chiropractic–West. In the modern age of health care, resources such as radiographic examination should not be used on every patient who enters the office. Routine radiography of any patient should not be performed without due regard for clinical need. Numerous conditions and clinical situations may require X-ray examinations in order to rule out pathology or trauma that may contraindicate many chiropractic approaches to treatment or referral.

Clinical necessity for radiography includes:

1. Significant recent trauma that may have resulted in fracture, dislocation, or substantial soft tissue injury
2. Clinical indications of active or aggressive bone or joint pathology, including chronic nocturnal pain, fever, warm and swollen joints or soft tissues, deformity or bony masses, and severe restriction of the active range of motion
3. No response to conservative care or worsening of condition after 2 to 4 weeks of care
4. A history of cardiac or pulmonary complaints with fever, dyspnea, or acute chest pain indicates the need for chest radiography
5. A history of malignancies that may metastasize to osseous structures (particularly the spine)
6. A significant or progressive scoliosis is felt to be present in a developing spine

Relative factors or indications for radiography are considered based on specific patient presentation and history. Radiography may be indicated in the following situations:

1. If the patient is over 50 years of age without recent relevant radiographic studies, or if the patient had films at another facility, have the patient get the films for the evaluation
2. If it is felt that the patient cannot provide an accurate clinical history, radiography may be indicated; if there is a history or suspicion of alcohol or drug abuse; the possibility of current mental or emotional impairment which would alter the patient's perception of symptoms or health history
3. If the patient has acute or progressive neurologic or neuromotor deficits
4. If there is clinical suspicion of peripheral joint or spinal instability
5. If the patient has clinical history that may point to serious medical or neoplastic conditions, such as unexplained weight loss, prolonged hormonal replacement or corticosteroid therapy or abuse
6. If there is a lack of physical, historical, or mechanical findings to explain the patient's symptoms (this would include patient symptoms that cannot be reproduced or exacerbated by clinical examination)
7. If the assessment or analysis of spinal articular malalignments, which might be indicative of subluxation, is a factor in determining the need for radiography. The chiropractor should have clear evidence that the outcome of the analysis of subluxation by additional radiographic studies in addition to the physical assessment is warranted. The suspicion of spinal malalignment should not routinely be the primary determining factor for performing radiographic studies.
8. If there are medical-legal issues that may be a factor in determining the need for X-rays (this should never be the *only* factor)
9. If for pre-employment or school admission screening or other administrative purposes

Re-examination of the patient radiographically may be indicated in certain circumstances. In such instances, the study should be limited to the views that best illustrate the abnormality. The indications for reexamination include:

1. In monitoring progressive idiopathic scoliosis, a P-A or A-P view is required. Follow-up studies should be done P-A on female patients. Lateral bending views are typically not taken as part of each reevaluation. If the curve is suspected of progressing, a follow-up should be performed during the first

3 months. If no progression is evident in the follow-up, scoliosis should be monitored by nonradiographic means, such as Moire screening, until changes are evident.

2. In cases of fracture to monitor healing. There are also times when a fracture is suspected but not seen on the initial films.

3. In cases when there is a failure to respond to conservative management, or where serious pathology is considered as a differential diagnosis.

4. In certain pathologic conditions, periodic reexamination may be indicated to monitor progression or to investigate a clinical suspicion of malignant degeneration.

Radiographic utilization guidelines were established by the American Chiropractic College of Radiology in 1984. These guidelines are based on the recognition that exposure to unnecessary ionizing radiation represents an unwarranted health hazard. The following policies have been adopted at Palmer College–West.

1. Routine radiography of any patient should not be performed without regard for clinical need.

2. Any offer or advertising for free or discounted X-rays to actual or potential patients shall be accompanied by a statement to avoid needless health hazards associated with ionizing radiation; no free X-rays will be given unless there is a prior observable clinical need.

3. Attenuation of radiation for the improvement of radiographic quality should be employed by means of filtration prior to the primary beam entering the patient.

4. Repeat radiographic evaluation should not be undertaken without significant, observable clinical need.

5. Pregnant women should not be radiographed unless the patient's symptoms are of such significance that proper care of the patient would be jeopardized without such radiographs. If the need for radiographs is determined, consultation with an orthopedist or obstetrician should be sought.

6. Radiographic procedures should not be undertaken without the use of appropriate compensating filters and gonadal shielding. Gonadal shielding should be used except where such shielding would exclude a clinically essential area from examination.

7. Collimation shall be used to restrict the primary beam to slightly smaller than the film size being used for the examination. When possible, the beam should be further restricted to just the area of clinical interest. The optimum radiograph will have at least three borders of collimation.

Other Sources of Assistance in the Decision-Making Process

There are algorithms formulated to assist the doctor with the decision-making process. These algorithms cover virtually all conditions that are likely to be seen in practice. *Differential Diagnosis and Management Protocols for the Chiropractor,* by Thomas Souza, DC, Aspen Publishers, can be of great help to guide one through the decision-making process.

What Constitutes a Complete Radiographic Examination?

It is important that the radiographic examination includes the views needed to demonstrate the area of clinical interest. For most areas of the body, community standards have established what views are essential. The minimum views of an area of the body should be opposing or right-angle views to produce an A-P or P-A view and a lateral view. When just these views are taken, the study will be referred to as a limited study. One can start with the limited study; and if pathology warranting a complete study is observed, one can take additional views.

In many cases, the views taken will be indicated by the patient's history. Histories that include recent trauma will typically call for a more complete study, as fractures or dislocations must be ruled out or diagnosed. In the shoulder, for example, there are special routine trauma views that should be taken. Pain referring or radiating to another area of the body may indicate a complete study in spinal evaluations.

One will ultimately be interpreting films or having them read by a radiologist. In either case, one will not want to miss a diagnosis because one took the wrong view or did an incomplete study. As an example, ordering a knee series for a patella injury has a high probability of missing a patella fracture. Owing to the fact that the patient is being exposed to ionizing radiation, unnecessary views and repeated films should be avoided. What would be worse would be to do multiple views that fail to demonstrate the cause of pain and then someone else clearly shows the problem. Besides being able to position precisely and use good technical factors, one must be able know what view or series of views will most likely demonstrate the cause of the patient's pain.

Typical Cervical Spine Studies

Limited C-spine: A-P lower C-spine, A-P open mouth for C-1 and C-2, neutral lateral C-spine

Complete C-spine: Add both posterior and anterior oblique views **or** hyper-flexion and hyper-extension lateral views.

Davis series: Add both anterior or posterior oblique views **and** hyper-flexion and hyper-extension lateral views.

Supplemental views: Fuchs, Pillar views, swimmers view

Thoracic spine: A-P, lateral views

Supplemental views: Swimmers, oblique views

Lumbar or Lumbopelvic Studies

Limited lumbopelvic: A-P or P-A and lateral lumbar views

Complete Lumbopelvic: A-P or P-A, both anterior or posterior oblique views, A-P sacral base and lateral spot film of L5/S1

Scoliosis survey: A-P full spine

Supplementary: Bending views

Spinal Surveys Used at Palmer–West

411 series: A-P full spine, APOM, lateral cervical, thoracic and lumbar spines

412 series: Limited cervical spine, thoracic spine, limited lumbopelvic

Supplementary views: Oblique views of cervical spine or lumbar spine, sacral base

Skull series: Towne's, P-A, both laterals of skull

Sinus series: Caldwell, Waters, lateral sinuses, SMV or basilar view

Sinus limited: Waters view

Extremity (finger, hand, wrist, elbow, foot, ankle): A-P or P-A, oblique, lateral

Limited extremity (finger, hand, wrist, elbow, foot, ankle, toes): A-P or P-A, lateral

Knee series: A-P, lateral, Camp-Coventry view

Knee limited: A-P, lateral recumbent or weight-bearing

Hip series (non-trauma): A-P and frog-leg lateral

Pelvis/hip series (trauma): A-P pelvis, frog-leg lateral

Femur, humerus, tibia-fibula: A-P, lateral

Patella series: P-A, Settegast view, lateral

Shoulder (non-trauma):   A-P view with internal and external rotation

Shoulder trauma: Grashey with internal rotation, outlet view, possible apical view

Shoulder unstable: Weighted and unweighted Grashey internal and external rotation, possible outlet view

Clavicle series: A-P or P-A and A-P or P-A axial

A-C joint: Weighted and non-weighted A-P or Zanca views

Developing a System or the Proper Sequence for Taking Films

Many mistakes can be avoided by developing a systematic approach to performing radiographic procedures. The time needed to do the study can also be optimized by using a systematic approach. There are many steps in accomplishing a radiographic examination. If any step is missed or performed in the incorrect order, mistakes can result in a repeated film or the exam will take longer to complete. In practice, either situation will cost both money and patient confidence.

This chapter discusses both the recommended sequence in taking views of the patient by body region and the steps of actually taking a single film. It is very important to learn the sequence before one practices positioning. Bad habits are hard to lose. A patient will be watching every step of the process. If one follows a logical sequence and does it with confidence, one will impress the new patient. Most patients will have horror stories about having X-rays taken. Do not let their experience with you add to the list.

3.1 What Views Come First?

The views needed of the area of clinical interest will determine the sequence of the views. If there are one or two views done with a 72-in. SID, get those out of the way first most of the time. If the study does not have a 72-in. view, start with the A-P view, followed by the lateral view. When multiple views are done on the same film (e.g., extremity studies), do the A-P or P-A view, the oblique projection, and the lateral view last.

Cervical Spine Studies

When the study is of the cervical spine, almost always do the neutral lateral cervical spine first. It is the only 72-in. view and the only Non-Bucky film in the routine or complete cervical spine. If possible, look at the view before attempting the A-P open mouth view. One will see the patient's cervical curve, and this will determine if a tube angle is needed. If this is a limited study, take the lateral view, followed by the A-P view. Do not forget the 15° cephalad tube angle on the A-P view. Look at the lateral view before taking the A-P open mouth view.

When the complete cervical spine exam is to be done, take the 72-in. Non-Bucky neutral lateral. Set the tube angle at 15° cephalad, and take the right and left posterior oblique views as the next two films. Once the horizontal central ray is set for the first oblique, it should not need to be adjusted for the other oblique. The A-P view is next because the same tube angle is required. The last view would be the A-P open mouth view.

The exception for doing the lateral view first would be for the acute patient immediately after a whiplash injury. In this case, neutral, flexion, and extension lateral views are indicated. Take the A-P view — the A-P open mouth views first. Then do the neutral lateral view. Evaluate these views before taking the flexion and extension lateral views. If the injury is not acute or the patient was seen and evaluated with X-rays in a hospital emergency room, the lateral views can be done first — but never have the patient exceed his/her limit on the flexion or extension view. The proper sequence for these views should be neutral lateral, followed by the extension lateral view. No adjustment of the film or central ray is required. The extension lateral view will require the film and central ray to be moved.

Thoracic Spine Studies

Because the film is set to the patient, the A-P view is generally done first. The top of the film is set 2-in. above C-7/T-1. Locate this landmark and the position the film. Set the tube to center the horizontal central ray to the film. To take the lateral view, the film and the tube should not be moved. This will make it easier to evaluate any pathology seen because the vertebrae will be at the same level on both views. Place the filters needed for each view on top of the collimator. After collimation is complete, install the filters before taking the view.

Lumbar Spine Studies

Start the exam with an A-P or P-A view. It will be the only view for which the horizontal central ray is placed below the iliac crest. It is also the only view for which the patient will wear the gonadal shield. If oblique views are needed, they are done next. Place the lateral gonad shield on top of the collimator so that one does not forget to use it on the view. Like the cervical spine, once the film and central ray are set for one side, they should not need to be moved for the other oblique view. The lateral view is taken last since the Bucky will need to be centered to the larger film size. If a spot view is needed of L-5/S-1, process the lateral lumbar view and look at it before positioning for the spot film. The amount of pelvic tilt and lordotic curve of the patient will dictate the placement of the horizontal and vertical central rays and film.

Studies That Include the A-P Full Spine

When the study includes the A-P full spine, it is generally the first view taken. It is a 72 to 84 in. SID Bucky view. The lateral cervical spine would be the next film taken. Because of the general poor quality, this text will not address the lateral full spine view. Unless the patient is very small, the image quality even with the use of added filtration is less than sectional views taken at 40 in. SID. It also requires much higher tube loads, so breathing or motion artifacts are more common. It can also lead to premature X-ray tube failure.

Film Sequence for Complete Spine Studies

Sectional series (may be called a 412 series)

1. Lateral C-spine
2. A-P C-spine
3. A-P open mouth
4. A-P thoracic
5. Lateral thoracic
6. A-P or P-A lumbopelvic
7. Lateral lumbar

Full spine series (also called a 411 series)

1. A-P full spine
2. Lateral C-spine
3. Lateral thoracic spine
4. Lateral lumbar
5. A-P open mouth

3.2 A Step-by-Step Approach to Taking Radiographs

1. Introduce yourself to the patient and explain to the patient what you are going to do.
2. Determine that the patient is not pregnant, using the Ten Day Rule. Give the gowning instructions.
3. Take the measurements needed to perform the necessary views. Record them on the X-ray Request Form. Locate gonadal shields for the first view. If apron is used, put on patient. If lateral gonadal shielding is needed, install on collimator after final collimation. If bell is used, put on patient before positioning for A-P lumbopelvic or A-P full spine.
4. Using the technique chart, enter the technique for the first film into the generator and record it on the request form.
5. Position tube, film, and patient.
   a. Set FFD.
   b. Put film into the Bucky with the correct anatomical marker and I.D. in recommended position.
   c. Position patient and central ray, and center film to central ray; *or*
   d. Position film to patient and center central ray to the film.
   e. Slide Bucky tray into Bucky.
   f. Fine-tune the positioning, monitoring patient stance, object to film distance, and appropriate planes (coronal, sagittal, or axial).
6. Collimate film to area of clinical interest or slightly less than film size, whichever is smaller.
7. Give breathing instructions and ask patient to hold very still.
8. Watch the patient during rotor prep and exposure. Repeat step 7 if needed.
9. Tell patient to breathe and relax while setting the technique for the next view. Change gonadal shield as needed.
10. Repeat steps 4 through 9 until the exam is complete. Separate unexposed and exposed films. Put exposed films outside room, yellow side up.
11. Process films with care.

Details of the Sequence for Taking Radiographs and Avoiding Mistakes

Step 1: *Introduction to the patient and explanation of why the X-rays are important.*

In practice and in the clinic, one needs to access the patient's condition and probably take a history and physical. After this is done, one can determine the need and value to the patient's care and radiographic procedures. Taking the time to explain to the patient why the radiographic study is needed provides valuable interaction with the patient and gains their assistance during the study. Radiographic studies are much easier when the patient is on one's team. They will hold still in uncomfortable positions better and follow instructions. One must be totally prepared to do the examination. Never read notes in front of the patient; it destroys the patient's confidence in one's abilities as a doctor or intern.

Step 2: *Determine that the patient is not pregnant using the Ten Day Rule. If not pregnant or possibly pregnant, proceed with the radiographic study. Make sure the patient signs the release for the study and documentation of LMP and not being pregnant. Give the patient gowning instructions. Refer to Section 3.3 for gowning instruction details.*

If the patient is of child-bearing age and potentially sexually active, the Ten Day Rule is used to determine the least dangerous time to do X-rays studies. If the patient is beyond the tenth day after the onset of menses, the risk of exposure must be weighed against the benefits of the study. The part of the body being exposed and the type of gonad protection available will be part of the decision-making process. A full-coat lead apron (0.5 mm of lead) can be used to provide total protection for extremity studies. In the worst case, the patient could take a pregnancy test or delay the examination.

Gowning instructions are very important. Most artifacts on films can be avoided by giving complete gowning instructions. It is very important that earrings and dentures are not overlooked. Some artifacts may be unavoidable but can be noted on the request form. Some body piercings and jewelry are not readily removable. Brassieres and hairbands are common artifact sources.

It is also important that shoes be removed for leg length evaluation. If prescribing orthotics, follow-up exams can be done with the shoes and orthotics in place. In both cases, have the patient stand with feet shoulder-width apart and knees locked during the exposure.

While the patient is changing into a gown, make sure that the cassettes and accessories needed to do the study are in the X-ray suite. Make sure the processor is on, all quality control tests are done, and the processor is properly operating. Locate the calipers so that measurements can be taken.

Set the equipment for the first view of the study. This will include the correct film size, SID, and Non-Bucky film holder, if needed. Also set collimation to film size and make sure the cassette is centered to the beam.

Step 3: *Take the measurements needed to perform all necessary views. Record them on the X-ray Request Form. Locate gonadal shields for the first view. If the X-ray generator is not anatomically programmed, record the technical factors for each view on the request form. Have the patient relax while this is done.*

If apron is used, put it on patient. If lateral gonadal sheilding is needed, install on collimator after final collimation. If bell is used, put it on patient before positioning for A-P lumbopelvic or A-P full spine.

Step 4:   *Using patient measurements or techniques recorded on the request form, enter the technique for the first film into the generator.*

With anatomically programmed generators, one will be able to quickly obtain the technical factors by entering the patient measurements. Record the factors on the request form for each view as it is done. Always make sure the technique is established and set before starting positioning. One is now ready to start positioning the patient.

Step 5:   *Position the patient.*

a.   Set FFD if not already done.

b   Put film into the Bucky with the correct anatomical marker and I.D. in recommended position, if not already done.

c.   Position patient and central ray; then center film to central ray, *or*

d.   Position film to patient and center central ray to the film.

e.   Slide Bucky tray into Bucky.

f.   Fine-tune the positioning, monitoring patient stance, object to film distance (OFD), and appropriate planes (coronal, sagittal, or axial).

If the patient changes into the gown quickly or does not need to be gowned, one will not have time to set the SID or FFD and film for the first view before bringing the patient into the room. These steps should be done before placing the patient in front of the Bucky. Any tube angle must also be set before the patient is placed in front of the Bucky.

The positioning of the patient will require either the film being centered to the anatomy, or the central ray set to the proper anatomical landmark and the film centered to the horizontal central ray. Once the film has been established, double-check the anatomical marker and the I.D. blocker location. Also make sure that the film is locked into the center of the Bucky tray. If the Bucky is used, it is now safe to slide the Bucky tray completely into the Bucky.

Fine-tune the patient positioning. Look for any patient rotation. Make sure the patient is as close to the Bucky as possible to minimize any magnification. When taking oblique views, make sure the pelvis and the shoulders are in the same plane. Check that intrapupillary and acanthomeatal lines are perpendicular to the film on cervical views.

Step 6:   *Collimate film to area of clinical interest or slightly less than film size, whichever is smaller.*

The patient's best protection against unnecessary radiation exposure is the operator's ability to collimate properly. If the collimation is set to slightly less than film size when starting to set up the view, this will ensure that all of the radiation is directed onto the film. There will be many opportunities to collimate smaller than film size; exposure beyond the skin of the area of interest is wasted exposure.

Collimation so restricted that clinically significant information is missed will result in repeated films and much higher radiation exposure than normally required; this is worse than not collimating less than film size. In any case, collimation is so important that in many states, failure to collimate is against the law.

X-ray units with automatic collimation to film size in clinical practice are rare. In medical facilities between the mid-1970s and early 1990s, this was required. The U.S. Food and Drug Administration found that the units were unreliable and radiographers were not collimating smaller than film size. It could be turned off with a key and did not operate when the tube was angled. It also would limit exposure to 40 in. or 72 in. SID. In 1992, the requirement was deleted from the Federal Code of Regulations. Both federal and state regulations require that the field size indicators on the collimator be accurate to within 2% of the SID. This makes the use of the dial indicators the most accurate means to set collimation slightly less than film size.

When tube angulation is used, the actual SID increases at a rate of approximately 0.5 in. for every 5° of tube angulation. To accurately collimate, the SID should be adjusted for the tube angulation. This is very important for angles greater than 20°.

When collimation is significantly less than film size, the anatomical markers must be moved closer to the center of the film. (Think about the actual film size and the area of exposure when placing the marker on the film.)

Step 7: Give breathing instructions and ask patient to hold very still.

The person being X-rayed must fully understand the breathing instructions; go over them with the patient before going into the control booth. The instructions should be in plain English or the patient's native language. The patient will probably be confused if one says, "Suspend inspiration" and takes the film. Always ask the patient to stand or remain still. See Section 3.4 on patient communications.

Step 8: Watch the patient during rotor prep and exposure. Repeat step 7 if needed.

As the rotor is prepared for exposure, give breathing instructions to the patient. Watch the patient through the window in the control booth for compliance. If the patient moves or does not follow the instructions, explain instructions again to the patient.

The ready light on the control panel of the machine will come on when the rotor is at the proper speed for exposure. If the patient is still and holding his/her breath appropriately for the view, press the exposure button. The exposure button will produce the actual exposure. The unit will make only one exposure without reinitiating the rotor preparation. This is very important because many repeated films may be the result of the operator lifting the exposure button prematurely.

Step 9: Tell patient to breathe and relax while one sets the technique for the next view. Place the exposed film outside the room. Get film for the next view and change gonadal shield as needed.

Step 10: Repeat steps 4 through 9 until the exam is complete. Separate unexposed and exposed films. Put exposed films outside room, yellow side up.

Step 11: Process films with care after all views are completed.

Make sure that the film processor is warmed up and functioning properly before attempting to process the first film. Some processors may take up to 30 minutes to warm up to operating parameters. Make sure the water is turned on and the rollers have been cleaned. If the equipment is available, daily sensitometry should be done before starting the examination.

Each film should be handled very carefully by the edges to avoid artifacts. The film needs to be permanently identified with at least the patient's name, date, and examination. Always feed the film into the processor lengthwise and toward the drive gear side of the feed tray.

Modification for Clinic Radiography

In school, one may have one or more interns assisting. One of the interns can process the films as they are taken. In practice, one can train an assistant to process the films.

The first steps in school

As a student, one must obtain the signed approval of a clinic clinician on the radiographic request form before the exam can be scheduled. When the patient arrives, obtain a route or charging slip from the clinic receptionist. A flash card is obtained from the X-ray department and completed prior to starting the exam. The patient's name is written in ink or typed — Last name, First Name, and Middle initial. The other information typed or written in ink on the flash card will include the patient's file number, age, date of service, ordering clinician and intern's name, and the exam being performed.

Review of the Sequence of Radiography

1. Explain
2. Pregnant?/gown
3. Measure/shield
4. Set technique for view
5. Position
   a. Tube and tube angle
   b. Film and I.D. location
   c. Marker
   d. Patient
6. Collimate
7. Breathing instructions and hold still
8. Observe and make exposure
9. Relax and remove exposed film from room
10. Steps 4 through 9 until exam is complete
11. Process films

3.3   Helpful Hints for Maintaining Image Quality

I. GOWNING INSTRUCTIONS: Proper gowning instructions are very important. They avoid artifacts on the films that result from metallic and other objects on the patient. Give the following instructions to the patient when taking films of the noted area.

Skull: Remove all hairpins, wigs, dentures, necklaces, eyeglasses, contact lenses, earrings, and all clothing that may be in or near the area being X-rayed. If necessary, have patient put on a gown with opening toward the back.

Cervical spine: Remove all hairpins, wigs, dentures, eyeglasses, necklaces, earrings, brassiere, and chewing gum. Remove all clothing in or near area being X-rayed and put on gown with opening toward the back.

Thoracic spine: Remove all necklaces and clothing (including brassiere) in the area being X-rayed. Put on a gown with the opening toward the back. Have patient remove shoes but leave socks on.

Lumbar spine: Remove orthopedic supportive devices and clothing above and below waist. Be sure to instruct patient that he/she may leave underwear on as long as there are no metallic clips or pins. Have patient put on gown with opening toward the back. Have patient remove shoes, but leave socks on. Proper gonadal shielding must be used on patients of reproductive potential except when it will obstruct an area of prime clinical interest.

Pelvis and hips: Remove all clothing in the area, including underwear if restrictive or bearing metallic clips, etc. Put on gown with opening toward the back. Proper gonadal shielding should be used, providing it does not obstruct visualization of an area of clinical interest.

Extremities: Remove any clothing and jewelry that may be in the area being X-rayed. If necessary, put on a gown with opening toward the back. When X-raying the torso, including the lumbar spine, pelvis, abdomen, thorax, and chest, the *Ten Day Rule* should be considered for females of reproductive potential. According to the NCRP 33, the least likely time to expose an embryo is in the first 10 days after the onset of menses. If it is essential that films be taken of these areas to ensure proper diagnosis of a patient, be sure to use correct technique, film/screen combinations, proper collimation, and as much shielding or filtration as possible. The LMP and questioning of the patient about the possibility of pregnancy must be documented on the X-ray Request Form. If there is a possibility of pregnancy, clinical judgment about delaying or canceling the X-rays must be exercised.

II. GONADAL SHIELD PLACEMENT

A. Female shield: The heart-shaped filter/shield should be placed so the *uppermost* margin is at the level of the ASIS and centered to the mid-sagittal plane. If properly positioned, it will overlie the inferior two thirds of the sacrum, the coccyx, and the inferior half of the sacroiliac joints. If these areas are of primary clinical interest, the gonad shield should be omitted. However, in all other instances, gonadal shielding shall be used on all patients of reproductive potential. This shield is for frontal views only (A-P full spine or A-P lumbopelvic). P-A lumbopelvic views are taken routinely on females of child-bearing age to reduce the exposure to the ovaries.

B. Male shield: The male shield is trapezoidal in shape. It should be positioned so the *uppermost* margin is just below the *lowermost* border of the pubic symphysis. The properly placed shield will overlie the scrotum, but not overlie any osseous structure. It is used on all male patients. This shield is also for frontal views only.

C. Shadow shield: The Nolan Filter System includes a quarter-spherically shaped *shadow shield,* which is used for lateral and oblique views of the lumbopelvic region. The filter is placed in the filter holder so the curved border is anterior and inferior to the spine for all views. *Females*: The uppermost margin of the shadow should be at the level or slightly below the level of the ASIS. *Males*: Same as female but the uppermost shadow should be 2 to 3 in. below the ASIS.

D. Lead apron: The half lead apron is tied around the waist of the patient for all studies other than lumbopelvic region exams. For thoracic spine studies, it must not be higher than the iliac crest.

III. OTHER HELPFUL HINTS

A. Preventing motion blurring: Motion blurring is the single greatest destroyer of anatomical detail. It is the result of the patient either breathing or moving during the exposure and can be avoided. When positioning the patient, have the patient spread his/her feet apart to get a good foundation for erect views. In giving final instructions to the patient before making the exposure, always include to remain perfectly still and give appropriate breathing instructions. Always look at the patient, through the window, before pressing the exposure button and make sure he/she is not moving. If the patient is not still, do *not* take the exposure. Either wait until the patient stops moving, or stop the rotor and go back into the room to give more instructions. One may need to reposition the patient into a wider stance and hold onto the Bucky. A sponge behind the head may help for A-P spine views. If the patient cannot stand still, one may need to take the view in a seated or recumbent position.

B. Tube tilt: Reducing the FFD or SID by 1 in. for every 5° of tube tilt will maintain the correct FFD for erect imaging. Lowering the tube 1 in. for every 5° tube tilt will achieve the correct FFD for recumbent studies. This is most important in any view with a tube tilt greater than 20°.

When the tube is tilted, be sure to align the cassette at the proper level, taking into account the angle of the central ray.

C. Collimation: The minimum acceptable standard for collimation is slightly smaller than film size; that is, to show three borders on the film. In many cases, the area being X-rayed will be smaller than the film. The rule then is to collimate to skin size. A film that cuts off the area of clinical importance due to too tight collimation will result in a repeated film and more radiation exposure to the patient. Proper collimation is a field as small as possible that shows the anatomy essential for the exam. Proper collimation is our standard. The collimation for each view will be discussed in the instructions on positioning.

D. When to adjust the technique from the technique chart: Additive and degenerative pathology and patient habitus will require adjustments to the techniques on the technique charts. Examples are:

Osteoporosis, found in women over age 55 and most males over age 60, requires a reduction in kVp of 6 to 10, with an increase in mAs for thoracic and lumbopelvic examinations.

Very muscular bodies require an increase of up to 10 kVp and an increase in mAs.

Overweight patients (excessive adipose tissue) will require a 40 to 60% increase in the mAs with the kVp left alone, or a reduction in kVp of 6 kVp and double the mAs.

IV. IDENTIFICATION

A. Identification blocker: The identification blocker is in a fixed position on the cassette. It is where the information typed or printed on the flash card is photographically imprinted on the film. Information that must be on the flash card includes the patient's name (Last, First); record number; age; date of study; facility name and address; the name of the doctor taking the films; and the study being performed. The blocker is moved by turning the cassette to get it out of the area being studied.

B. Anatomical lead markers: R or L anatomical markers are placed on the film on the side closest to the film. An arrow can be used to identify any nonroutine position of the part being X-rayed, such as internal or external rotation or flexion and extension views. They are usually placed at the outer border of the cassette or the outer field of collimation. The placement is determined by the anatomy being radiographed, as one must avoid placing the marker over the area of interest. For any Anterior-Posterior (A-P) type view, including posterior obliques, the marker is face-up so that one can read the letter. For Posterior-Anterior (P-A) views, including anterior obliques, the marker is pronated or turned so that one cannot read the letter. Recommended marker and ID locations are taught in positioning classes. For extremities, they are turned upside down to the patient.

3.4   Communications with the Patient during Radiography

In radiography, the image is everything. This not only refers to the film, but also to the operator's demeanor, confidence, and communication skills with the patient. The patient has come to one for their care. Reward that patient with the care. Treat the patient as if they were the mother, father, or best friend. This will also help build your practice, and it makes good business sense.

Before Scheduling the Radiograph

For female patients of child-bearing age, one must determine if the patient is potentially pregnant. The Ten Day Rule will be the guide. The safest time to radiograph a female patient is within 10 days of the onset of menses. Performing studies outside this window has potentially greater risks to the patient and child. Discuss this with the patient before scheduling the X-ray exam.

One of the keys to gaining the cooperation of the patient is explaining to the patient why he/she needs the X-ray and how it will benefit his/her care, how many views will be taken, and how long the study will take. After the study has been explained, the patient can give informed consent and become part of the decision-making process. Remember that the patient is not a low back pain, but a human being with pain who wants to be treated for that pain. From a risk management standpoint, the full cooperation of the patient is very important.

When the Patient Arrives

When the patient arrives for an X-ray procedure, it is important that he/she receive accurate instructions about what clothing needs to be removed before the study can begin. For female patients, document the LMP (last menstrual period) date and have the patient sign a statement that she believes she is not pregnant. If there is a possibility of pregnancy, clinical judgment about delaying or canceling the X-ray must be exercised.

Gowning instructions for cervical spine or skull studies will require the patient to remove any earrings, necklaces, hairpins, wigs, eyeglasses, contact lenses, dentures, chewing gum, and brassiere. The patient should put on a gown with the opening to the back. The patient's hair should be clean, dry, and not tightly braided. Wet hair or hair with oil or mousse will potentially produce artifacts on the films.

Thoracic region studies require the removal of the brassiere, necklaces, earrings, and clothing from the waist up. Have patient put gown on with the opening to the back. The patient should remove shoes prior to taking the film unless the study is a follow-up exam after orthotic treatment.

The abdomen and lumbar regions will require the removal of any orthopedic supportive devices and clothing above and below the waist. Underwear excluding the brassiere may be left on if they contain no metallic clips or pins. Have patient put on a gown with the opening toward the back. The patient should remove shoes, but leave socks on. Body jewelry such as nipple rings or umblicus rings are generally not removable.

Extremity studies require the removal of jewelry and clothing adjacent to the area being X-rayed. It is tempting to just roll up the pants for a knee study, but the rolled-up pants will make an artifact on the film. It is better to have the patient remove the clothing and put on a gown with opening toward the back.

During the X-ray Examination

One will need to take measurements of the patient using calipers. Explain what is being done and that the metal calipers may be cold to the skin. Ask the patient to point to the landmarks needed for the measurements, or ask to locate it for the patient. Approach the patient from the back for torso measurements. It is generally most accurate to locate anatomical landmarks after having explained their importance.

The gonad radiation protection shields require very accurate placement. If they are placed too high, they will obscure clinical information. If they are placed too low, they will be ineffective. The placement of protective devices will require the location of the base and top of the symphysis pubis and the ASIS. The bell shield should be placed just below the most inferior border of the symphysis pubis. The heart-shaped shield requires location of the top of the pubis and the ASIS. The lateral gonadal shield requires location of the ASIS.

When taking films erect, all adjustments of the positioning will require the patient to move. Do not have the patient lean to achieve the proper position. Have the patient stand with feet at shoulders width apart. This can help avoid motion. Make sure the feet are an equal distance apart and in the proper plane. Having the patient lock or fully extend his/her knees will provide a more accurate assessment of leg length. All of these movements will require effective communication with the patient. Let the patient know when and where one will be touching them for landmark location.

When ready to make the exposure, give the patient concise breathing instructions and watch the patient through the leaded glass window of the control booth. By watching the patient, one can verify compliance with instructions. One will also know if the patient is having difficulty staying still for the view. Always instruct the patient to remain still. For expiration views, say "Please remain in this position. Take a little breath in; now blow it all the way out and hold it out." For inspiration views, one will generally get better inspiration by taking the film on the second breath in. Instructions should be, "Please remain as one are positioned. Take a little breath in and blow it out. Now take a deep breath in and hold it in." If the view just requires suspended respiration, say, "Don't breathe, move, or swallow." Always tell the patient to breathe and relax after the exposure is complete.

When leaving to process the films, make sure that the patient is comfortable. Inform the patient of the duration of your absence. This way, the patient will not feel abandoned — without their clothes. As soon as the films have been checked, let the patient get dressed if no further examinations are needed. Upon review of the films, communication skills will be further tested as one explains the findings to the patient. It may be that a more complete history is needed in order to be able to fully evaluate the films. Document the history. If films are sent out to a radiologist, explain that to the patient, and let the patient know when the results will be available.

By treating a patient with dignity and respect, the patient will gain more respect for you. A good recommendation from a patient to a friend is the best form of advertising one can get. Also make sure that everyone in the office is patient focused.

Chapter 4

Spinal Positioining
Quick Reference Charts

The following pages are charts that cover the basic elements of radiographic positioning. The more detailed instructions for positioning are in the following chapters by body region. These charts are not a substitute for studying the detailed information.

The charts are designed for the student that assimilates this type of information better in chart form. They will assist in learning films sizes, tube angulations, and I.D. locations.

4.1 Cervical Spine

View	Measure	Film Size I.D./R or L	FFD	Tube Tilt	Central Ray	Filter/ Shielding	Positioning	Collimation TB = Top to Bottom SS = Side to Side	Essential Anatomy
A-P cervical spine	A-P at C-4 or top of Adam's apple.	I.D. down 8 × 10	40 in. Bucky	15° Cephalad	H: @ C-4, Thyroid Cart. and film center to horizontal; V: Mid-sagittal	Lead apron	Pt. standing with mid-sagittal plane perpendicular to Bucky, chin is slightly elevated (acanthiomeatal line perpendicular to film).	TB: Mastoid tips to T-1 SS: skin of C-spine Suspend respiration	A-P view of C-2 to T-1
APOM	A-P at C-4 or top of Adam's apple.	I.D. down 8 × 10	40 in. Bucky	None 90°	H: Perpendicular to C-1 (through middle of mouth) 1 in. inferior to upper incisors. Center to film; V: Mid-sagittal.	Lead apron	Pt. standing with mid-sagittal plane perpendicular to Bucky. Mouth open wide with lower border of upper incisors and mastoid tip perpendicular to film.	5 in. square box or smaller Vert. comp. just below nose. Suspend respiration or say "ah" to lower tongue	Atlas and axis of C-1 and C-2 seen in open mouth, free of occipital bone and teeth.
Fuches projection of dens	A-P at C-4	I.D. down 8 × 10 Regular	40 in. Bucky	None 90°	H: parallel to ramus of the mandible. Center film to H: CR; V: Mid-sagittal plane.	Lead apron	Pt. stands A-P. Pt. extends head until the ramus of the mandible is perpendicular to the film. Make sure mid-sagittal plane of the patient is perpendicular to film.	TB: 5 in. SS: 5 in. Suspend respiration	View of dens when not seen on APOM. Do not take view as part of any recent trauma evaluation.
Cervical posterior obliques RPO LPO Standard	A-P at C-4 or top of Adam's apple.	I.D. down 8 × 10	40 in. Bucky	15° Cephalad	H: at C-4 or Thyroid Cart. and film center to horizontal. V: 1 in. anterior to EAM with head straight with spine. V: through EAM with head turned.	Lead apron	Pt. standing. Facing tube. Mid-coronal plane 45 to film. Chin slightly extended. Head turned parallel to Bucky. RPO: Rt. shoulder to Bucky. LPO: Lt. shoulder to Bucky.	TB: EAM to T-1 SS: to skin of neck or slightly less than film size. Suspend respiration	Oblique view of entire cervical spine. IVFs must be open. LPO to see Rt. IVFs. RPO to see Lt. IVFs.

View	Centering	I.D. / Film	Distance	CR Angle	H / V	Shield	Patient Position	TB / SS / Respiration	Comments
Cervical anterior obliques RAO LAO Optional	A-P at C-4 or top of Adam's apple.	I.D. Down Pronate marker. 8 × 10	40 in. Bucky	15° Caudal	H: at C-4 or Thyroid Cart. and film center to horizontal. V: 1 in. posterior to EAM with head straight. V: through EAM with head turned.	Lead apron	Pt. standing. Facing Bucky. Mid-coronal plane 45° to film. Chin slightly extended. Head turned parallel to Bucky. RAO: Rt. shoulder to Bucky. LAO: Lt. shoulder to Bucky.	TB: EAM to T-1. SS: skin of neck or slightly less than film size. Suspend respiration	Oblique view of entire cervical spine. IVFs must be open. RAO: to see Rt IVFs. LAO to see Lt. IVFs.

Lateral Cervical Spine Views

View	Centering	I.D. / Film	Distance	CR Angle	H / V	Shield	Patient Position	TB / SS / Respiration	Comments
Neutral lateral cervical spine	Lateral at C-4 or top of Adam's apple	I.D. down 8 × 10	72 in. Non-Bucky	None 90°	H: At C-4 with film centered to CR. V: Through EAM.	Lead apron	Pt. standing with Lt. side next to Bucky. Chin raised until the acanthomeatal line is parallel to floor. Mid-coronal plane is perpendicular to film. Have pt. hold sandbags to drop shoulders.	TB: from EAM to T-1 SS: Skin of neck or film size Suspend expiration	Neutral lateral view of the cervical spine to include EAM to T-1. Trachea and posterior skin is also very important.
Flexion lateral cervical spine	Lateral at C-4 or top of Adam's apple	I.D. up 10 × 8	72 in. Non-Bucky	None 90°	H: At C-4 with film centered to CR. V: through C-4 EAM will align between the horizontal or vertical CR, depending on amount of flexion.	Lead apron	Pt. standing with Lt. side next to Bucky. Chin tucked into chest, head dropped forward as far as the pt. can tolerate. Have pt. hold the sandbags to drop shoulders.	TB: from EAM to T-1 SS: from EAM to T-1 Suspend expiration	Flexion lateral view of C-spine and upper aspect of T-1. Amount of flexion will impact the vertical CR. Must show C-1 to T-1.
Extension lateral cervical spine	Lateral at C-4 or top of Adam's apple	I.D. down 8 × 10	72 in. Non-Bucky	None 90°	H: at C-4 with film centered to CR. V: through C-4.	Lead apron	Pt. standing with Lt. side next to Bucky. Elevate chin and extend head backward as far as pt. can tolerate. Pt. holds sandbags to drop the shouldrs.	TB: EAM to T-1 SS: to skin of neck or to film size Suspend expiration	Extension lateral view of C-spine and upper aspect of T-1. Careful centering required so entire C-spine is well visualized.

Pillars Views of Cervical Spine

View	Measure	Film Size I.D./R or L	FFD	Tube Tilt	Central Ray	Filter/ Shielding	Positioning	Collimation TB = Top to Bottom SS = Side to Side	Essential Anatomy
P-A oblique pillar views of cervical spine Done in pairs optional	A-P at C-4 or top of Adam's apple.	I.D. down Pronate marker 8 × 10	40 in. Bucky	35° Cephalad	H: At C-5 spinous process and film center to horizonal. V: Rt. 1 in. lateral to mid-sagittal. V: Lt. 1 in. lateral to mid-sagittal.	Lead apron	Pt. standing facing Bucky. For Right, have patient turn head 60 to 70° to right. For Left, have patient turn head 60 to 70° to left.	TB: EAM to T-1 or to film size. SS: to skin of neck of film size. Use sandbags to pull shoulders down. Suspend respiration.	Must see entire cervical spine. Shows the articular processes and the apophyseal joints. Rt. obl. for left joints. Lt. obl. for right joints.
A-P oblique pillar views of cervical spine Right Left Optional	A-P at C-4 or top of Adam's apple.	I.D. down 8 × 10	40 in. Bucky	35° Caudal	H: At C-5 or 1 in. below the thyroid cartiledge. V: Rt. 1 in. lateral to mid-sagittal. V: Lt. 1 in. lateral to mid-sagittal. Center film to horizontal central ray.	Lead apron	Pt. recumbent on table. For Right, have patient turn head right 60 to 70°. For Left, have patient turn head to left 60 to 70°.	TB: EAM to T-1 or to film size. SS: To skin of neck of film size. Use strap to pull shoulders down. Suspend respiration.	Must see entire cervical spine. Shows the articular processes and the apophyseal joints. Rt. head turn for left joints.
A-P pillar view of cervical spine	A-P at C-4 or top of Adam's apple.	I.D. down 8 × 10	40 in. Bucky	25° Caudal	H: At C-5 or 1 in. below the thyroid cartiledge. V: Mid-sagittal plane. Center film to horizontal central ray.	Lead apron	Pt. recumbent on table. Have patient hyperextend head as far as possible. If patient cannot tolerate hyperextension, do oblique views.	TB: EAM to T-1 or to film size. SS: To skin of neck of film size. Use straps to pull shoulders down. Suspend respiration.	Demonstrates the lateral masses, the articular facets, the laminae, and spinus processes of the cervical spine.

4.2 Thoracic Spine

View	Measure	Film Size I.D./R or L	FFD	Tube Tilt	Central Ray	Filter/ Shielding	Positioning	Collimation TB = Top to Bottom SS = Side to Side	Essential Anatomy
A-P thoracic spine	A-P at sternum. Over shoulder.	I.D. down 7 × 17	40 in. Bucky	None 90°	H: centered to film. Film 2 in. above C-7. V: mid-sagittal plane (through mid-sternal notch and umbilicus).	40 in. Thyroid or cervico-thoracic filter. Slide down from top until light is seen at the top, then up to close the light. Apron	Pt. standing facing tube. Top of filme 2 in. above C-7. Bottom 3 in. below the xiphoid process. Mid-sagittal plane is perpendicular to the film. Chin slightly elevated. Full inspiration.	TB: C-7 to L-1 or film size. SS: ~6 in. or wide enough to visualize spine and the rib articulations.	A-P view of C-7 to L-1. Full thoracic spine Filter use essential to equalize the densities for upper thoracic spine. (Above heart.)
Lateral thoracic spine	Lateral at subaxillary (from post. aspect)	I.D. up 7 × 17 or 14 × 17	40 in. Bucky	None 90°	H: at center of film. Top of film is 1 in. above C-7. V: between mid-coronal plane and posterior skin.	Point filters per chart below horizontal to CR. Apron	Film 2 in. above C-7. Pt. standing Lt. side to the Bucky. Arms flexed in prayer position with elbows pulled together. Full inspiration.	TB: C-7 to L-1 or film size to see entire T-spine. SS: from mid-coronal plane to posterior skin. Pay close attention to the vertical collimation if pt. is not standing true vertical, open if needed.	True lateral thoracic spine and upper lumbar. Lower cervical if possible. Filters essential to equalize density of entire film.
Swimmer's lateral cervico-thoracic spine	Lateral at subaxillary (from post. aspect)	I.D. up 10 × 12	40 in. Bucky	None 90° optional; 5° caudal for larger pt.	H: through the mid-sternal notch. Center film to the horizontal CR. V: anterior humeral head or mid-clavicular of Rt side of patient.	Lead apron	Pt. standing with Lt. side next to Bucky. Rotate the body 10° posteriorly (toward Bucky). Lt. arm flexed and on top of head. Rt. arm is extended and holding sandbag or grasping thigh. Suspend inspiration.	TB: from C-6 to T-6 or slightly less than film size. SS: slightly smaller than film size.	Unobstructed view of lower cervical and upper thoracic spine. Used also when C-7 is not seen on C-spine with history of trauma.

4.3   Chest, Ribs, Sternum

View	Measure	Film Size I.D./R or L	FFD	Tube Tilt	Central Ray	Filter/ Shielding	Positioning	Collimation TB = Top to Bottom SS = Side to Side	Essential Anatomy
Chest P-A	A-P at mid-sternum	I.D. up 14 × 17	72 in. Bucky	None 90° Pronate marker	H: top of film 2 in. above shoulder. H: CR to Film. V: mid-sagittal plane.	Lead apron	Pt. standing facing Bucky. Hands on hips, shoulders rolled forward to Bucky. Full inspiration.	TB: film size SS: film size	P-A view of lungs, ribs, and heart. Use high kVp to improve lung detail.
Chest lateral	Lateral at subaxillary	I.D. up 14 × 17	72 in. Bucky	None 90°	H: top of film 1 in. above C7/T1. H: CR center to film; V: Mid-coronal plane.	Lead apron	Pt. standing, Lt. shoulder to Bucky. Arms crossed over head. Full inspiration.	TB: film size SS: film size or skin	Lateral view of lungs and heart. Use high kVp to improve lung detail.
Ribs A-P or P-A	A-P at mid-sternum; Pronate marker for P-A views	I.D. up 14 × 17	40 in. Bucky	None 90°	Top of film 2 in. above the shoulder. H: CR center to film; V: centered between mid-sagittal and lateral skin of affected side.	Lead apron	A-P: Standing facing tube. P-A: Standing facing Bucky. Mid-coronal parallel to film. Hands at sides. Inspiration for above the diaphragm injury. Expiration for below the diaphragm injuries.	TB: film size SS: film size or skin *Note:* For below the diaphram injuries, films should be taken recumbent.	View of ribs to r/o rib fractures. P-A is for anterior injury. A-P is for posterior rib injury. Use kVp range of 70 to 80 to improve rib detail.
Ribs oblique anterior or posterior	A-P at mid-sternum Pronate marker for P-A views 12 HD I.D. to spine for lower ribs	I.D. up 14 × 17	40 in. Bucky	None 90°	Above diagram injury top of film 1 in. above shoulder. Below diaphragm injury: bottom of film at iliac crest. H: center to film; V: center between mid-sag. and the lateral borders of ribs.	Lead apron	Patient rotated 30° from A-P or P-A. For anterior obliques, center on side away from film. For posterior obliques, center to side next to film. Use full inspiration for above the diaphragm injury and expiration for below diaphragm injury.	TB: film size SS: film size or skin	Oblique view of ribs. Anterior obliques, i.e., LAO and RAO done for anterior injury and of the affected side. Posterior likewise. Use low kVp for rib detail.

View	Measure	Film Size I.D./R or L	FFD	Tube Tilt	Central Ray	Filter/ Shielding	Positioning	Collimation TB = Top to Bottom SS = Side to Side	Essential Anatomy
Sternum RAO	A-P at mid-sternum	I.D. up 10 × 12	40 in. Bucky	None 90°	H: to film and mid-sternum. V: through sternal long axis. Top of film 1–1.5 in. above episternal notch.	Lead apron	Pt. standing facing Bucky. Mid-coronal plane turned 20 to 30°. Suspend inspiration.	TB: film size SS: film size	View of sternum free of heart and spine.
Sternum lateral	Lateral at mid-sternum	I.D. up 10 × 12	40 in. Bucky	None 90°	Top of film 1.5 in. above sternal notch. H: CR centered to film; V: long axis of sternum.	Lead apron	Pt. standing. Lt. side to the Bucky. Arms locked behind the back with shoulders as far back as possible. Full inspiration.	TB: film size SS: less than film size	Lateral view of the sternum. Vertical collimation essential to reduce scatter and see sternum.

4.4 Extremities

View	Measure	Film Size I.D./R or L	FFD	Tube Tilt	Central Ray	Filter/ Shielding	Positioning	Collimation TB = Top to Bottom SS = Side to Side	Essential Anatomy
Wrist: P-A for scaphoid	A-P at carpals	I.D./R or L 1/2 of 8 × 10 Extremity cassette	40 in. Bucky	15 – 20° Cephalad	H: at scaphoid Center film to H: CR; V: mid-carpals or scaphoid	Coat Apron	Pt. seated next to table. Wrist P-A on film	TB: 5 in. or less SS: 5 in. or less	Carpal bone with the joint spaces around scaphoid open
Elbow: Coyle trauma	Lateral 1 in. distal to medial epicondyle	8 × 10 Extremity cassette	40 in. Bucky	45° Cephalad	H: 1 in. distal to medial epicondyle. Center film to H: CR; V: 1 in. distal to medial epicondyle	None	Pt. is kneeling next to the table. Elbow in lateral position and flexed 90°	TB: Slightly less than film size. SS: Slightly less than film size.	Radial head will be clear of ulna.

4.5 Lumbar Spine and A-P Full Spine

View	Measure	Film Size I.D./R or L	FFD	Tube Tilt	Central Ray	Filter/ Shielding	Positioning	Collimation TB = Top to Bottom SS = Side to Side	Essential Anatomy
Lumbopelvic A-P: Male P-A: Female	A-P at the umbilicus	I.D. up 14 × 17	40 in. Bucky	None 90°	H: not more than 1.5 in. below the iliac crest or midway between the ASIS, crest and iliac crest, whichever is higher. Do not get the ASIS and iliac crest confused. V: mid-sagittal plane.	Gonadal shields: Bell shield used on males. No shield for female when taken P-A.	Pt. is standing with the mid-sagittal plane perpendicular to the Bucky and mid-coronal plane parallel to film. Arms are away from the body, hands holding onto the Bucky. Feet apart. Suspend expiration.	TB: trochanters to T-12. SS: to film size. Gonadal shielding: Male: bell goes at inferior aspect of pubic symphysis. Female: top of heart to level of ASIS for A-P view. None if done P-A.	A-P view of T-12/L-1 to pubic symphysis. It is essential that all lumbar vertebrae be seen. Always try to get the ischeal tuberosities.
Lateral lumbopelvic	Lateral at umbilicus	I.D. up 14 × 17	40 in. Bucky	None 90°	H: 1 in. above the iliac crest. Center film to the horizonal CR. V: mid-coronal plane or halfway between the ASIS and PSIS	Lateral gonadal filter. Spot filters for small-waist female patients.	Pt. standing with Lt. side to Bucky. Mid-sagittal plane parallel to Bucky. Mid-coronal plane perpendicular to film. Arms crossed with hands on shoulders. Suspend expiration.	TB: film size. SS: mid-coronal to skin posteriorly. Gonadal shielding: Top of shield not higher inferior aspect of ASIS with curved side to spine.	True lateral lumbar pelvic spine. Must see from T-12/L-1 to coccyx. Watch object to film distance!
A-P full spine	A-P at umbilicus	I.D. up 14 × 36	72 in. Bucky	None 90°	H: to film. V: mid-sagittal plane. Gonad protection: Bell shield used for male patients. Heart shield used for female patients for A-P films.	Gonadal shields. Filters: 1. Lung to xiphoid process 2. Thyroid 3. Point filters to xiphoid.	Pt. standing with mid-sagittal plane perpendicular to film and arms to sides holding the Bucky. Chin elevated. Bottom of film is 1 in. below the gluteal fold with top at pinna of ear. Xiphoid process should be close to CR when correctly positioned. Full inspiration.	TB: from EAM to just below gluteal fold. SS: to include both trochanters. Make sure that the patient is centered to CR with back in contact with Bucky.	A-P view of the entire spine. Filter placement is key to good film quality. Install filters in order. Point filter per the technique chart from top to xiphoid process or horizontal CR.

Lumbar Spine Obliques and S.I. Joints

Lumbar posterior obliques RPO LPO	A-P at umbilicus	I.D. down 10 × 12	40 in. Bucky	None 90°	H: 1 in. above iliac crest. Film centered to the horizonal CR. V: 2 in. medial to ASIS that is closest to tube.	Gonadal filter same as lateral	Pt. is standing facing the tube. Mid-coronal plane is 40 to 45° to film. Elbow nearest tube is flexed with hand on head. Other arm forward and holding Bucky. Suspend expiration. RPO: Rt. shoulder to Bucky. LPO: Lt. shoulder to Bucky.	TB: T-12 to S-1 or film size. SS: ~6 in. less than film size. Gonadal filter placement. Be careful to not have the gonadal filter above ASIS. Place the curved side toward the spine.	Oblique views of the lumbar spine. Angle of the body is critical. ROP for R facets, Pars and L SI Joint. LPO for L facets, Pars and R SI joint. Best done recumbent.
Lumbar anterior obliques RAO LAO	A-P at umbilicus	I.D. down Pronate markers 10 × 12	40 in. Bucky	None 90°	H: 1 in. above iliac crest. Center film to the horizonal CR. V: laterally or toward tube 1 to 1.5 in. from spinous processes.	Gonadal filter same as lateral	Pt. standing facing Bucky. Mid-coronal plane is 40 to 45° to film. Arm nearest Bucky is behind patient and holding the Bucky. Arm nearest the tube on head. Suspend expiration.	TB: T-12 to S-1 or film size. SS: ~6 in. less than film size. Gonadal filter placement. Be careful to not have the gonadal filter above ASIS. Place the curved side toward the spine.	Oblique views of the lumbopelvic spine. RAO for L facets and Pars and R SI joint. LAO for R facets and Pars and L SI joint.
Sacroiliac joints posterior obliques	A-P at trochanter	I.D. down 8 × 10	40 in. Bucky	None 90°	H: 1 in. below the ASIS nearest the tube. V: 1 in. medial to ASIS closest to tube. Film centered to horizontal CR.	Gonadal filter same as lateral	Pt. standing facing tube. Mid-coronal plane 25 to 30° to Bucky. Arm nearest tube flexed and extended above head. Other arm forward. Suspend expiration	TB: Slightly less than film size. SS: slightly less than film size. If pt. is large, use 10 × 2.	Oblique view to open the sacral iliac joints. Angle of the obl. is critical. Do not use more than 30° rotation of patient.

4.6 Sacrum and Coccyx

View	Measure	Film Size I.D./R or L	FFD	Tube Tilt	Central Ray	Filter/ Shielding	Positioning	Collimation TB = Top to Bottom SS = Side to Side	Essential Anatomy
Sacroiliac joints anterior obliques	A-P at the trochanter	I.D. down Pronate markers 8 × 10	40 in. Bucky	None 90°	H: 1 in. below the PSIS nearest the Bucky. Film centered to H: CR. V: 1 in. medial to PSIS nearest the Bucky.	Gonadal filter same as lateral	Pt. is standing facing the Bucky. Mid-coronal plane is 25 to 30° to Bucky. Elbow nearest tube is flexed with hand on head or shoulder. Other arm away from body and holding Bucky. Suspend expiration.	TB: slightly less than film size. SS: slightly less than film size. For large pt., 10 × 12 film can be used.	Oblique to open the sacroiliac joints. Angle critical not greater than 30°. RAO for R SI joint. LAO for L SI joint. Both obliques always done.
Sacral base A-P spot	A-P at trochanter	I.D. up 8 × 10	40 in. Bucky	30° Cephalad	H: 30° cephalad through inferior aspect of ASIS. Film center to H: CR. V: mid-sagittal plane.	Gonadal shield for males; none for females	Pt. standing facing tube. Mid-sagittal perpendicular to film. Mid-coronal parallel to film. Hands holding Bucky.	TB: 5 in. SS: 5 in.	A-P view of base of sacrum and articulation with L-5.
Sacral base lateral spot L5/S1	Lateral at trochanter	I.D. up 8 × 10	40 in. Bucky	None 90°	H: 1 to 2 in. below iliac crest. Film center to H: CR. V: 1 in. posterior to mid-coronal plane.	Gonadal filter	Pt. standing with Lt. side to Bucky. Mid-coronal plane perpendicular to Bucky. Arms crossed with hands on shoulders.	TB: 5 in. SS: 5 in.	Lateral spot of the L-5/S-1 space and upper sacrum.
A-P sacrum	A-P at trochanter	I.D. up 8 × 10	40 in. Bucky	15° Cephalad	H: 15° ceph. midway between ASIS and pubic symphysis. Film centered to H: CR. V: mid-sagittal plane.	Shield for men; none for women	Pt. standing facing tube. Mid-sagittal plane is perpendicular to film.	TB: slightly less than film size. SS: slightly less than film size.	A-P view of sacrum.
A-P coccyx	A-P at trochanter	I.D. up 8 × 10	40 in. Bucky	10° Caudal	H: 10° caudal, 2 in. superior to pubic symphysis. Film centered to H: CR. V: mid-sagittal plane.	Same as sacrum	Pt. standing facing tube. Mid-sagittal plane perpendicular to film.	TB: slightly less than film size. SS: slightly less than film size.	A-P view of coccyx.
Lateral sacrum and coccyx	Lateral at trochanter	I.D. up 10 × 12	40 in. Bucky	None 90°	H: between ASIS and pubic symphysis. Film to H: CR. V: 2 to 3 in. posterior to mid-coronal plane.	Lateral gonadal filter	Pt. standing with Lt. side to Bucky. Arms crossed with hands on shoulders. Feet in wide stance.	TB: slightly less than film size. SS: slightly less than film size.	True lateral view of sacrum and coccyx.

4.7 Special Chest and Abdomen

View	Measure	Film Size I.D./R or L	FFD	Tube Tilt	Central Ray	Filter/Shielding	Positioning	Collimation TB = Top to Bottom SS = Side to Side	Essential Anatomy
Chest lateral decubitus view	A-P at mid-chest	14 × 17 Regular; arrow to side up.	72 in. Bucky	None 90°	H: mid-sagittal plane (spinus process). CR: to film center. Side of film 1 in. above the shoulder.	Lead apron	Pt. lies on affected side on table with towels or sponge between tabletop and ribs. Arms over head. May be done A-P or P-A. Note for visceral fluid have affected side up and use expiration. Routine would be inspiration.	TB: slightly less than film size. SS: slightly less than film size.	View of chest to evaluate fluid in the lungs or hilar area. Fluid in the plural cavity should gravitate and be seen as a layer on the film.
Chest obliques RAO LAO	A-P at mid-chest	14 × 17 Regular	72 in. Bucky	None 90°	Top of film 2 in. above shoulder. CR to film center. V: 2 to 3 in. lateral to the spine furthest from film. (Pt. centered to see all of lung fields on film.)	Lead apron	Pt. stands P-A with arm closest to the film on hip and arm furthest from film over head. For RAO, the pt. is turned 45°. For LAO, patient is turned 60° from P-A. Full inspiration.	TB: slightly less than film size. SS: slightly less than film size.	Oblique chest views will show those structures that the spine or aorta may obscure on the P-A view.
Chest axial or apical lordotic	A-P at mid-chest	10 × 12 Regular	72 in. Bucky	15 to 20° cephalad	Top of film 1.5 in. above shoulders. H: mid-sagittal plane. V: to film center.	Lead apron	Pt. standing 1 foot from Bucky in A-P position. Pt. arches back until shoulders are in contact with Bucky. Full inspiration.	TB: slightly less than film size. SS: slightly less than film size.	View of apices of lungs free of overlying clavicles.
Abdomen KUB	A-P at umbilicus	14 × 17 Regular	40 in. Bucky	None 90°	H: 1 in. below the iliac crest. V: mid-sagittal plane. Film center to H: CR.	Bell for men	Pt. recumbent on table. Legs may be bent for comfort. Full expiration.	TB: slightly less than film size. SS: slightly less than film size.	A-P view of abdomen to include kidneys, lower portion of liver, and the psoas muscle.
Abdomen upright w/o P-A chest	A-P at umbilicus	14 × 17 Regular	40 in. Bucky	None 90°	H: 1.5 to 2 in. above iliac crest if P-A chest not done. H: at level of iliac crest if P-A chest is done. V: mid-sagittal plane. Center film to H: CR.	Bell for men	Pt. stands facing tube. If P-A chest is done, position like A-P lumbopelvic. If chest is not done, upright view must include diaphrams to detect free air. Full expiration.	TB: slightly less than film size. SS: slightly less than film size.	Upright abdomen to visualize, air fluid levels, masses, and possible free air under diaphrams. Free air may indicate a rupture in GI tract.

Acute abdomen series should include an erect P-A chest, KUB, and upright abdomen.

Chiropractic Radiography and Quality Assurance Handbook

4.8 Skull

View	Measure	Film Size I.D./R or L	FFD	Tube Tilt	Central Ray	Filter/ Shielding	Positioning	Collimation TB = Top to Bottom SS = Side to Side	Essential Anatomy
Skull base posterior (SMV)	A-P at glabella	10 × 12 Regular	40 in. Bucky	None (see positioning)	H: through EAM. Center film to H: CR. V: mid-sagittal plane of skull.	Lead apron	Pt. seated A-P with head extremely extended until the infraorbitalmeatal line is parallel to film. Tube angulation may be used if patient has difficulty extending head.	TB: slightly less than film size. SS: slightly less than film size.	Axial view of dens and foramen magnum of skull. Also good to evaluate zygomatic arches.
Skull towne's or half-axial	A-P at glabella	10 × 12 Regular	40 in. Bucky	35° Caudal to the canthomeatal line of skull	H: 2 in. above glabella passing through both EAMs. Center top of film to the vertex of skull. V: mid-sagittal plane of skull.	Lead apron	Pt. seated A-P. With occiput of skull on the Bucky, tuck the chin down until the canthomeatal line is perpendicular to film. May be done P-A with 30° cephalad tube angle. Horizonal CR through AM.	TB: slightly less than film size. SS: slightly less than film size.	Occipital region of skull petrous bone and the atlas in the foramen magnum.
Skull P-A	A-P at glabella	10 × 12 Regular	40 in. Bucky	None 90°	H: to exit at the level of the glabella. Film center to H: CR. V: mid-sagittal plane of skull.	Lead apron	Pt. seated facing Bucky. Forehead and nose on Bucky center line. Make sure there is no rotation of the mid-sagittal plane.	TB: slightly less than film size. SS: slightly less than film size.	Frontal view of skull.
Skull lateral	Lateral at AM	12 × 10 Regular	40 in. Bucky	None	H: 1 in. above the AM. V: 1 in. in front of the AM. Center film to H: CR.	Lead apron	Pt. seated P-A with the head turned so the affected ear is on the center line of Bucky. Interpupillary line perpendicular to the film. Central ray should be through the sella turcica or sella depression.	TB: slightly less than film size. SS: slightly less than film size.	Lateral view skull, sella turcica, and sinuses.

4.9 Facial Bones, Sinuses, and TMJ

View	Measure	Film Size I.D./R or L	FFD	Tube Tilt	Central Ray	Filter/ Shielding	Positioning	Collimation TB = Top to Bottom SS = Side to Side	Essential Anatomy
Facial/sinus Water's view	A-P at glabella	8 × 10 Regular	40 in. Bucky	None 90°	H: through the mentomeatal line of skull. Center film to H: CR; V: mid-sagittal plane.	Lead apron	Pt. seated P-A facing Bucky. With chin resting on the Bucky, extend head until the mentomeatal line is perpendicular to the film. The mid-sagittal plane of the patient is also perpendicular to film. Nose will be about 3 cm from Bucky.	TB: slightly less than film size. SS: slightly less than film size.	View of maxillary sinuses, orbits, frontal sinuses. With mouth open, sphenoid sinus can be seen.
Sinus submental vertex (SMV)	A-P at glabella	8 × 10 Regular	40 in. Bucky	None (see positioning)	H: through angles of the mandible. Center film to H: CR; V: mid-sagittal plane of skull.	Lead apron	Pt. seated A-P with head extremely extended until the cantomeatal line is 100° to tube or the acanthiomeatal line is parallel to the film. The angulation may be used to achieve angles.	TB: slightly less than film size. SS: slightly less than film size.	Axial view of sphenoid sinus, zygomatic arches.
Caldwell P-A	A-P at glabella	8 × 10 Regular	40 in. Bucky	15° Caudal	H: to exit at the level of the glabella. Film center to H: CR; V: mid-sagittal plane of skull.	Lead apron	Pt. seated, facing Bucky. Forehead and nose on Bucky center line. Make sure there is no rotation of the mid-sagittal plane.	TB: slightly less than film size. SS: slightly less than film size.	Frontal view of frontal sinus, superior orbital fissure, ethmoid sinus and greater wing of the sphenoid.
Sinus/facial lateral	Lateral at AM	8 × 10 Regular	40 in. Bucky	None	H: outer canthus of eye. V: outer canthus of eye. Center film to H: CR.	Lead apron	Pt. seated P-A with the head turned so the affected ear is on center line of Bucky. Interpupillary line perpendicular to the film.	TB: slightly less than film size. SS: slightly less than film size.	Lateral view of sinuses.

View	Measure	Film Size I.D./R or L	FFD	Tube Tilt	Central Ray	Filter/Shielding	Positioning	Collimation TB = Top to Bottom SS = Side to Side	Essential Anatomy
Schuller's view of the TM joints open and closed mouth	Lateral at AM	8 × 10 Regular	40 in. Bucky	25° Caudal	H: exits through TMJ next to the film (1 in. in front of EAM). V: exits through TMJ next to the film. Center film to H: CR.	Lead apron	Pt. seated P-A with head turned so affected TMJ is on center line of Bucky. Interpupillary line perpendicular to film. Views taken with mouth open and closed bilaterally. 4 views per series.	TB: slightly less than film size. SS: slightly less than film size.	View of the TM joint with full open and closed mouth.

Special reference lines for skull and sinus positioning. Cantomeatal line: An imaginary line that runs from the outer canthus of the eye to the external auditory meatus. Acanthiomeatal line: An imaginary line that runs from the acanthion or tip of the nasal spine to the EAM. Interpupillary or interorbital line: An imaginary line that joins the orbits or pupils of the eyes. Intraorbital-meatal line: An imaginary line running from the inferior rim of the orbit to the EAM.

4.10 Sacrum, Sacral Base and Coccyx Female of Child-Bearing Age

View	Measure	Film Size I.D./R or L	FFD	Tube Tilt	Central Ray	Filter/Shielding	Positioning	Collimation TB = Top to Bottom SS = Side to Side	Essential Anatomy
Sacral Base P-A	A-P at trochanters	8 × 10 Reg. I.D. Up marker pronated	40 in. Bucky	30° Caudal	H: level of the PSIS Center film to H: CR; V: mid-sagittal.	None	Pt. is standing facing the Bucky with feet shoulder's width apart.	TB: slightly less than film size. SS: slightly less than film size.	L5/S1 disc space and sacral illiac joints.
Sacrum P-A	A-P at trochanters	8 × 10 Reg. I.D. Up marker pronated	40 in. Bucky	15° Caudal	H: 2 in. below PSIS Center film to H: CR; V: mid-sagittal.	None	Pt. is standing facing the Bucky with feet shoulder's width apart.	TB: slightly less than film size. SS: slightly less than film size.	Sacrum and S.I. joints.
Coccyx P-A	A-P at trochanters	8 × 10 Reg. I.D. Up marker pronated	40 in. Bucky	10° Caudal	H: midway between PSIS and trochanter. Film center to H: CR; V: mid-sagittal.	None	Pt. is standing facing the Bucky with feet shoulder's width apart.	TB: slightly less than film size. SS: slightly less than film size.	Coccyx.

5

Cervical Spine Radiography

5.1 Cervical Spine Radiography: Introduction

All cervical spine views are taken on 8 in. × 10 in. Regular Speed cassettes. The identification blocker should be down for all views, especially the lateral views. The lateral views are taken at a 72 in. SID or FFD using a Non-Bucky cassette holder. The 72 in. SID is needed to reduce magnification because of the width of the shoulders. The distance between the shoulders and film produces an air gap, so the Bucky is not needed. The use of the Bucky would result in a fivefold increase in unnecessary radiation exposure.

Sandbags (5 to 10 lb) are used to lower the shoulders to better visualize the 7th cervical and 1st thoracic vertebrae on the lateral and upright pillars projections. Expiration is also used for the same reason because patients will typically lower their shoulders on expiration. Another technique that can be used is to have the patient pull their shoulders back.

The measurements for the technique selection are taken at the level of the 4th cervical vertebra. This is approximately at the level of the top of the Adam's apple. This is also the location for placement of the horizontal central ray for all views except those taken for the dens.

For all cervical spine views except the Fuchs projection, the chin of the patient should be elevated until the acanthameatal line is perpendicular to the film. For lateral views, the extension can be increased until the occiput and the chin are parallel to the film. A very common mistake is to not raise the chin. This results in the mandible overlying the upper cervical vertebrae on the lateral view and centering the central ray too low. When the chin is not raised on A-P and oblique views, the mandible will again obscure visualization of the upper cervical spine. It is equally important to check the interpupillary line on the lateral views to make sure that it is also perpendicular to the film.

A 15 to 20° cephalad tube angle is used on A-P lower cervical and posterior oblique views. This will open the disc spaces. Anterior oblique views need a 15 to 20° caudal tube angle. There are at least three different SIDs recommended for the oblique views of the cervical spine. Oblique views can be taken using the air gap method at 60 in. SID or 72 in. SID using the Non-Bucky film holder. The oblique views can also be taken at 48 in. SID using the Bucky. In all of the optional combinations, the increased SID will reduce magnification distortion. The 60 in. or 72 in. Non-Bucky view can be taken with comparable technical factors to the 40 in. Bucky technique. The skin radiation dose is significantly reduced.

The lateral views should always have the tube perpendicular to the film. Routine views of the dens use no tube angle, but patients with abnormal cervical curves may need a 5° cephalad tube angle. A patient in a cervical collar may need a 5° caudal tube angle to see the dens.

While there should be no exposure to the patient's gonads from cervical spine radiography, the lead apron is used primarily for patient reassurance. The cervical spine views should be vertically collimated to the skin of the neck. This will almost always be less than film size and will reduce exposure to the patient. The A-P open mouth or Fuchs projection uses a 5-in. square as collimation. The upper border for collimation for the lateral view is the EAM.

Cervical Spine Studies

Limited Cervical Spine	Neutral lateral view, A-P lower cervical spine, A-P open mouth
Complete Cervical Spine*	Neutral lateral view, right and left posterior, or anterior oblique views, A-P lower cervical spine, and A-P open mouth.
	*Flexion and extension lateral views may be substituted for oblique views.
Davis Series	Complete cervical spine series and flexion and extension lateral views.
Supplemental views:	Fuchs, right and left pillars oblique views, base posterior skull, A-P pillar view, swimmers view to see C-7.

Cervical spine oblique views can be performed as anterior or posterior oblique. For a tall patient, the patient may need to be seated due to the 15 to 20° caudal tube angulation. The anterior oblique will have the patient closer to the film. Posterior oblique can be quickly incorporated into the routine cervical spine study because the same tube angulation (15 to 20° cephalad) as the A-P lower cervical spine view is used. In either case, the patient should be 40 to 45° oblique. The chin must be elevated and the head turned lateral to get a clear view of the upper cervical spine. If an increased SID is employed, posterior oblique views will probably be the only option.

RAO will demonstrate the right foramina (the side closest to the film). The right marker is pronated and placed behind the body and spinous process.

LAO will demonstrate the left foramina. The left marker is pronated and placed behind the spinous process.

RPO will demonstrate the left foramina (the side furthest from the film). The right marker is placed in front of the body and spinous process.

LPO will demonstrate the right foramina. The left marker is placed in front of the body.

Important skull and cervical spine positioning lines are depicted in Figure 5.1.

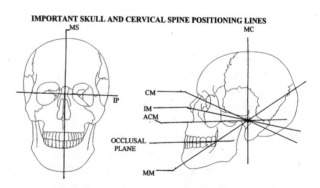

IMPORTANT SKULL AND CERVICAL SPINE POSITIONING LINES

FIGURE 5.1
Important skull and cervical spine positioning lines.

MS- MID-SAGITTAL PLANE
IP- INTER- PUPILLARY LINE
IM- INFERIOR ORBITAL-MEATAL LINE
ACM- ACANTHA-MEATAL LINE

MC- MID CORONAL PLANE
CM- CANTOMEATAL LINE
MM-MENTA-MEATAL

5.2   Cervical Spine Positioning: A-P Open Mouth View

Measure

A-P at C-4

Protection

Lead apron

SID

40 in. using Bucky

Tube Angulation

No tube angulation; anterior weight-bearing or patients lacking a normal curve may require a 5° cephalad tube angulation.

Film

8 in. × 10 in. regular speed rare-earth cassettes with I.D. down

Positioning

1. Patient standing, facing the tube. The intra-orbital or interpupillary line parallel to floor with the mid-sagittal plane perpendicular to film.
2. Align the mastoid tips and upper incisors or the acanthiomeatal line perpendicular to film. The acanthiomeatal line is usually parallel to the mastoid tips and upper incisors.
3. Horizontal CR 1 in. below upper incisors.
4. Center film to horizontal CR. Vertical CR to mid-sagittal plane.
5. Have patient open mouth as far as possible without moving head.

Collimation

5-in. square

Breathing Instructions

Say "ah" or suspend respiration.

Image Critique

There should be a clear view of C-1 and C-2 through the open mouth. The mastoid tips should be in line with the upper teeth. There should be no rotation of the patient's head. If the dens is not well demonstrated, other views such as the Fuchs or base posterior view can be done.

Optimum kVp

75–80 kVp

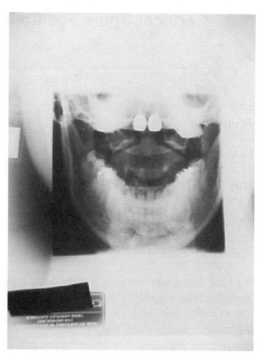

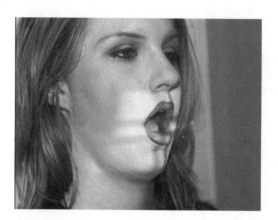

FIGURE 5.2
APOM positioning.

FIGURE 5.3
APOM image.

5.3   Troubleshooting the A-P Open Mouth (APOM) View

The APOM view is the most challenging view of the cervical spine. A number of factors will impact the quality of the view. Factors include:

1.   The shape of the skull. Round or brachycephalic skull is the most challenging.

2.   The degree of anterior weight-bearing will impact how close one can get the patient to the Bucky and if a tube angulation will be needed. With the anterior shift of the cervical spine, it is very easy to get the teeth to obscure the dens.

3.   The ability of the patient to open the mouth wide without extending the head. It is very important to take the view as soon as the proper position is obtained. Make sure the technical factors are set before positioning the patient.

Positioning techniques that can help improve the view include:

1.   Minor adjustments in positioning will result in significant changes on the film. At 40 in. SID, a change in position of 0.25 in. will result in a 0.5-in. change on the film.

2.   Precise positioning of the patient. The mid-sagittal plane must be perpendicular to the film; slight rotation will impair image quality.

3.   Patients that are anterior weight-bearing will generally need a sponge placed behind the head.

4. Communicate with the patient; having the patient open the mouth as wide as possible without raising the head is very important.

5. Sometimes it is necessary to use a 5° cephalad tube angle to raise the incisors above the dens. The 5° tube angle will raise the teeth 0.5 in.

6. One may also find that placing the horizontal central ray 1 in. below the incisors will help raise the teeth above the dens due to the divergent rays.

Problem: Caps obscuring view of dens (Figure 5.4)

This image is of a patient with porcelain caps on the front teeth. Note that the mastoid tips and upper teeth are aligned. Positioning is therefore correct.

Solutions

1. A slight or less than 5° cephalad tube angulation may throw the caps clear of the dens without getting the base of the skull in the way.

2. Have the patient extend the head back about 1/8 in. to move the incisors above the dens.

Problem: Base of skull obscuring dens (Figure 5.5)

The teeth are clear of the dens but the base of the skull is obscuring the view. The acantha meatal or mastoid tips to upper incisors line is not perpendicular to the film.

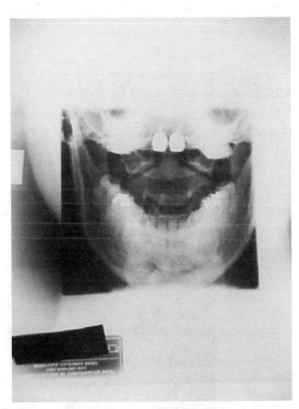

FIGURE 5.4
APOM caps.

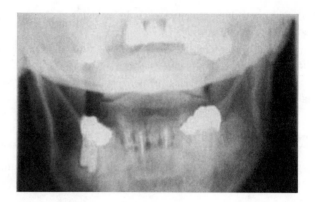

FIGURE 5.5
APOM head back too far.

Solutions

1. Lower the teeth and raise the base of the skull by having the patient tuck the head down about 0.5 in. (1 cm).
2. Make sure that the patient does not raise head when opening the mouth.
3. If everything else has been tried, try a 5° caudal tube angle or proceed with a Fuchs projection.

Problem

Base of skull covers superior part of lateral masses; dens is clear of teeth with base of skull slightly covering the top (Figure 5.6)

Solutions

1. Angle tube less than 5° cephalad.
2. Lower chin by 1/8 in.
3. This view is acceptable.

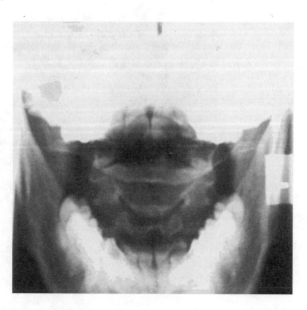

FIGURE 5.6
APOM OK.

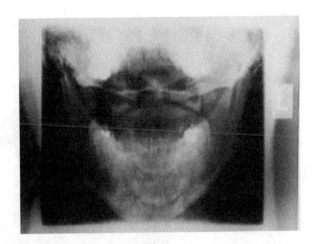

FIGURE 5.7
APOM tube angled.

Problem

Base of skull covers dens (Figure 5.7)

Solutions

1. Lower chin by 1/4 in. if patient can tolerate position and open mouth wide.
2. If tube angulation was used, retake with no tube angulation.

Problem

Upper teeth totally obscure the view. (Figure 5.8)

Solutions

1. The most common solution if the teeth are in proper alignment with mastoid tips is a 5° cephalad tube angle.
2. If alignment is off, raise chin until the mastoid tips and incisors are perpendicular to film.

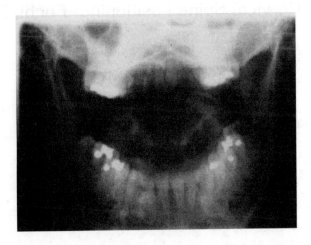

FIGURE 5.8
APOM teeth block view.

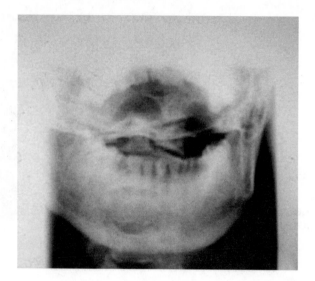

FIGURE 5.9
APOM rotated.

Problem

Head rotated (Figure 5.9)

Solutions

1. Closely observe patient to make sure the mid-sagittal plane is perpendicular to the film.
2. Try to compare distance from Bucky to EAM bilaterally to correct rotation.

Note: *When using the 5-in. square for collimation, the upper border should be just below the nose. One can use this as a guide to check the acanthiomeatal line. Follow the light from the bottom of the nose to the EAM. This line usually runs parallel to the upper incisors and mastoid tip.*

5.4   Cervical Spine Positioning: Fuchs Projection

Measure

A-P at C-4

Protection

Lead apron

SID

40 in. using Bucky

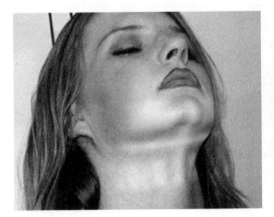

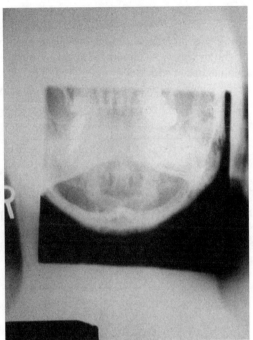

FIGURE 5.10
Fuchs positioning.

FIGURE 5.11
Fuchs film.

Tube Angulation

No tube angulation

Film/Markers

8 in. × 10 in. regular speed rare-earth cassette with I.D. down. R or L anatomical.

Positioning

1. Patient standing, facing the tube. The intra-orbital line parallel to floor with the mid-sagittal plane perpendicular to film.
2. Have patient extend head back until the mentameatal line is perpendicular to the film.
3. Align horizontal central ray just below angle of the mandible.
4. Center film to horizontal central ray; Vertical CR to mid-sagittal plane.
5. Have patient suspend respiration

Collimation

5 in. square

Breathing Instructions

Suspend respiration.

Image Critique

The Fuchs projection should provide a clear view of the dens. It will be seen in the foramen magnum. This view should not be taken immediately post-trauma. The view can be taken P-A with chin in contact with Bucky and nose 0.5 in. off of the Bucky. The patient position would be similar to the Water's sinus with the central ray directed at C-2.

Optimum kVp

75–80 kVp

5.5   Cervical Spine Positioning: A-P Lower Cervical Spine View

Measure

A-P at C-4

Protection

Lead apron

SID

40 in. using Bucky

Tube Angulation

15° cephalad

Film/Marker

8 in. × 10 in. regular speed rare-earth cassette with I.D. down. R or L anatomical.

Positioning

1. Patient stands in front of Bucky, facing the tube.
2. Chin elevated until the acanthiomeatal line is perpendicular to film.
3. Mid-sagittal plane should be perpendicular to film with no rotation of head or body.
4. Center horizontal central ray to C-4 and then center film to horizontal central ray.
5. Center patient so vertical central ray aligns with the mid-sagittal plane.

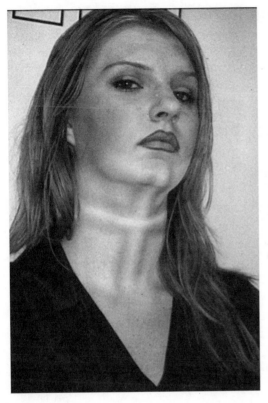

FIGURE 5.12
AP C-spine positioning.

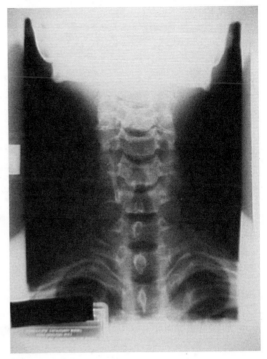

FIGURE 5.13
AP C-spine film.

Collimation

Top to Bottom: mastoid tips to T-2; Side to Side: skin of neck

Breathing Instructions

Suspend respiration

Image Critique

Occiput and mandible should be superimposed. Disc spaces should be open. There should be no rotation of body or skull. Check sternoclavicular joints and mandible for rotation. Optional modification of A-P lower cervical spine view is lateral bending views to check for stability.

Optimum kVp

70–75 kVp

5.6   Cervical Spine Positioning: Posterior Oblique View

Measure

A-P at C-4

Protection

Lead apron

SID

40 in. using Bucky; optional 60–72 in. Non-Bucky; optional 48 in. using Bucky

Tube Angulation

15 to 20° cephalad

Film

8 in. × 10 in. regular speed rare-earth cassette with I.D. down. R or RPO and L or LPO anatomical.

Positioning

1. Patient turned 40 to 45° from A-P. The shoulder next to the Bucky will determine if the view is RPO or LPO. Mark the film appropriately. The chin should be extended until the acanthiomeatal and interpupillary lines are perpendicular to film.
2. Place horizontal central ray at level of C-4 and center film to the horizontal central ray.
3. With the head in the same plane as the body, the vertical central ray will be 1 in. anterior to EAM.
4. Turn head to true lateral and the vertical central ray will pass through the EAM.
5. Have patient suspend respiration. Expose film. Repeat steps with the other shoulder next to the film.

Collimation

Side to Side: Skin of neck; Top to Bottom: EAM to T-1 or T-2

Breathing Instructions

Suspend respiration

Image Critique

The disc spaces and intravertebral foramens should be open. The body of the vertebra should be the same. If angle of obliquity is more than 45°, the body will appear small, like the lateral view. If the angle is too shallow or less than 40°, the body will be large, similar to A-P view. The RPO

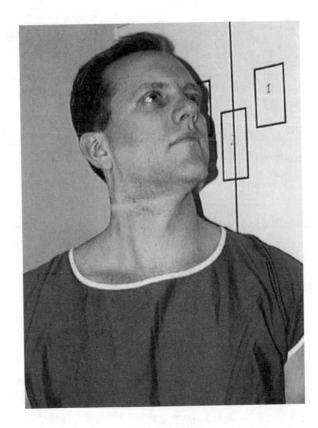

FIGURE 5.14
Posterior oblique positioning.

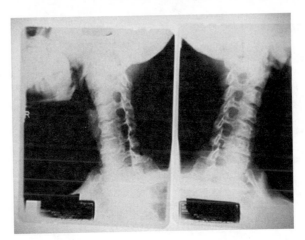

FIGURE 5.15
Posterior oblique films.

will demonstrate the left intravertebral foramens. The LPO will demonstrate the right intravertebral foramens. If head is not properly positioned, mandible will obscure upper cervical spine.

Optimum kVp

70–80 kVp

5.7   Cervical Spine Positioning: Anterior Oblique View

Measure

A-P at C-4

Protection

Lead apron

SID

40 in. using Bucky; optional 48 in. using Bucky; optional 60 in. to 72 in. Non-Bucky

Tube Angulation

15 to 20° caudal

Film

8 in. × 10 in. regular speed rare-earth cassette with I.D. down

Marker

Pronated R and L, or RAO and LAO

Positioning

1. Patient is seated on stool and turned 40 to 45° from P-A. The shoulder next to the Bucky will determine if the view is the RAO or LAO. Chin should be extended so the acanthiomeatal and interpupillary lines are perpendicular to film.
2. Place horizontal central ray at level of C-4 and center film to horizontal central ray.
3. Turn the head to true lateral and align the vertical central ray with the EAM.
4. Have patient suspend respiration and make exposure.
5. Repeat steps 1 through 4 with other shoulder to film.

Collimation

Side to Side: Skin of neck; Top to Bottom: EAM to T-1 or T-2

Breathing Instructions

Suspend respiration

Image Critique

1. The disc spaces and IVFs should be open.
2. The body of the vertebra should look the same. If rotation is too great, the body will be small. If too shallow, it will be too large, similar to A-P.

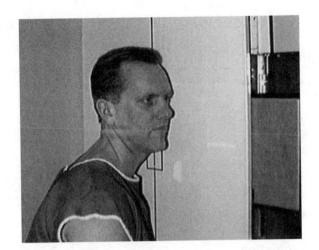

FIGURE 5.16
Anterior oblique positioning.

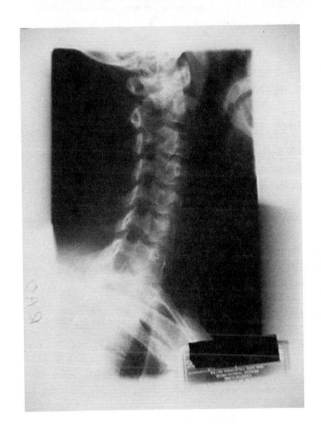

FIGURE 5.17
Anterior oblique film.

3. RAO will demonstrate the right IVFs and LAO will show the left IVFs.

4. If chin is not extended, mandible will obscure upper vertebra.

5. Must demonstrate C-1 to T-1.

Optimum kVp

75–80 kVp

5.8   Cervical Spine Positioning: Neutral Lateral View

Measure

Lateral at C-4

Protection

Lead apron

SID

72 in. Non-Bucky

Tube Angulation

None

Film

8 in. × 10 in. regular speed rare-earth cassette with I.D. down

Positioning

1. Center Non-Bucky film holder and film to vertical central ray.
2. Have patient stand with left shoulder next to film.
3. Have patient raise chin until the acanthiomeatal line is perpendicular to film. Check interpupillary line and make sure the skull is in a true lateral.
4. Place horizontal central ray at the level of C-4 or top of Adam's apple and center film to horizontal central ray.
5. Align the vertical central ray with the EAM.
6. Give patient sandbags to hold to lower shoulders. Recheck the positioning. For very large shoulder, pull shoulder back to better clear C-7.

Collimation

Side to Side: skin of neck; Top to Bottom: EAM to T-1

Breathing Instructions

Full expiration

Image Critique

Must see all seven cervical vertebrae. The head should be in true lateral with mandibles superimposed. Need to see the entire airway. I.D. is placed down to avoid covering C-1 and C-2 in the lateral projection. In order to evaluate McGregor's line, the hard palate must be seen.

Optimum kVp

70–75 kVp

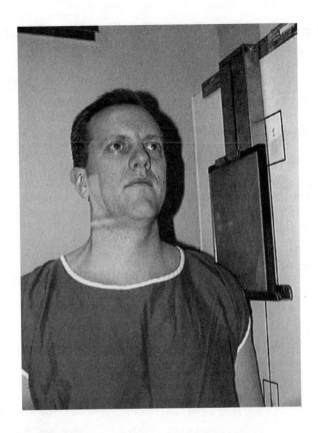

FIGURE 5.18
Neutral lateral C-spine positioning.

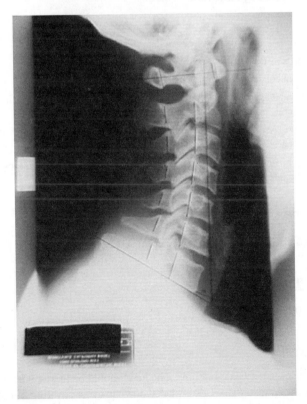

FIGURE 5.19
Neutral lateral film.

5.9   Cervical Spine Positioning: Extension Lateral View

Measure

Lateral at C-4

Protection

Lead apron

SID

72 in. Non-Bucky

Tube Angulation

None

Film

8 in. × 10 in. Lanex regular with I.D. down

Marker

L and arrow pointing backward, or EXT

Positioning

1.   Center Non-Bucky film holder and film to vertical central ray.
2.   Have patient standing with left shoulder next to the film.
3.   Have patient extend neck as far as possible. Check interpupillary line and make sure the skull is in a true lateral.
4.   Place horizontal central ray at the level of C-4 and center film to horizontal central ray.
5.   Align the vertical central ray with EAM.
6.   Give patient sandbags to hold to lower shoulders. Recheck the positioning. For very large shoulder, pull shoulder back to better clear C-7.

Collimation

Side to Side: skin of neck; Top to Bottom: EAM to T-1

Breathing Instructions

Full expiration

Image Critique

Must see all seven cervical vertebrae. The head should be in true lateral with mandibles superimposed. Need to see the entire airway. I.D. is placed down to avoid covering C-1 and C-2 in the lateral projection.

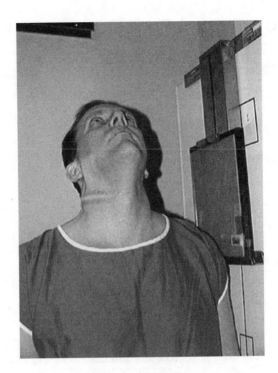

FIGURE 5.20
Extension lateral C-spine positioning.

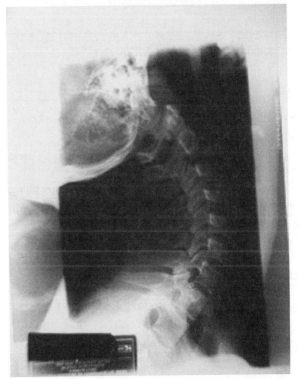

FIGURE 5.21
Extension lateral film.

Optimum kVp

70–75 kVp

Caution: *Do not force patient beyond their motion limit.*

5.10   Cervical Spine Positioning: Flexion Lateral View

Measure

Lateral at C-4

Protection

Lead apron

SID

72 in. Non-Bucky

Tube Angulation

None

Film

10 in. × 8 in. regular speed rare-earth cassette with I.D. down

Marker

L and arrow pointing forward, or FLEX marker

Positioning

1. Center Non-Bucky film holder and film to vertical central ray.
2. Have patient standing with left shoulder next to film.
3. Have patient tuck chin into chest as neck flexes forward. Check interpupillary line and make sure the skull is in a true lateral.
4. Place horizontal central ray at the level of C-4 and center film to horizontal central ray.
5. Align the vertical central ray with the C-4. Make sure that EAM to T-1 is in the field of view.
6. Give patient sandbags to hold to lower shoulders. Recheck the positioning. For very large shoulder, pull shoulder back to better clear C-7.

Collimation

Side to Side: EAM to T-1; Top to Bottom: EAM to T-1

Breathing Instructions

Full expiration

Image Critique

Must see all seven cervical vertebrae. The head should be in true lateral with mandibles superimposed. Need to see the entire airway. I.D. is placed up on left lateral to avoid covering C-1 and

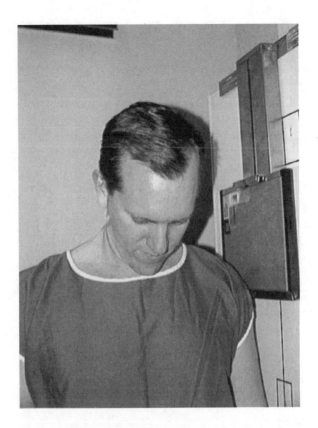

FIGURE 5.22
Flexion lateral positioning.

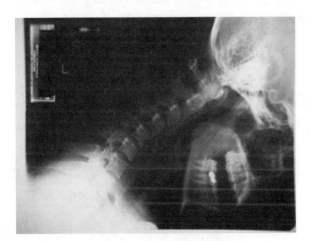

FIGURE 5.23
Flexion lateral film.

C-2 in the lateral projection. If patient has very limited flexion, change cassette orientation to 8 in. ×
10 in. with I.D. down.

Optimum kVp

70–75 kVp

Caution: *Do not force patient beyond their motion limit.*

5.11   Cervical Spine Positioning: A-P Pillars View

Measure

A-P at C-4

Protection

Lead apron

SID

40 in. using Table Bucky

Tube Angulation

25 to 30° caudal

Film

8 in. × 10 in. regular speed rare-earth cassette with I.D. down

Positioning

1. Patient supine on table. Place a large-angle sponge under the shoulders. Have patient extend head as far as possible. Make sure that the interpupillary line is straight and the mid-sagittal plane is perpendicular to film.
2. Align the mentameatal line at least perpendicular to film.
3. Horizontal central ray through C-5. The film is centered to the horizontal central ray.
4. Vertical central ray to mid-sagittal plane.
5. Have patient suspend respiration. Make exposure.

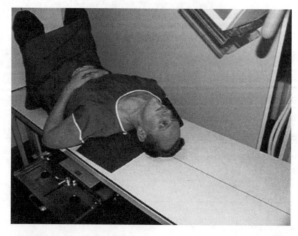

FIGURE 5.24
Pillars A-P positioning.

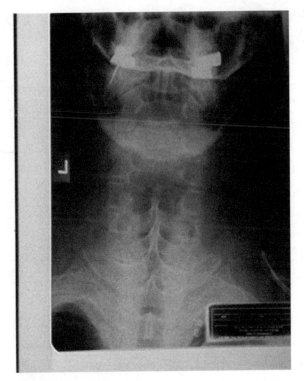

FIGURE 5.25
Pillars film.

Collimation

Top to Bottom: C-2 to T-4 or slightly less than film size; Side to side: skin of neck

Breathing Instructions

Suspend respiration

Image Critique

The success of this view will depend on the patient's ability to hyperextend head. If the patient has pain with extension of the neck, the oblique pillars views would be better tolerated by the patient and provide better visualization of the lateral masses. The view will demonstrate the cervical lateral masses, the laminae, and the spinous processes of the cervical and upper thoracic spine.

Optimum kVp

75–80 kVp

5.12   Cervical Spine Positioning: Posterior Oblique Pillars View

Measure

A-P at C-4

Protection

Lead apron

SID

40 in. using Table Bucky or seated on wall Bucky

Tube Angulation

35 to 40° caudal

Film

8 in. × 10 in. regular speed rare-earth cassettes with I.D. down.

Positioning

1. Patient supine on table. Have patient extend chin until the acanthameatal line is perpendicular to film. Make sure that the interpupillary line is straight and have patient turn head to side 45 to 50°.
2. Horizontal central ray through C-5. The film is centered to the horizontal central ray.
3. Vertical central ray to long axis of cervical spine.
4. Have patient suspend respiration. Make exposure.
5. Repeat with head turned to other side. These views are always done in pairs.

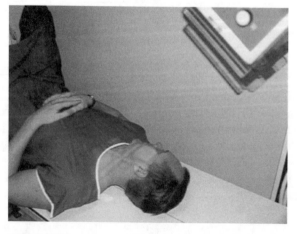

FIGURE 5.26
Pillars A-P oblique positioning.

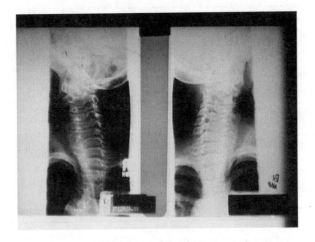

FIGURE 5.27
Pillars A-P film.

Collimation

Top to Bottom: C-2 to T-4 or slightly less than film size; Side to Side: skin of neck

Breathing Instructions

Suspend respiration

Image Critique

The oblique views are always done in pairs. The 45 to 50° head rotation will generally demonstrate the articular facets of C-2 to C-7 and of the first thoracic vertebrae. Sometimes, the head rotation will need to be increased to 60 to 70° for C-7 to T-4. These views are generally done post-whiplash involving a rotation and extension mode of injury.

Optimum kVp

75–80 kVp

5.13   Cervical Spine Positioning: Anterior Oblique Pillars View

Measure

A-P at C-4

Protection

Lead apron

SID

40 in. using Bucky

Tube Angulation

35 to 40° cephalad

Film

8 in. × 10 in. regular speed rare-earth cassette with I.D. down

Positioning

1. Patient standing, facing the Bucky. Have patient extend chin until the acanthameatal line is perpendicular to film. Make sure that the interpupillary line is straight. Have patient turn head to side 45 to 50° and rest cheek on Bucky.
2. Horizontal central ray through C-5. The film is centered to the horizontal central ray.
3. Vertical central ray to long axis of cervical spine.
4. Have patient suspend respiration. Make exposure.
5. Repeat with head turned to other side.

Collimation

Top to Bottom: C-2 to T-4 or slightly less than film size; Side to side: skin of neck

Breathing Instructions

Suspend respiration

Image Critique

The oblique pillars views are always done in pairs. The 45 to 50° head rotation will generally demonstrate the articular facets of C-2 to C-7 and of the first thoracic vertebrae. Sometimes, the

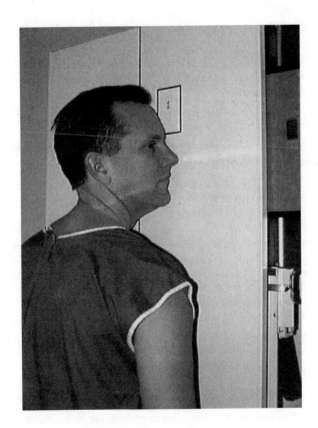

FIGURE 5.28
Pillars P-A oblique positioning.

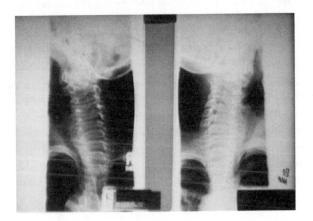

FIGURE 5.29
Pillars oblique film.

head rotation will need to be increased to 60 to 70° for C-7 to T-4. These views are generally done post-whiplash involving a rotation and extension mode of injury. The P-A version is the only method that can be performed relatively easily erect.

Optimum kVp

75–80 kVp

5.14   Review of Cervical Spine Positioning

1. Measurements for cervical spine technical factors are usually taken at the level of the 4th cervical vertebra. With the acathiomeatal line parallel to the floor, the 4th cervical vertebra lies at the top of the Adam's apple.

2. For all views except flexion and extension lateral cervical views and the Fuchs's projection, the acanthiomeatal line should be parallel to the floor.

3. The interpupillary line should be parallel to the floor for all erect cervical spine views.

4. It is very important to have the cassette identification blocker down on lateral and oblique cervical spine views.

5. Lateral cervical spine views should be taken Non-Bucky with a SID of 72 in. The use of the Bucky will result in unnecessary radiation exposure to the patient. The air gap with 72 in. SID will control the scatter radiation.

6. When positioning the A-P open mouth view, the upper border of the 5 in. square collimation is at the acanthion. One can use the upper border of the collimation to help align the acanthiomeatal line perpendicular to the film. If the teeth obstruct the view of the dens, the head was tucked down too low. If the base of the skull is seen in the view, the head was not tucked down low enough. Patients with a reversal of the cervical curve or anterior weight-bearing will usually need a 5° cephalad tube angulation. They may also need a sponge placed behind the head for stability.

7. Lateral views of the cervical spine should be taken on suspended expiration, with the patient holding sandbags to retract the shoulders below the 7th cervical vertebra. Expiration is important because the patient will not raise the shoulders. The shoulders can be pulled back to further help visualize the 7th cervical vertebra.

8. The Fuchs projection may demonstrate the dens when it cannot be visualized on the APOM.

9. Pillars oblique views are taken to evaluate the lateral masses of the cervical and upper thoracic spine.

10. Oblique views of the cervical spine are taken with the patient positioned 40 to 45° to the film. Posterior oblique views use a 15° cephalad tube angle, while anterior oblique views employ a 15° caudal angle. The right posterior oblique view will demonstrate the same anatomy as the left anterior oblique.

11. For patients that are post significant whiplash injuries, lateral bending films may be helpful in evaluating stability. The patient is positioned exactly like the routine A-P view with the same tube angulation. The patient is asked to bend the head laterally. Both right-side and left-side bending views are taken.

12. To evaluate the posterior arch of the upper cervical spine, the base posterior view of the skull can be very helpful. Positioning of this view is covered in skull radiography.

13. On the A-P view, the sternal-clavicular joints should be equally distant from the thoracic spine and the base of the skull aligned with the mandible.

14. The mandible should be clear of the upper cervical spine, with the mastoid tips and mandible super-imposed on the lateral cervical spine view. Close attention to head rotation and the interpupillary line is important for accurate positioning of the lateral cervical spine.

Chapter 6

Thoracic Spine, Chest, and Bony Thorax Radiography

6.1 Thoracic Spine, Chest, and Bony Thorax Radiography: Introduction

The bony thorax is a region of the body where one generally places the film to a landmark and then centers the tube to the film. This brings use to one of the old rules from radiographic physics. At a 40 in. SID, the anatomy at the top or bottom of the film will be projected 2 in. up and down on the film due to the divergent rays. Using anatomical landmarks such as the shoulder or the 7th cervical vertebra, one can ensure that the essential anatomy will be on the film.

When radiographs of the thoracic spine are taken, one must deal with variation of tissue density and the effects of air in the lungs. The A-P view has the air-filled lung, aorta, and heart muscle superimposed on the spine. One needs to adjust the exposure to adequately visualize the thoracic spine behind the heart without burning out the upper thoracic spine. This is done using a cervico-thoracic or thyroid filter. The lateral thoracic spine has the density of the shoulders at the top and just air-filled lungs at the bottom of the image. For the lateral view, point or compensating filters are used, based on the size of the patient.

Patient measurements are different for the thoracic spine and the rest of the thoracic views. The A-P measurement is taken over the shoulder with the calipers in contact with the sternum and thoracic spine. For P-A chests or ribs, the measurement is made at the middle of the chest, taking breast and muscle tissue into account. The lateral thoracic spine measurements are taken just under the axilla, while the chest measurements are taken laterally at the middle of the chest.

The kVp is in the 70 to 80-kVp range when looking for bone detail. This provides more contrast and a shorter gray scale. The exams where this relatively low kVp is used include the thoracic spine, sternum, and ribs. For chest films, high values, in excess of 110 kVp, are used. This provides a lower contrast film with more shades of gray. This is important as one wants to see minor changes in lung tissue density.

The breathing instructions for chest, thoracic spine, and rib above the diaphragm views are to have the patient hold a deep inspiration. This pulls the diaphragms down and fully inflates the lungs. Ribs below the diaphragm, sternum, and swimmer's projections use full expiration. This pulls the diaphragms up so that one can visualize the lower ribs with the technique adjusted for viewing the abdominal region of the body. The swimmer's view is taken on full expiration to keep the patient from raising the shoulders.

Rib studies should always have the injured ribs as close to the film as possible. An anterior rib injury will need P-A and anterior oblique views as the minimum study. The anterior oblique view will have the beam and film centered to the side away from the film. This will still have the anterior ribs closer to the film than with a posterior oblique view. Posterior rib injuries will use A-P and posterior oblique as the minimum routine views. Ribs above the diaphragm are best taken erect. Lower ribs should be taken recumbent. A small lead marker or metal washer can be taped to the patient over the painful area to assist in the intrepretation of the films. It will help bring attention to the ribs in question and ensure that they are adequately seen on the film.

6.2 Thoracic Spine Positioning: A-P Thoracic Spine View

Measure

A-P over shoulder in contact with thickest part of sternum and T-spine.

Protection

Lead apron

SID

40 in. using Bucky

Tube Angulation

None

Film

7 in. × 17 in. regular speed rare-earth cassette with I.D. down

Positioning

1. Patient standing, facing tube with back in contact with Bucky.
2. Place top of film 2 in. above C-7.
3. Center horizontal central ray to center of film.
4. Align mid-sagittal plane with vertical central ray.
5. Collimate to film size, top to bottom.
6. Place cervicothoracic filter so it just covers the top of the field. Thickest part of filter to top of film. Bottom of the filter will be at horizontal central ray.
7. Make exposure with full inspiration.

Collimation

Top to Bottom: C-7 to L-1 or film size; Side to Side: 6 in. or less.

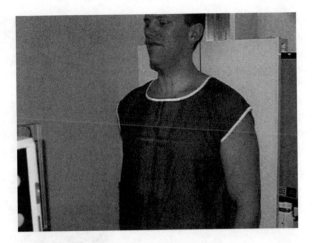

FIGURE 6.1
A-P thoracic spine positioning.

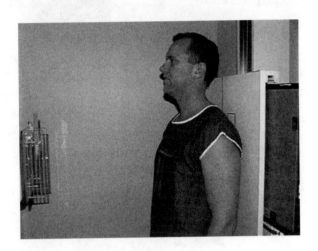

FIGURE 6.2
A-P thoracic spine with filter.

Filtration

40 in. cervicothoracic (thyroid)

Breathing Instructions

Full inspiration

Image Critique

Must include entire thoracic spine and rib articulations. There should be no rotation of patient in positioning. Exposure should be sufficient to see entire spine with adequate contrast and density.

Optimum kVp

75–80 kVp

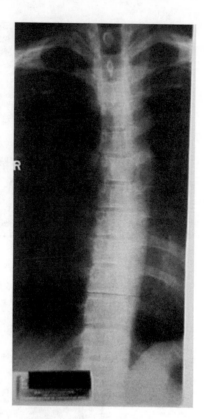

FIGURE 6.3
A-P thoracic spine film.

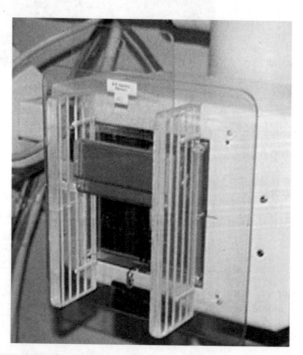

FIGURE 6.4
40 in. Cervicothoracic filter placement.

6.3   Thoracic Spine Positioning: Lateral Thoracic Spine View

Measure

Laterally subaxillary

Protection

Lead apron

SID

40 in. using Bucky

Tube Angulation

None

Film

14 in. × 17 in. or 7 in. × 17 in. with I.D. up

Positioning

1.   Patient standing with left shoulder next to Bucky and mid-coronal plane perpendicular to Bucky.
2.   Top of film is 2 in. above C-7. Center horizontal central ray to film.
3.   Align vertical central ray slightly posterior to humeral head.
4.   Patient assumes a prayer position with arms parallel to floor.
5.   Collimate and then place point filters from horizontal central ray down so the area below axilla is filtered.
6.   Have patient pull elbows together just prior to exposure.

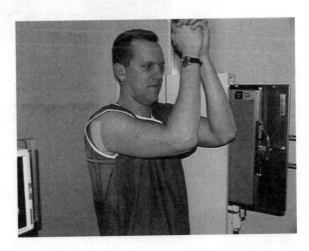

FIGURE 6.5
Lateral T-spine positioning.

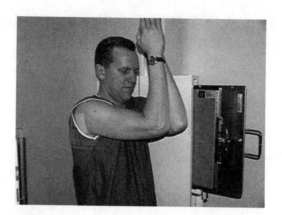

FIGURE 6.6
Lateral T-spine with elbows together.

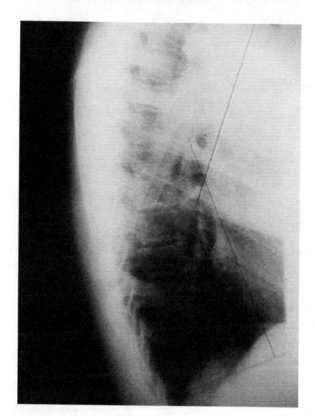

FIGURE 6.7
Lateral T-spine film.

Collimation

Top to Bottom: film size or T-1 to L-1; Side to Side: mid-coronal plane to posterior skin.

Filtration

Point filters per technique chart

Breathing Instructions

Full inspiration

Image Critique

The positioning in true lateral is important. The posterior ribs should be superimposed. Visualization of upper thoracic spine depends on having patient pull elbows together. This moves the shoulder anterior to the thoracic spine.

Optimum kVp

80–85 kVp

6.4   Thoracic Spine Positioning: Swimmer's Lateral View

Measure

Laterally subaxillary

Protection

Lead apron

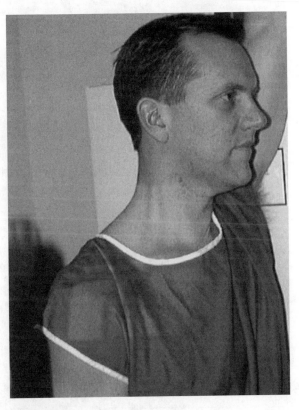

FIGURE 6.8
Swimmer's positioning.

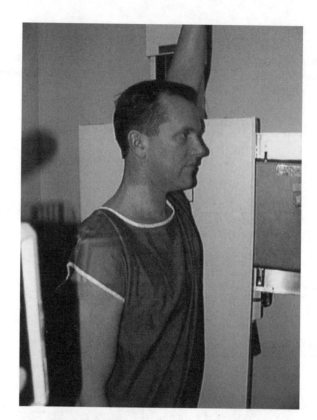

FIGURE 6.9
Swimmer's film.

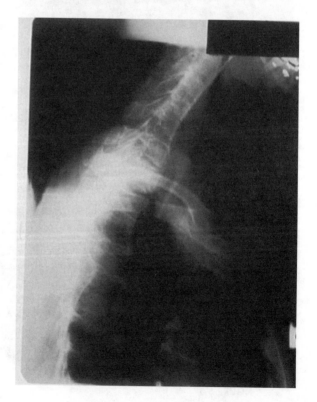

FIGURE 6.10
Swimmer's film.

SID

40 in. using Bucky

Tube Angulation

None; large patients may need a 5° caudal tube angle

Film

10 in. × 12 in. (or 24 cm × 30 cm) regular speed rare-earth cassette with I.D. up

Positioning

1. Patient standing with left shoulder next to Bucky and mid-coronal plane perpendicular to Bucky. The left arm is extended over head of patient.
2. The horizontal central ray is placed at the level of the sternal notch. The film is centered to horizontal central ray.
3. Rotate the patient 5 to 10° posteriorly off of true lateral position.
4. Have the patient hold the sandbag in right hand to retract the right shoulder. Align the vertical central ray with the head of the right humerus.
5. Collimate and make exposure.

Collimation

Top to Bottom: film size or C-5 to T-5; Side to Side: film size.

Breathing Instructions

Full expiration

Image Critique

The view should clearly demonstrate the upper thoracic and lower cervical vertebrae. The key to obtaining a good image is the degree of separation of the shoulders. Tube angulation tends to close the disc spaces. The amount of patient rotation will also impact the image. Try to keep the patient as lateral as possible.

Optimum kVp

80 kVp

6.5   Chest Positioning: P-A View

Measure

A-P at mid-chest

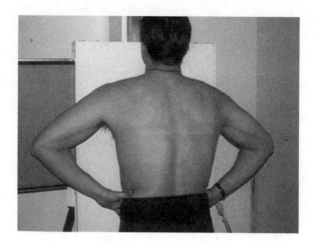

FIGURE 6.11
Chest P-A positioning.

Protection

Lead apron

SID

72 in. using Bucky

Tube Angulation

None

Film

14 in. × 17 in. regular speed rare-earth cassette with I.D. up

Positioning

1. Patient standing P-A with hands on hips and shoulders rolled forward. Do not let patient turn head.
2. Place top of film 2 in. above shoulder.
3. Center horizontal central ray to center of film, or 2 in. above film center for small patients.
4. Align mid-sagittal plane of patient to the vertical central ray.
5. Make sure that the patient is not rotated.
6. Collimate to slightly less than film size.
7. Make exposure with full inspiration.

Collimation

Top to Bottom: apex of lungs to base of lungs; Side to Side: skin of chest side to side.

Breathing Instructions

Full inspiration unless for pneumothorax; then full expiration

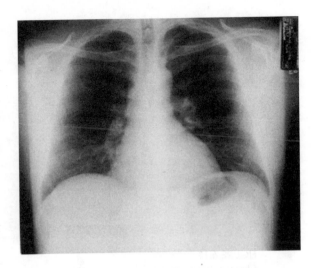

FIGURE 6.12
Chest P-A film.

Image Critique

Must include entire lung field. Respiratory effort should be down to 10th ribs or lower. There should be no rotation of patient, as indicated by sternoclavicular joints being equidistant from spine. The scapula must be clear of lung fields. The adequately exposed chest will allow visualization of body of thoracic spine behind heart.

Optimum kVp

110–125 kVp

6.6 Chest Positioning: Lateral View

Measure

Lateral at mid-chest

Protection

Lead apron

SID

72 in. using Bucky

Tube Angulation

None

Film

14 in. × 17 in. regular speed cassettes with I.D. up

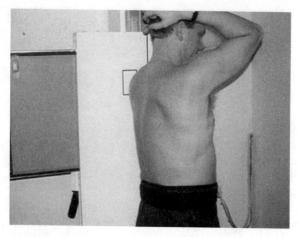

FIGURE 6.13
Chest lateral positioning.

Positioning

1. Patient standing with left side to Bucky.
2. Place top of film 2 in. above shoulder.
3. Center horizontal central ray to center of film.
4. Align mid-coronal plane of patient to the vertical central ray.
5. Make sure that the patient is not rotated and have patient raise arms over head and grasp elbows or lock hands behind head.
6. Collimate to slightly less than film size.
7. Make exposure with full inspiration.

Collimation

Top to Bottom: apex of lungs to base of lungs; Side to Side: skin of chest side to side.

Breathing Instructions

Full inspiration

Image Critique

Must include entire anterior lung field. Respiratory effort should be down to 10th ribs or lower. There should be no rotation of patient, as indicated by the superimposition of the posterior ribs. The arms must be clear of lung fields.

Optimum kVp

110–125 kVp

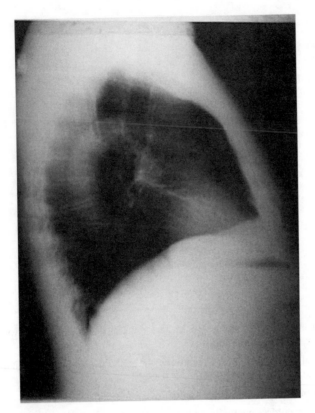

FIGURE 6.14
Chest lateral film.

6.7 Chest Positioning: Apical Lordotic View

Measure

A-P at mid-chest

Protection

Lead apron

SID

72 in. using Bucky

Tube Angulation

10 to 20° cephalad. Use greater angle if patient can not arch back very well.

Film

14 in. × 17 in., or 12 in. × 10 in. regular speed rare-earth cassette with I.D. up

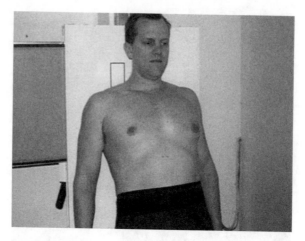

FIGURE 6.15
Apical lordotic film positioning.

Positioning

1. Patient standing about 12 in. from the Bucky, facing the tube. Patient is asked to extend backward until the shoulders are touching the Bucky.
2. Center horizontal central ray midway between the xiphoid process and manubrium. Center film to horizontal central ray.
3. Align vertical central ray with the mid-sagittal plane of the patient.
4. Have patient roll shoulders internally with hands on hips to help clear scapulas from lung field.
5. Make exposure with full inspiration.

Collimation

Top to Bottom: apex of lungs to base of lungs, or less than film size for 12 in. × 10 in.; Side to Side: skin of chest side to side or film size.

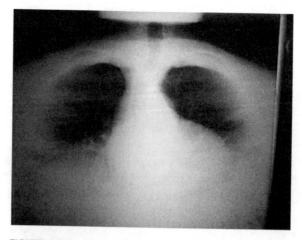

FIGURE 6.16
Apical lordotic film.

Breathing Instructions

Full inspiration

Image Critique

The medial ends of the clavicle must be projected superior to the first ribs and apices of lungs. The posterior and anterior aspects of the first four ribs should be nearly superimposed.

Optimum kVp

110–125 kVp

6.8   Chest Positioning: Right Anterior Oblique View

Measure

A-P at mid-chest

Protection

Lead apron

SID

40 in. using Bucky

Tube Angulation

None

Film

14 in. × 17 in. regular speed rare-earth cassette with I.D. up

Positioning

1. Patient standing facing the Bucky. Patient rotated 45° with right shoulder to film.
2. Place top of film 2 in. above shoulder.
3. Center horizontal central ray to center of film.
4. Align patient so the sternum is centered to the Bucky center line.
5. Patient may raise left arm over head or grasp the Bucky. The right hand should be on hip.
6. Make exposure with full inspiration.

Collimation

Top to Bottom: shoulder to base of lungs; Side to Side: slightly less than film size.

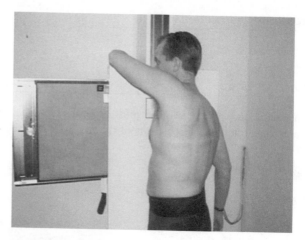

FIGURE 6.17
Chest right anterior oblique positioning.

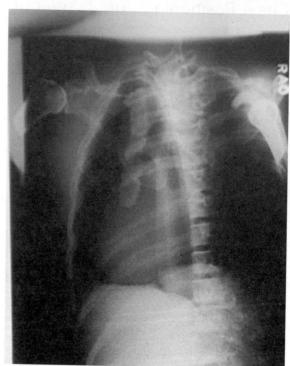

FIGURE 6.18
Chest RAO film (phantom).

Breathing Instructions

Full inspiration

Image Critique

Must include entire lung field. The RAO will give a clear view of the sternum and left lung field. The heart should be clear of the thoracic spine.

Optimum kVp

100–125 kVp

6.9   Chest Positioning: Left Anterior Oblique View

Measure

A-P at mid-chest

Protection

Lead apron

SID

72 in. using Bucky

Tube Angulation

None

Film

14 in. × 17 in. regular speed rare-earth cassette with I.D. up

Positioning

1.   Patient standing, facing the Bucky. Patient rotated 60° with left shoulder to film.
2.   Place top of film 2 in. above shoulder.
3.   Center horizontal central ray to center of film.
4.   Align patient so both lung fields will be within the collimated field of view.
5.   Have patient raise right arm over head or grasp the Bucky. The left hand should be on hip.
6.   Make exposure with full inspiration.

Collimation

Top to Bottom: apex of lungs to base of lungs; Side to Side: skin of chest side to side.

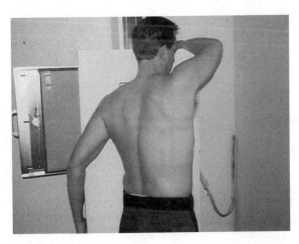

FIGURE 6.19
Chest left anterior oblique positioning.

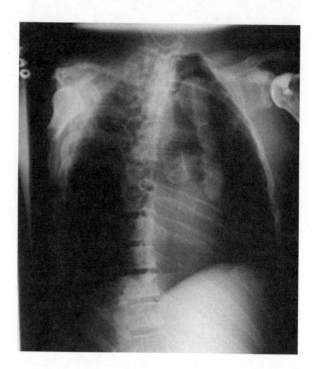

FIGURE 6.20
Chest LAO film (phantom).

Breathing Instructions

Full inspiration

Image Critique

Must include entire lung field. Respiratory effort should be down to 10th ribs or lower. The view will demonstrate the right lung, trachea, heart, aorta, and the bony thorax and sternum. The sternoclavicular joints will be clear of the spine. The heart shadow should be seen without spinal involvement if the obliquity is 60°.

Optimum kVp

110–125 kVp

6.10   Chest Positioning: A-P Posterior Ribs
Above Diaphragm

Measure

A-P at mid-chest

Protection

Lead apron

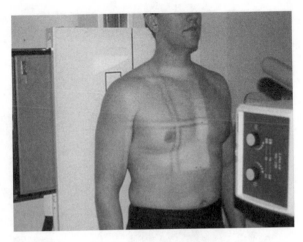

FIGURE 6.21
A-P upper posterior ribs positioning.

SID

40 in. using Bucky

Tube Angulation

None

Film

14 in. × 17 in. regular speed rare-earth cassette with I.D. up

Positioning

1. Patient standing, facing tube with back in contact with Bucky.
2. Place top of film 2 in. above shoulder.
3. Center horizontal central ray to center of film.
4. Align ribs of affected side to the vertical central ray.
5. Collimate to film size top to bottom.
6. Have patient internally rotate shoulders to get the scapulas clear of the ribs.
7. Make exposure with full inspiration.

Collimation

Top to Bottom: shoulder to 12th rib; Side to Side: skin of affected ribs to sternum.

Breathing Instructions

Full inspiration

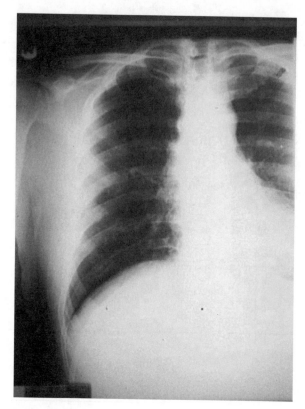

FIGURE 6.22
A-P upper ribs film.

Image Critique

Must include entire posterior rib cage of the affected side. The scapula should be clear of ribs. A small steel or copper ball (or BB) can be taped to the area of injury to assist in identification of the site of injury. Exposure should be sufficient to see ribs with adequate contrast and density.

Optimum kVp

70–75 kVp

6.11   Chest Positioning: A-P Oblique Posterior Ribs Above Diaphragm

Measure

A-P at mid-chest

Protection

Lead apron

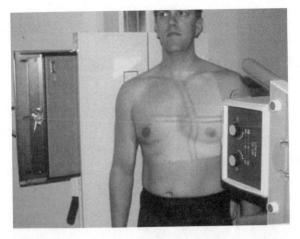

FIGURE 6.23
Upper posterior ribs oblique positioning.

SID

40 in. using Bucky

Tube Angulation

None

Film

14 in. × 17 in. regular speed rare-earth cassette with I.D. up

Positioning

1. Patient rotated 45° to Bucky with shoulder of affected side touching the Bucky.
2. Place top of film 2 in. above shoulder.
3. Center horizontal central ray to center of film.
4. Align ribs of affected side to the vertical central ray.
5. Collimate to film size top to bottom.
6. Have patient internally rotate shoulders to get the scapulas clear of the ribs.
7. Make exposure with full inspiration.

Collimation

Top to Bottom: shoulder to 12th rib; Side to Side: skin of affected ribs to sternum.

Breathing Instructions

Full inspiration

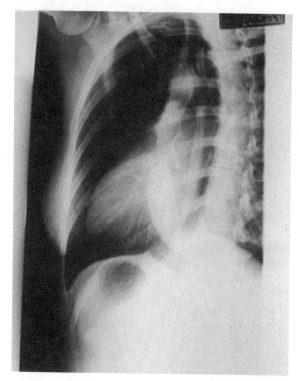

FIGURE 6.24
Upper posterior ribs film.

Image Critique

Must include entire posterior ribs cage of the affected side. The scapula should be clear of ribs. A small steel or copper ball (or BB) can be taped to the area of injury to assist in identification of the site of injury. Exposure should be sufficient to see ribs with adequate contrast and density.

Optimum kVp

70–75 kVp

6.12   Chest Positioning: P-A Anterior Ribs Above Diaphragm

Measure

P-A at mid-chest

Protection

Lead apron

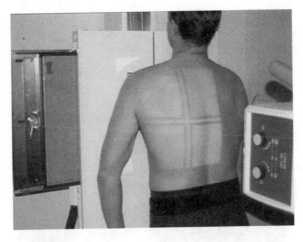

FIGURE 6.25
P-A anterior ribs positioning.

SID

40 in. using Bucky

Tube Angulation

None

Film

14 in. × 17 in. regular speed rare-earth cassette with I.D. up

Positioning

1. Patient standing P-A with hands on hips and shoulders rolled forward.
2. Place top of film 2 in. above shoulder.
3. Center horizontal central ray to center of film.
4. Align ribs of affected side to the vertical central ray.
5. Collimate to film size top to bottom.
6. Have patient raise arm on affected side to clear ribs.
7. Make exposure with full inspiration.

Collimation

Top to Bottom: shoulder to 12th rib; Side to Side: skin of affected ribs to sternum.

Breathing Instructions

Full inspiration

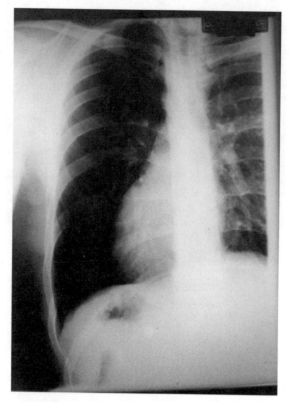

FIGURE 6.26
P-A anterior ribs film.

Image Critique

Must include entire anterior ribs cage above the diaphragm of the affected side. The scapula should be clear of ribs. A small steel or copper ball (or BB) can be taped to the area of injury to assist in identification of the site of injury. Exposure should be sufficient to see ribs with adequate contrast and density.

Optimum kVp

70–75 kVp

6.13   Chest Positioning: P-A Oblique for Anterior Ribs Above Diaphragm

Measure

P-A at mid-chest

Protection

Lead apron

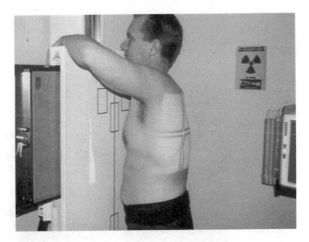

FIGURE 6.27
Oblique anterior ribs positioning.

SID

40 in. using Bucky

Tube Angulation

None

Film

14 in. × 17 in. regular speed rare-earth cassette with I.D. up

Positioning

1. Patient standing P-A and rotated 45° to Bucky with shoulder of unaffected side touching the Bucky. The injured ribs will be away from the film.
2. Place top of film 2 in. above shoulder.
3. Center horizontal central ray to center of film.
4. Align ribs of affected side to the vertical central ray.
5. Collimate to film size top to bottom.
6. Have patient raise arm on affected side to clear ribs.
7. Make exposure with full inspiration.

Collimation

Top to Bottom: shoulder to 12th rib; Side to Side: skin of affected ribs to sternum.

Breathing Instructions

Full inspiration

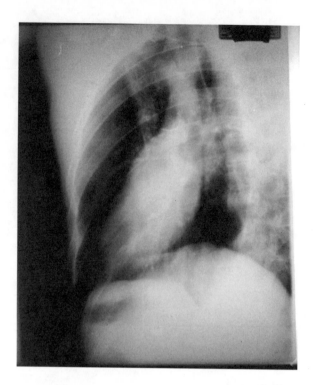

FIGURE 6.28
Oblique anterior ribs film.

Image Critique

Must include entire anterior ribs cage above the diaphragm of the affected side. The scapula should be clear of ribs. A small steel or copper ball (BB) can be taped to the area of injury to assist in identification of the site of injury. Exposure should be sufficient to see ribs with adequate contrast and density.

Optimum kVp

70–75 kVp

6.14   Chest Positioning: A-P Lower Ribs
      Below Diaphragm

Measure

A-P at mid-chest

Protection

Lead apron

SID

40 in. using Bucky

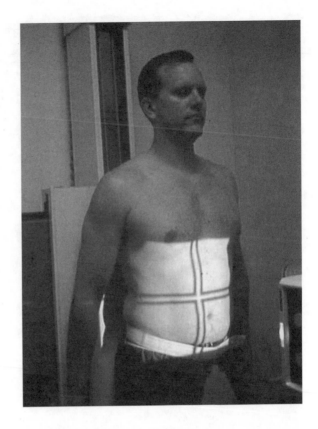

FIGURE 6.29
Lower ribs A-P erect positioning.

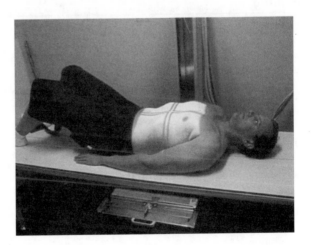

FIGURE 6.30
Lower ribs A-P supine positioning.

Tube Angulation

None

Film

14 in. × 17 in. regular speed rare-earth cassette with I.D. up

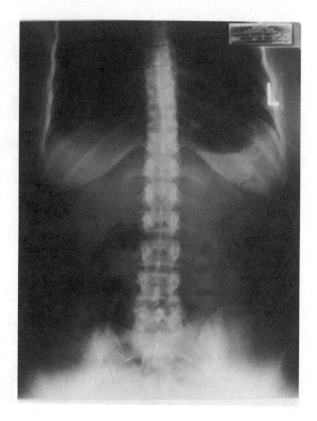

FIGURE 6.31
Lower ribs A-P film.

Positioning

1. Patient standing, facing the tube or recumbent.
2. Center horizontal central ray to the xiphoid process or place bottom of film 2 in. above the iliac crest.
3. Center horizontal central ray to film.
4. Align vertical central ray with the mid-sagittal plane of the patient or 1 to 2 in. toward the affected side.
5. Make exposure with full expiration.

Collimation

Top to Bottom: slightly less than film size; Side to Side: skin of chest side to side.

Breathing Instruction

Full expiration

Image Critique

Must demonstrate 12th ribs and superiorly as high as possible. The domes of the diaphragm should be up to the 8th rib or higher. The diaphragm may be higher on the recumbent views.

Optimum kVp

70–80 kVp

6.15   Chest Positioning: A-P Oblique View of Lower Ribs Below Diaphragm

Measure

A-P at mid-chest

Protection

Lead apron

SID

40 in. using Bucky

Tube Angulation

None

Film

12 in. × 10 in. or 30 cm × 24 cm regular speed rare-earth cassette with I.D. to spine

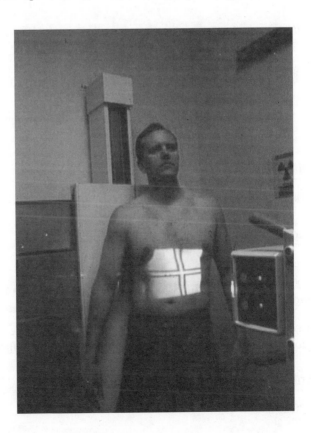

FIGURE 6.32
Oblique lower ribs erect positioning.

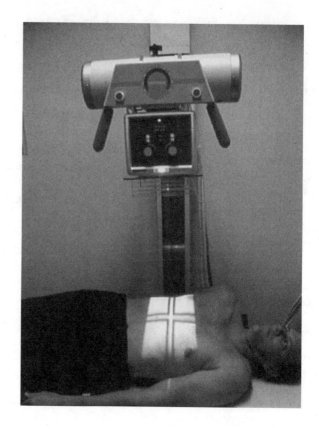

FIGURE 6.33
Oblique lower ribs supine positioning.

Positioning

1. Patient standing, facing the tube or recumbent. The patient is rotated 30 to 45° toward the affected side.
2. Place bottom of film 2 in. above the iliac crest.
3. Center horizontal central ray to film.
4. Align vertical central ray so the collimated field will demonstrate ribs of the affected side.
5. Make exposure with full expiration.

Collimation

Top to Bottom: slightly less than film size; Side to Side: skin of chest of the affected side.

Breathing Instructions

Full expiration

Image Critique

Must demonstrate 12th ribs and superiorly as high as possible. The domes of the diaphragms should be up to the 8th ribs or higher. The diaphragms may be higher on the recumbent views

Optimum kVp

75–80 kVp.

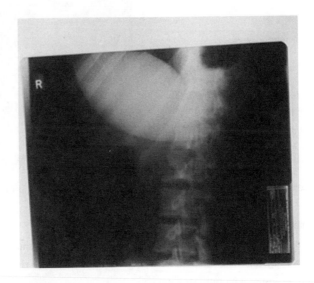

FIGURE 6.34
Oblique lower ribs film.

6.16   Chest Positioning: Right Anterior Oblique View of Sternum

Measure

A-P at mid-chest

Protection

Lead apron

SID

40 in. using Bucky

Tube Angulation

None

Film

10 in. × 12 in. regular speed rare-earth cassette with I.D. up

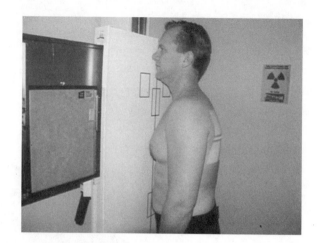

FIGURE 6.35
Sternum right anterior oblique positioning.

Positioning

1. Patient standing, facing the Bucky. Patient rotated 20 to 25° with right shoulder to film.
2. Place top of film 2 in. above sternoclavicular joints.
3. Center horizontal central ray to center of film.
4. Align patient so the sternum is centered to the Bucky center line.
5. Patient may raise left arm over head or grasp the Bucky. The right hand should be on hip.
6. Make exposure with full inspiration.

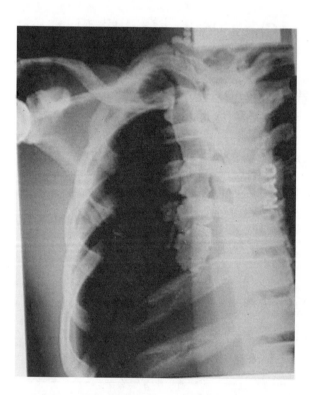

FIGURE 6.36
Sternum RAO film (phantom).

Collimation

Top to Bottom: sternoclavicular joints to xiphoid process; Side to Side: skin of chest side to side.

Breathing Instructions

Full expiration

Image Critique

Must include entire sternum. The sternum should be clear of the heart border. Excessive rotation of the patient will distort view. Optional views of sternoclavicular joints can be taken with shallow RAO and LAO views.

Optimum kVp

75–85 kVp

6.17   Chest Positioning: Lateral Sternum View

Measure

Lateral at mid-chest

Protection

Lead apron

SID

40 in. using Bucky

Tube Angulation

None

Film

10 in. × 12 in. regular speed rare-earth cassette with I.D. up

Positioning

1.   Patient standing with left side to Bucky.
2.   Place top of film 2 in. above sternoclavicular joints.

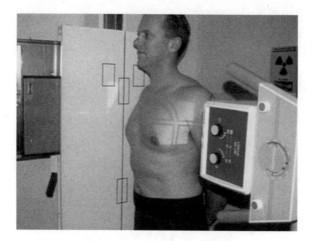

FIGURE 6.37
Sternum lateral positioning.

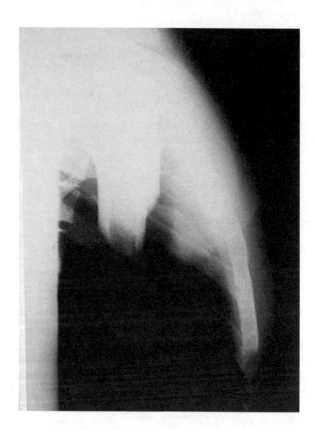

FIGURE 6.38
Sternum lateral film (phantom).

3. Center horizontal central ray to center of film.
4. Align the patient so the vertical central ray passes through the sternum, or about 2 to 3 in. anterior to mid-coronal plane.
5. Make sure that the patient is not rotated and have patient lock hands behind back.
6. Collimate to slightly less than film size.
7. Make exposure with full inspiration.

Collimation

Top to Bottom: sternoclavicular joints to xiphoid process; Side to Side: skin of chest side to side.

Breathing Instructions

Full inspiration

Image Critique

Must include entire sternum.

Optimum kVp

85–90 kVp

6.18   Review of Thoracic Spine and Chest Radiography

Key Thoracic Spine Positioning Notes

1. Because there is no reliable anterior landmark for the thoracic spine, the top of the film is placed 2 in. above C-7/T-1. Most texts recommend 1 in., which often misses T-1. The tube is then centered to the film.

2. Additional or compensating filters are used to better equalize exposure on thoracic spine films. Always complete positioning and collimation before installing added filtration. The Nolan filtration system is highly recommended.

3. Compensating filters should be used for the A-P view of the thoracic spine. On the A-P view, the 40-in. cervical-thoracic filter is used. When properly installed, it will close off the collimator light at the top of the film. The thicker part of the filter will be toward the center of the film. If filters are not available, consider the anode heel effect. The top of the thoracic spine should be positioned toward the anode side of the tube.

4. The point filters are used on the lateral view of the thoracic spine, based on the size of the patient. The technical factors can be adjusted for the use of point or compensating filters. This will result in a greater change of visualizing the upper thoracic spine. The point filters are placed below the axilla to reduce exposure to the lower thoracic spine.

5. When positioning the lateral thoracic spine, the film can be left at the same height as used for the A-P view. The patients's arms should be raised until they are parallel to the floor, with the elbows flexed 90°. The hands are together in a "prayer position." Just before making the exposure, have the patient pull elbows together. This will move the shoulders anterior to the upper thoracic spine, providing better visualization.

6. The vertical central ray should be just posterior to the head of the humerus on the lateral thoracic spine.

7. Breathing instructions for all thoracic spine views is full inspiration.

8. A swimmer's view may be needed when the upper thoracic or lower cervical spine is not seen on the lateral view. This is typically due to the size of the shoulders. The object of the view is to separate the shoulders by raising the arm closest to the Bucky and dropping the other shoulder using weights. The patient is rotated posteriorly 5 to 10° off of lateral.

Chest Positioning Review

9. All chest views are taken with a 72 in. SID.

10. All chest views use high kVp to extend the gray scale for better visualization of the many tissue types in the chest.

11. The top of the film is placed 2 in. above the shoulder for chest views.

12. The apical lordotic view is taken to visualize the apices of the lungs clear of any superimposition of the clavicles.

13. Oblique views of the chest are typically taken as anterior oblique views. The heart border should be clear of the thoracic spine on oblique views of the chest. The LAO is taken with a 60° oblique. The RAO is taken with a 45° oblique. The LAO will demonstrate the right lung field, and the RAO will visualize the left lung field.

14. The arms are raised and locked over the patient's head for the lateral view of the chest.

Ribs and Sternum Review

15. Ribs and sternum views are taken at 40 in. SID. Relatively low kVp is used to provide a short contrast scale for better bone visualization.

16. A 20° RAO will provide the frontal view of the sternum. Both RAO and LAO views can be taken to evaluate the sterno-clavicular joints.

17. The arms are positioned behind the back for the lateral sternum.

18. Anterior rib injuries will require P-A and an anterior oblique view to evaluate the injury. The affected side should be away from the film for the oblique view. Ribs studies above the diaphragm are taken with full inspiration. The first rib should be seen on both views.

19. Posterior rib injuries will require A-P and a posterior oblique view to evaluate the injury. The affected side is next to the Bucky for the posterior oblique view. Ribs studies above the diaphragm are taken with full inspiration. The first rib should be seen on both views.

20. Rib injuries below the diaphragm will require A-P and posterior oblique view taken recumbent if possible. The breathing instructions would be full expiration. The 12th ribs should be seen on both views.

7

A-P Full Spine and Lumbar, Sacrum, and Coccyx Views

7.1 A-P Full Spine

Measure

A-P at umbilicus

Protection

Bell for males; heart for females

SID

72 in. using Bucky

Tube Angulation

None

Film

14 in. × 36 in. regular or high-speed rare-earth cassette with I.D. up

Positioning

1. Patient stands in front of Bucky, facing the tube.
2. Make sure that the lead bell is not higher than below the inferior border of the pubis on males. Heart filter should be below the ASIS on female.
3. Locate the gluteal fold and place bottom of film 1 in. below gluteal fold. Locate xiphoid process and place central ray at the xiphoid process. Adjust film center if necessary.

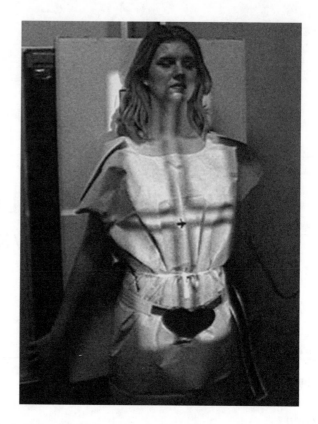

FIGURE 7.1
A-P full spine positioning.

4. Collimate top to bottom to include from EAM to trochanter. Top of bell may be used to assist with lower collimation limit.

5. Collimate side-to-side to film size. Have patient hold onto side of Bucky.

Collimation

Top to Bottom: EAM to trochanter; Side to Side: film size or to include both trochanter.

Filters

Para-spinal shield down to horizontal CR; 72 in. thyroid down to close light at top; point filters per technique chart placed down to level of xiphoid process.

Breathing Instructions

Full inspiration

Image Critique

This view requires precise positioning to avoid rotation of the patient. Make sure feet are shoulder-width apart. Have patient lock knees prior to exposure. P-A views are not done routinely on females due to divergent ray impact on cervical disc spaces. For serial studies for scoliosis, follow-up views should be done P-A. to reduce exposure.

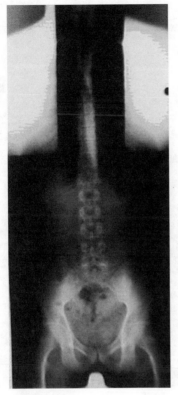

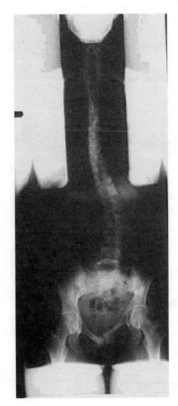

FIGURE 7.2
A-P full spine film.

FIGURE 7.3
A-P full spine film.

Optimum kVp

80–85 kVp

7.2 A Step-by-Step Positioning of the A-P Full Spine

Step 1: Positioning of the patient radiation protection

Start by placing the gonadal shield or filter on the patient. This will establish where the symphysis is located — one of the major landmarks for positioning the patient. (Figure 7.4.)

Step 2: Position the patient, film, and central ray

Have patient stand in front of the Bucky, facing the tube with feet shoulder-width apart. Make sure feet are parallel to the film and the patient is as close to the Bucky as possible. Make sure that there is no rotation of the patient. Find gluteal fold and place bottom of film 1 to 2 in. below the gluteal fold. Next, locate the xiphoid tip and place central ray on the tip. Have the patient raise chin until the acanthameatal line is perpendicular to film. Instruct the patient to remain in this position until the study is complete. (Figure 7.5.)

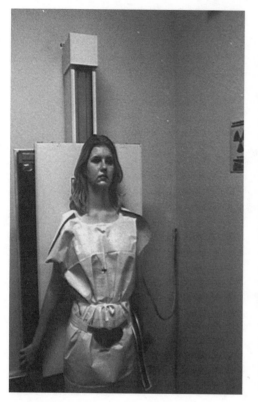

FIGURE 7.4
A-P full spine, step 2.

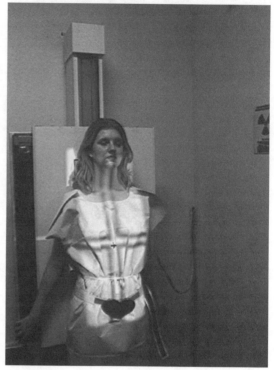

FIGURE 7.5
A-P full spine, step 3.

Step 3: Collimation

Set the side-to-side collimation to slightly less than 14 in. Open the top-to-bottom collimation until it covers from EAM to 1 in. below the symphysis pubis. The horizontal central ray and film may need a minor adjustment to set these limits. Make sure that the film is centered to the horizontal central ray and the film is pushed completely into the center of the Bucky.

Step 4: Paraspinal Shield

The paraspinal shield contains lead and will block exposure to the lung and breast tissue. (Nolan also makes a partial shield that has brass and aluminum filters that will reduce exposure; this one is not used at Palmer.) There are two of these shields. One is designed for 40 in. SID and one for 72 in. SID. We use the 40 in. shield because the 72 in. unit is too narrow for most patients. This shield is placed in the first slot nearest the collimator. It is taken down to the level of the xiphoid process or to the horizontal central ray. If seeing the abdominal structures is not important or one is doing serial studies, the shield can be pushed down further to the top of the iliac crest. (Figures 7.6 and 7.7.)

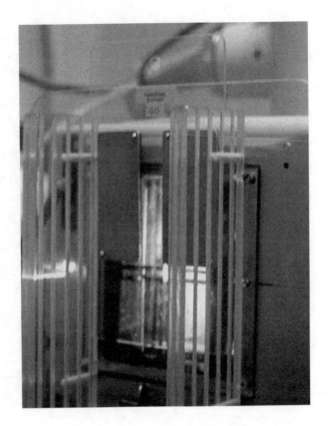

FIGURE 7.6
Paraspinal shield.

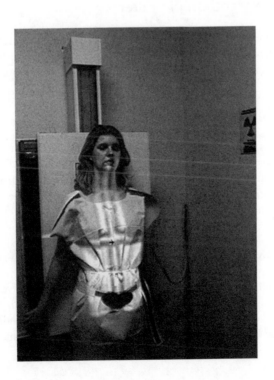

FIGURE 7.7
A-P full spine, step 4.

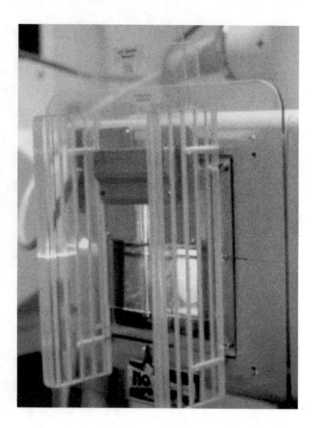

FIGURE 7.8
72 in. thyroid filter, step 5.

Step 5: Cervicothoracic Filter

The cervicothoracic filter or thyroid filter is placed in the second slot of the filter holder. It is installed with the thickest part toward the cervical spine or skull. It is pushed down from the top until light is seen at the top of the collimated field and then moved up to close off the light. (Figures 7.8 and 7.9.)

Step 6: Point Filters

The point filters are used to further reduce exposure in the cervical and thoracic spine regions. The filtration is based on sex and body size. Typically, two point filters are used. Skip a slot to avoid contact with the thyroid filter. The point filters are installed from the top in the last two slots of the collimator. They are pushed down to the level of the xiphoid process or diaphragms. (Figures 7.10 and 7.11.)

Step 7: Exposure

Have the patient lock knees to ensure the legs are straight. Have patient hold onto the sides of the Bucky. Instruct the patient to take a deep breath in and hold breath. Make the exposure. It is imperative that one hold both exposure buttons down until the exposure audible tone or beep has stopped. The exposure time for the A-P full spine is the longest exposure time that one typically experiences.

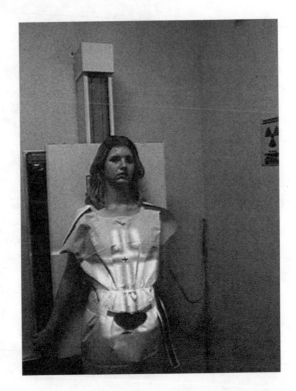

FIGURE 7.9
A-P full spine, step 5.

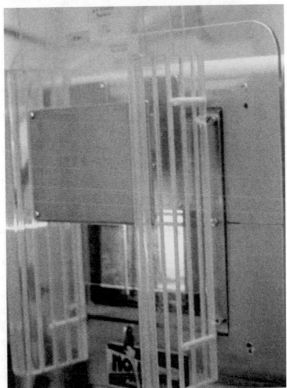

FIGURE 7.10
A-P full spine with point filters.

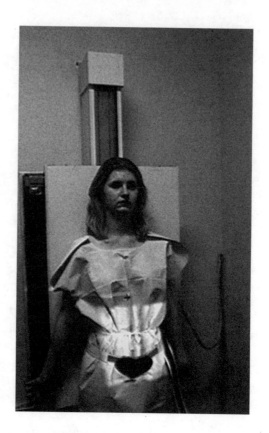

FIGURE 7.11
Point filters placement.

7.3   Lumbar Spine Radiography: Introduction

Radiography of the lumbar spine region will provide the greatest radiation exposure to the patient. For this reason, accurate positioning, measurements, and gonadal protection is very important. The technique is based on measurements at the umbilicus. The A-P full spine is included in the lumbar region because the basic technical factors are established to visualize the lumbar spine and pelvis. The male patient will use the bell-shaped gonadal shield. A belt with Velcro to hold the bell is placed on the patient. The placement of the bell is critical. If it is above the most inferior border of the symphysis pubis, it will obstruct the view of the bottom of the pelvis.

Two options are available for the female patient. When the film is taken A-P, a heart-shaped filter can be used to reduce exposure to the ovaries. It is placed so that the top of the heart is at the level of the ASIS. The other option is to turn the patient P-A. The bones of the pelvis will absorb much of the exposure and reduce the exposure to the ovaries. The A-P image will have the filter partially blocking the image of the sacroiliac joints and the pubic area. The P-A image will have increased magnification but will better visualize the disc spaces because the lordotic curve will more closely match the divergent rays. Unless the patient is very large, the P-A view is probably best. These modifications are needed only during the potential child-bearing years.

The A-P or P-A lumbopelvis view is used only by chiropractors. It is the only lumbar spine view that has the horizontal central ray 1 to 1½ in. below the iliac crest. The horizontal central ray should not be placed below the ASIS. The inexperienced intern may get the iliac crest and the ASIS mixed up if the patient is approached anterior to posterior. Feel the patient from posterior to anterior and one will be able to accurately locate the iliac crests. On male patients, if the collimated field hits more than the very top of the bell, the horizontal central ray is either too low or the bell placed too high.

Patients should lock knees and remove shoes for the lumbar spine and full spine studies. They should also have their feet placed at about shoulder-width apart to minimize motion. Wide placement of the feet and locking the knees will make the assessment of leg length much more accurate. The feet should also be parallel to the Bucky for A-P views, and perpendicular for lateral views. Have the patient side-step for centering, and not just lean. Also make sure the buttocks are placed on the Bucky to reduce the possibility of rotation. Concise positioning will yield accurate information about the patient's spine.

When oblique views of the lumbar spine are needed, upright oblique views come out better with anterior oblique positioning. As far as image quality is concerned, recumbent oblique views are generally superior to erect views. The lordotic curve is flattened on recumbent views, getting the complete lumbar spine in the same plane. In either case, the patient should be in a 40 to 45° oblique, with the shoulders and the pelvis in the same plane. It is easy to have the shoulders at the correct degree of rotation and still have the pelvis improperly positioned. Ask the patient to turn or roll like a log; the use of a radiographic 45° sponge will assist in accurate positioning.

With the exception of female patients in the lateral position, the tissue density is relatively uniform in the lumbar region. For female patients, lateral measurements at the trochanter and at the umbilicus are taken. The umbilical measurement is used for the technique and is subtracted from the trochanteric measurement to determine how much compensating filtration is needed.

A shadow shield shaped like a quarter of a circle is placed in the filter holder on the collimator for lateral and oblique views of the lumbar spine. The curve of the shield should follow the curve of the sacrum. It is placed about 2 in. below the ASIS for male patients, and at the level of the ASIS for female patients. It is referred to as the lateral gonadal shield.

The optimum kVp for A-P lumbar spine views is about 75 kVp. Oblique views need the low 80-kVp range. The lateral lumbar spine is adequately visualized at 90 kVp. Lower kVp generally will just increase the ionization and patient exposure.

The A-P full spine is taken in the 80-kVp range. When the Nolan filtration system is used, good quality A-P full spine studies can be taken on patients weighing up to about 230 pounds. The key is filtration to reduce the exposure in the thoracic and cervical regions. This view will put the greatest load on the X-ray tube. Make sure that it has been properly warmed up. It will also have the longest exposure time and has the greatest potential for motion artifacts.

There is generally a significant amount of scatter radiation coming off the patient's body when full spine views are taken. Even with the use of a paraspinal lead shield, the lungs and breast tissue will receive some exposure. When serial studies are needed to monitor scoliosis, after the initial film, the follow-up studies on female patients should be taken P-A to reduce breast tissue exposure.

As mentioned earlier, oblique views of the lumbar spine can be very challenging when taken erect. The degree of difficulty depends on patient size and the amount of lordotic curve. If a table is not available and the patient is not very large, anterior oblique views will provide less distortion because the divergent rays will better follow the lordotic curve.

It is imperative to keep the spine in the same plane on obliques. The shoulders and hips of the patient should be at a 40 to 45° angle to the film.

The Scotty dog is a good way to recognize the anatomy on the lumbar oblique:

Eye: Pedicle
Nose: Transverse process
Ear: Superior articular facet
Legs: Inferior articular facet
Neck: Pars interarticularis
Body: Lamina
Tail: Opposing side transverse process

RAO: Demonstrates the left facets and pars interarticularis (side farthest from film) and right sacroiliac joint. Right marker is pronated and placed behind the spinous process.

LAO: Demonstrates the right facets and pars interarticularis and left sacroiliac joint. Left marker is pronated and placed behind the spinous process.

RPO: Demonstrates the right facets and pars interarticularis and left sacroiliac joint. Right marker placed in front of the spinous process.

LPO: Demonstrates the left facets and pars interarticularis and right sacroiliac joint. Left marker placed in front of spinous process.

7.4   Lumbar Spine Positioning: A-P Lumbopelvic View

Measure

A-P at umbilicus

Protection

Lead bell (males); heart filter (females)

SID

40 in. using Bucky

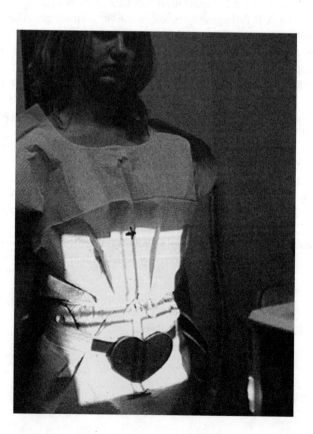

FIGURE 7.12
Lumbopelvic A-P female positioning.

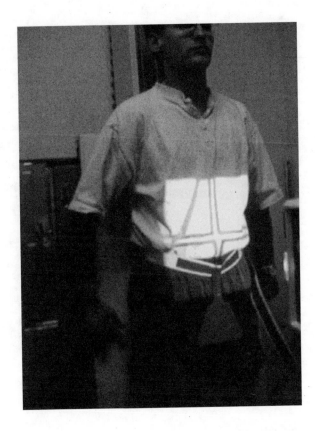

FIGURE 7.13
Lumbopelvic A-P male positioning.

Tube Angulation

None

Film

14 in. × 17 in. regular speed rare-earth cassette with I.D. up

Positioning

1. Patient stands in front of Bucky, facing the tube.
2. Make sure that the lead bell is not higher than below the inferior border of the pubis on males. Heart filter should be below the ASIS if A-P is done on female.
3. Locate the top of the iliac crest and place horizontal central ray from 1 in. to 1½ in. below crest. Center the film to the horizontal central ray.
4. Align mid-sagittal plane with the vertical central ray. Umbilicus may be used.
5. Make sure there is no rotation of the patient. Have patient lock knees. Make exposure.

Collimation

Top to Bottom: inferior border T-12 to pubis; Side to Side: slightly less than film size.

Breathing Instructions

Full expiration

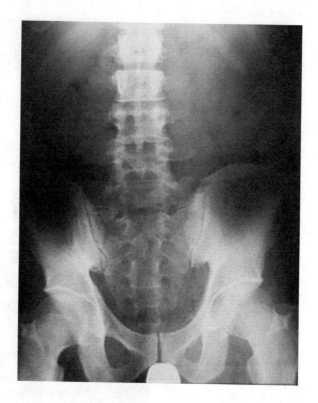

FIGURE 7.14
Lumbopelvic A-P film.

Image Critique

Must see from L-1 to as much of the pelvis as possible. Getting patients as close to Bucky as possible and with no rotation is also very important. Not placing shielding too high is also very important. If there is a concern about leg length, having patient lock knees will provide greater accuracy. Most female patients should be imaged P-A to reduce radiation exposure.

Optimum kVp

70–75 kVp

7.5 Lumbar Spine Positioning: P-A Lumbopelvic View

Measure

A-P at umbilicus

Protection

None; pelvic bone and distance from beam point of entry will reduce exposure.

SID

40 in. using Bucky

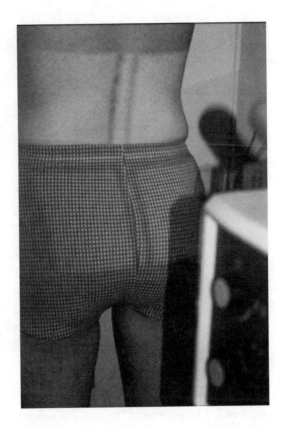

FIGURE 7.15
Lumbopelvic P-A positioning.

Tube Angulation

None

Film

14 in. × 17 in. regular speed rare-earth cassette with I.D. up

Positioning

1. Patient stands, facing the Bucky.
2. Locate the top of the iliac crest and place horizontal central ray from 1 in. to 1½ in. below crest.
3. Center film to the horizontal central ray.
4. Align mid-sagittal plane with the vertical central ray. Spinus processes may be used.
5. Make sure there is no rotation of the patient. Make sure shoulders and feet are parallel to film.
6. Have patient lock knees. Make exposure.

Collimation

Top to Bottom: inferior border T-12 to pubis; Side to Side: film size.

Breathing Instructions

Full expiration

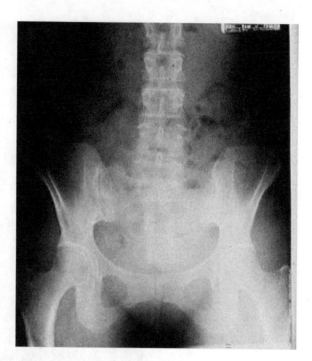

FIGURE 7.16
Lumbopelvic P-A film.

Image Critique

One must see from L-1 to as much of the pelvis as possible. Getting patients as close to Bucky as possible and with no rotation is also very important. The disc spaces and SI joints will be seen better than in the A-P view. If there is a concern about leg length, having patient lock knees will provide greater accuracy. Any rotation of the patient will severely degrade the image due to the increased distance the spine is away from the film.

Optimum kVp

75 kVp

7.6   Lumbar Spine Positioning: Lateral View

Measure

Laterally at umbilicus; female patients will be measured laterally at trochanter for filtration only

Protection

Lateral gonad shield

SID

40 in. using Bucky

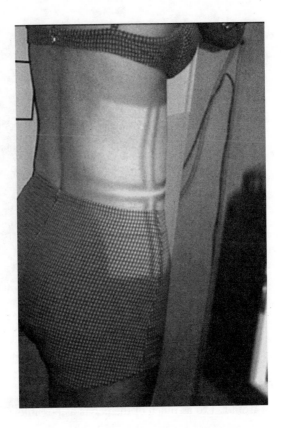

FIGURE 7.17
Lumbar lateral positioning.

Film

14 in. × 17 in. regular speed rare-earth cassette with I.D. up

Positioning

1. Patient stands with left side to Bucky. If patient has scoliosis with convexity to right, a right lateral is done.
2. Locate the top of the iliac crest and place horizontal central ray 1 in. above the crest. Center film to horizontal central ray.
3. Find mid-coronal plane by determining the midpoint between the PSIS and ASIS. Center vertical central ray to mid-coronal plane.
4. Collimate and position the lateral gonad shield. For male patients, it should be 2 to 3 in. below ASIS. For female patients, it should be just below ASIS.

Collimation

Top to Bottom: film size or T-10 to coccyx; Side to Side: posterior skin.

Filtration

Point filter from top to horizontal central ray for female patients; one point for every centimeter difference between umbilicus and trochanter measurement minus 5. If the difference is less than 5, no point filters are needed.

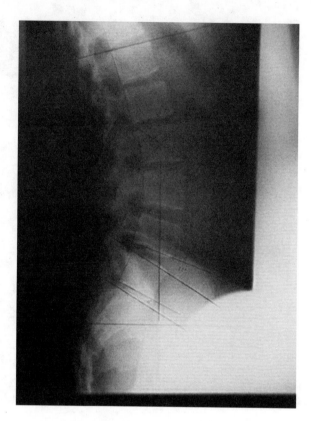

FIGURE 7.18
Lumbar lateral film.

Breathing Instructions

Full expiration

Image Critique

The image should be free of any rotation of the patient. Lower thoracic and lumbar vertebrae to lumbar sacral junction must be seen. Laterally, there should be evidence of collimation and this will help visualization of spinous processes. If patient has scoliosis, aim central ray into the convexity to better visualize disc spaces.

Optimum kVp

90–95 kVp

7.7 Lumbar Spine Positioning: Posterior Oblique View

Measure

A-P at umbilicus

Protection

Lateral gonadal shield

SID

40 in. using Bucky

Tube Angulation

None

Film

10 in. × 12 in. regular speed rare-earth cassette with I.D. down

Marker

R and L, or RPO and LPO

Positioning

1. Patient stands in front of Bucky, facing the tube.
2. Have patient turn entire body 40 to 45° with the right shoulder next to Bucky. This would be a right posterior oblique (RPO).
3. Locate the top of the iliac crest and place horizontal central ray from 1 in. above the crest. Center the film to the horizontal central ray.
4. Place the vertical central ray 1 to 1½ in. medial to the ASIS closest to the X-ray tube.
5. Make sure the shoulders and hips are in the same plane. Make exposure.
6. Repeat process with left shoulder to Bucky.

Collimation

Top to Bottom: film size or L-1 to S1; Side to Side: film size or 8 in.

Breathing Instructions

Full expiration

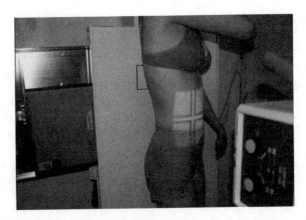

FIGURE 7.19
Lumbar posterior oblique positioning.

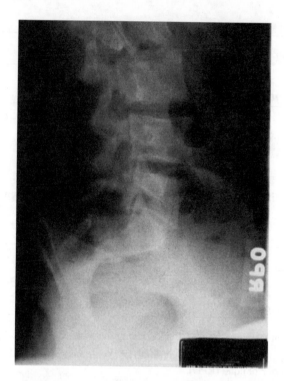

FIGURE 7.20
Lumbar posterior oblique film.

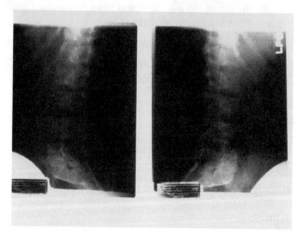

FIGURE 7.21
Lumbar posterior oblique film supine.

Image Critique

One must see from L-5/S-1 to L-1. Getting patients as close to Bucky as possible and with no rotation is also very important. The shoulders and hips should be in the same plane. Obliquity of 40 to 45° will produce the best results. The lateral gonadal shield should not be higher than the most inferior aspect of the ASIS. Anterior oblique views will have greater object to film distance, but are easier to accurately position. On very large patients, posterior oblique views should be taken. Patients with significant lordotic curves should be imaged recumbent.

Optimum kVp

80–85 kVp

7.8   Lumbar Spine Positioning: Anterior Oblique View

Measure

A-P at umbilicus

Protection

Lateral gonadal shield

SID

40 in. using Bucky

Tube Angulation

None

Film

10 in. × 12 in. regular speed rare-earth cassette with I.D. down

Marker

Pronated R and L, or RAO and LAO

Positioning

1. Patient stands in front of Bucky, facing the Bucky.
2. Have patient turn entire body 40 to 45°, with the right shoulder next to Bucky. This would be a right anterior oblique (RAO).
3. Locate the top of the iliac crest and place horizontal central ray from 1 in. above the crest. Center the film to the horizontal central ray.

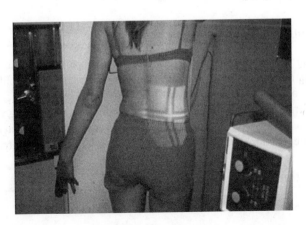

FIGURE 7.22
Lumbar anterior oblique positioning.

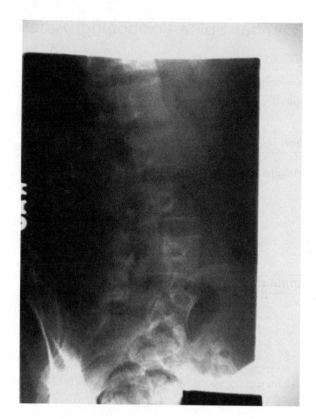

FIGURE 7.23
Lumbar anterior oblique film.

4. Palpate the spinous processes and adjust patient position until the vertical central ray is 1 to 1½ in. lateral (toward the tube) from the spinous processes.

5. Make sure there is no rotation of the patient. Have patient lock knees. Make exposure. Repeat process with left shoulder to Bucky.

Collimation

Top to Bottom: film size, or L-1 to S1; Side to Side: film size or 8 in.

Breathing Instructions

Full expiration

Image Critique

One must see from L-5/S-1 to L-1. Getting patients as close to Bucky as possible and with no rotation is also very important. The shoulders and hips should be in the same plane. Obliquity of 40 to 45° will produce best results. The lateral gonadal shield should not be higher than the most inferior aspect of the ASIS. Anterior obliques will have greater object to film distance, but are easier to accurately position. On very large patients, posterior oblique views should be taken. Patients with significant lordotic curves should be imaged recumbent.

Optimum kVp

80–85 kVp

7.9   Impact of Positioning on Lumbar Oblique Views

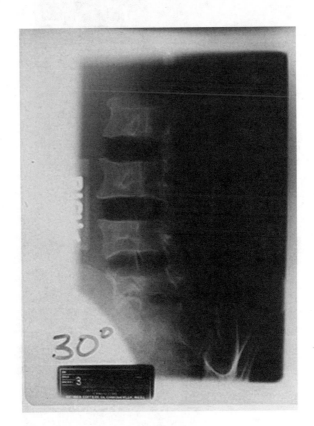

FIGURE 7.24
30° oblique view.

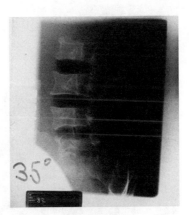

FIGURE 7.25
35° oblique view.

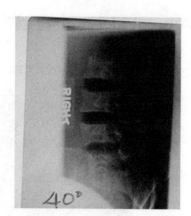

FIGURE 7.26
40° oblique view.

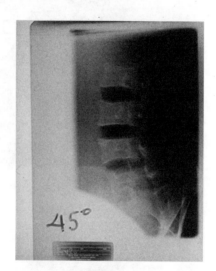

FIGURE 7.27
45° oblique view.

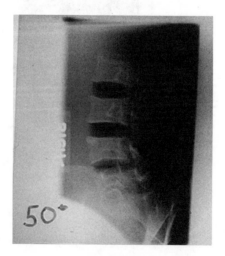

FIGURE 7.28
50° oblique view.

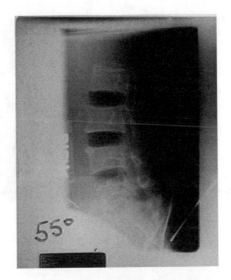

FIGURE 7.29
55° oblique view.

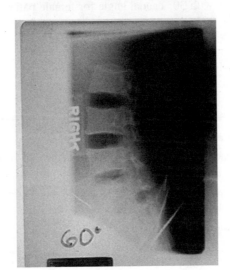

FIGURE 7.30
60° oblique view.

7.10   Lumbar Spine Positioning: A-P Sacral Base View

Measure

A-P at trochanter

Protection

Bell for males; optional P-A for female patients

SID

40 in. using Bucky

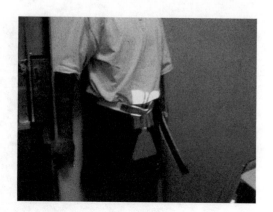

FIGURE 7.31
A-P sacral base positioning.

Tube Angulation

30° cephalad; optional P-A with 30° caudal angle for female patients

Film

8 in. × 10 in. regular speed rare-earth cassette with I.D. up

Positioning

1. Patient stands in front of Bucky, facing the tube.
2. Locate the ASIS and place horizontal central ray at level of the ASIS. Center film to horizontal central ray.
3. Position patient so the vertical central ray is aligned with the mid-sagittal plane of patient.
4. Make sure there is no rotation of the patient. Check the position of the gonadal shield on male patients to ensure that it is not above the most inferior aspect of the symphysis pubis.
5. Give breathing instructions. Make exposure.

Collimation

Top to Bottom: 5 in. unless interested in SI joints; film size for SI joints; Side to Side: 5 in. unless interested in SI joints.

Breathing Instructions

Full expiration

Image Critique

One must see from sacroiliac joint space open to disc space for L-5/S-1. Getting patients as close to the Bucky as possible, with no rotation, is also very important. The shoulders and hips should be in the same plane. If the gonadal shield is too high, it will obscure L-5/S-1.

Optimum kVp

80–85 kVp

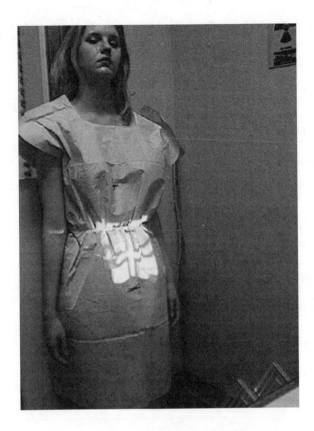

FIGURE 7.32
A-P sacral base positioning.

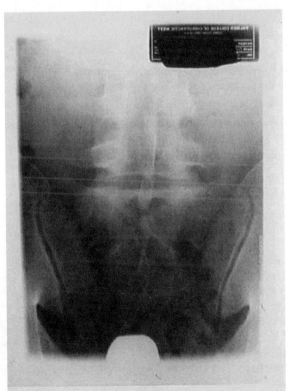

FIGURE 7.33
A-P sacral base film.

7.11   Lumbar Spine Views: P-A Sacral Base View

Measure

A-P at the trochanter

Protection

The purpose of this view is to reduce radiation exposure to the ovaries in women of child-bearing age.

SID

40 in. using Bucky

Tube Angulation

30° caudal

Film Size

8 in. × 10 in. regular rare-earth cassette with I.D. up

Markers

Pronated R or L

Positioning

1. Female patient stands facing Bucky with feet at shoulder-width apart and parallel; she should be as close to the Bucky as possible.
2. Locate the PSIS. Place horizontal central ray at the PSIS.
3. The vertical central ray should be aligned down the spinous processed of the lumbar spine. Make sure that there is no rotation of the body.
4. Center the film to the horizontal central ray.

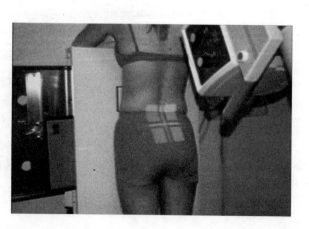

FIGURE 7.34
P-A sacral base positioning.

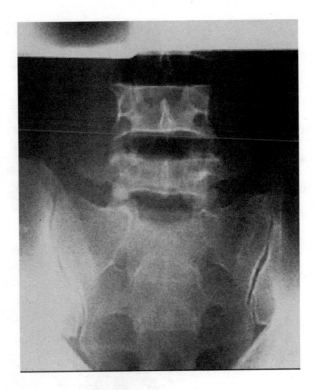

FIGURE 7.35
P-A sacral base film.

Collimation

Slightly less than film size instead of the 5-in. square due to magnification.

Image Critique

This view is a compromise to reduce radiation exposure on females of child-bearing age. The small focal spot should be used to help compensate for the magnification caused by increased object to film distance. The information on the view will be the same as the A-P sacral base, with the exception of the magnification. Do not take this view on obese patients.

Optimum kVp

80 kVp

7.12 Lumbar Spine Positioning: Lateral Spot View of L-5 and S-1 Disc Space

Measure

Laterally at trochanter

Protection

Lateral gonad shield

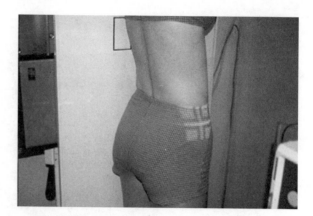

FIGURE 7.36
Spot lateral L-5/S-1 positioning.

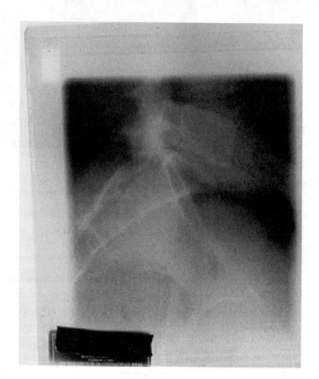

FIGURE 7.37
Spot lateral film.

SID

40 in. using Bucky

Film

8 in. × 10 in. regular speed rare-earth cassette with I.D. up

Positioning

1. Patient stands with left side to Bucky. If patient has scoliosis with convexity to right, a right lateral is done.
2. Locate the top of the iliac crest and place horizontal central ray 2 in. below the crest. Center film to horizontal central ray.

3.　Find mid-coronal plane by determining the mid-point between the PSIS and ASIS. Center vertical central ray 1 in. posterior to mid-coronal plane.

4.　Collimate and position the lateral gonad shield. For male patients, it should be 2 to 3 in. below ASIS. For female patients, it should be just below ASIS.

Collimation

Top to Bottom: 5 in.; Side to Side: 5 in.

Breathing Instructions

Full expiration

Image Critique

The image should be free of any rotation of the patient. If time permits, take the routine lateral and look at the film before taking the spot film. The amount of pelvic tilt and posture will impact positioning. If there is a leg length discrepancy or scoliosis, taking the full lateral with the beam aimed into the convexity may avoid the need for the spot film.

Optimum kVp

100–110 kVp

7.13　Lumbar Spine Positioning: Posterior Oblique View of Sacroiliac Joints

Measure

A-P at trochanter

Protection

Lateral gonadal shield

SID

40 in. using Bucky

Tube Angulation

None

Film

8 in. × 10 in. regular speed rare-earth cassette with I.D. down

Markers

R and L, or RPO and LPO

Positioning

1. Patient stands in front of Bucky, facing the tube.
2. Have patient turn entire body 20 to 30° with the right shoulder next to Bucky. This would be a right posterior oblique.
3. Locate the top of the ASIS and place horizontal central ray 1 in. below the ASIS. Center the film to the horizontal central ray.
4. Palpate the ASIS away from the Bucky and adjust patient position until the vertical central ray is 1 to 1½ in. medial (toward the Bucky) from the ASIS.
5. Make sure there is no rotation of the patient. Have patient lock knees. Make exposure. Repeat process with left shoulder to Bucky.

Collimation

Top to Bottom: film size, or SI joint; Side to Side: film size, or 6 in.

Breathing Instructions

Full expiration

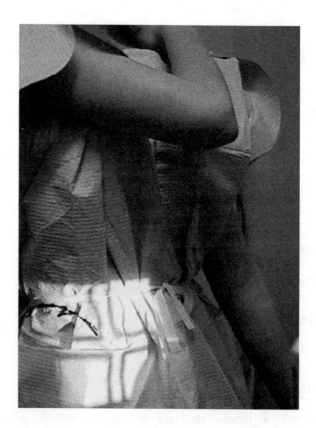

FIGURE 7.38
SI joint posterior oblique positioning.

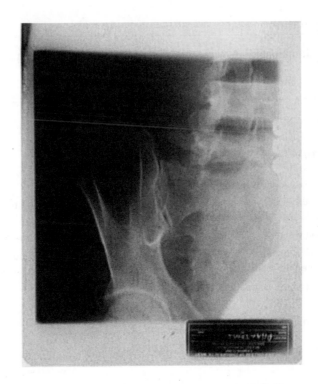

FIGURE 7.39
SI joint film.

Image Critique

One must see from sacroiliac joint space open. Getting patients as close to Bucky as possible and with no rotation is also very important. The shoulders and hips should be in the same plane. Obliquity of 25 to 30° will produce the best results. The lateral gonadal shield should not be higher than the most inferior aspect of the ASIS. Anterior obliques will have greater object to film distance but are easier to accurately position. On very large patients, posterior oblique views should be taken.

Optimum kVp

80–85 kVp

7.14   Lumbar Spine Positioning: A-P Sacrum View

Measure

A-P at trochanter

Protection

Bell for males

SID

40 in. using Bucky

Tube Angulation

15° cephalad; optional P-A view with 15° caudal angle for female patients

Film

8 in. × 10 in. regular speed rare-earth cassette with I.D. up

Positioning

1. Patient stands in front of Bucky, facing the tube.
2. Locate the ASIS and symphysis pubis, and place horizontal central ray midway between these landmarks. Center film to horizontal central ray.
3. Position patient so the vertical central ray is aligned with the mid-sagittal plane of patient.
4. Make sure there is no rotation of the patient. Check the position of the gonadal shield on male patients to ensure that it is not above the most inferior aspect of the symphysis pubis.
5. Give breathing instructions and make exposure.

Collimation

Top to Bottom: slightly less than film size; Side to Side: slightly less than film size.

Breathing Instructions

Full expiration

Image Critique

Must see entire sacrum and S.I. joint space open. Getting patients as close to Bucky as possible and with no rotation is also very important. The shoulders and hips should be in the same plane. If the gonadal shield is too high, it will obscure lower sacrum.

Optimum kVp

75–85 kVp

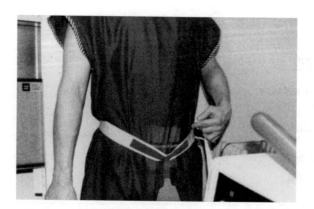

FIGURE 7.40
Sacrum A-P positioning.

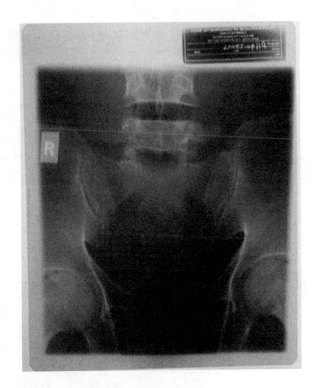

FIGURE 7.41
Sacrum A-P film.

7.15   Lumbar Spine Positioning: P-A Sacrum View

Measure

A-P at trochanter

Protection

The purpose of this view is to reduce radiation exposure to the ovaries in women of child-bearing age.

SID

40 in. using Bucky

Tube Angulation

15° caudal

Film Size

8 in. × 10 in. regular speed rare-earth cassette with I.D. up

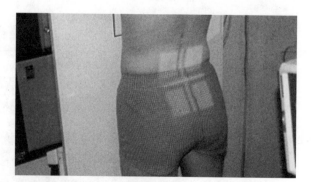

FIGURE 7.42
Sacrum P-A positioning

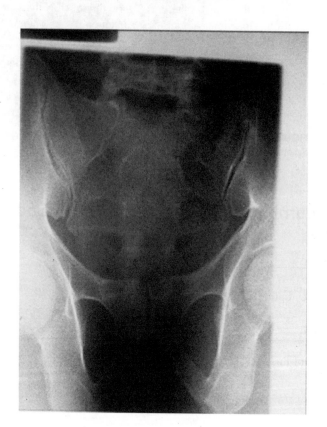

FIGURE 7.43
Sacrum P-A film.

Markers

Pronated R and L

Positioning

1. Female patient stands facing Bucky with feet shoulder-width apart and parallel. She should be as close to the Bucky as possible.

2. Locate the PSIS or the spinous process of the 5th lumbar vertebrae. Place horizontal central ray 2 in. below the PSIS.

3. The vertical central ray should be aligned down the spinous process of the lumbar spine. Make sure that there is no rotation of the body.

4. Center the film to the horizontal central ray.

Collimation

Slightly less than film size.

Image Critique

This view is a compromise to reduce radiation exposure on females of child-bearing age. The small focal spot should be used to help compensate for the magnification caused by increased object to film distance. The information on the view will be the same as the A-P sacrum, with the exception of the magnification. This view should not be taken on obese patients. Bowel gas will degrade the image more than the A-P view.

Optimum kVp

70–74 kVp

7.16   Lumbar Spine Positioning: A-P Coccyx View

Measure

A-P at trochanter

Protection

Bell for males optional, P-A view for female patient

SID

40 in. using Bucky

Tube Angulation

10° caudal; optional P-A angle 10° cephalad

Film

8 in. × 10 in. regular speed rare-earth cassette with I.D. up

Positioning

1. Patient stands in front of Bucky, facing the tube.

2. Locate the ASIS and symphysis pubis, and place horizontal central ray midway between these landmarks. One can also center the horizontal central ray 2 in. superior to the symphysis. Center film to horizontal central ray.

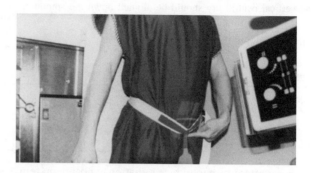

FIGURE 7.44
Coccyx A-P positioning.

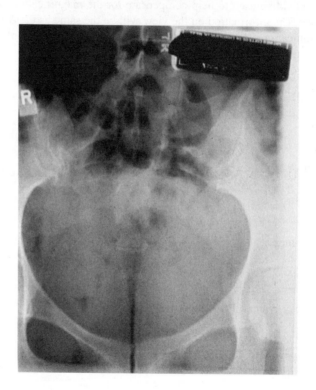

FIGURE 7.45
Coccyx A-P film.

3. Position patient so the vertical central ray is aligned with the mid-sagittal plane of patient.
4. Make sure there is no rotation of the patient. Check the position of the gonadal shield on male patients to ensure that it is not above the most inferior aspect of the symphysis pubis.
5. Give breathing instructions and make exposure.

Collimation

Top to Bottom: slightly less than film size; Side to Side: slightly less than film size.

Breathing Instructions

Full expiration

Image Critique

One must see entire coccyx. Getting patients as close to Bucky as possible and with no rotation is also very important. The shoulders and hips should be in the same plane. If the gonadal shield is too high, it will obscure lower coccyx. The P-A view will have significant magnification distortion.

Optimum kVp

75–80 kVp

7.17   Lumbar Spine Positioning: P-A Coccyx View

Measure

A-P at trochanter

Protection

The purpose of this view is to reduce radiation exposure to the ovaries in females of child-bearing age.

SID

40 in. using Bucky

Tube Angulation

10° cephalad

Film Size

8 in. × 10 in. regular speed rare-earth cassette with I.D. up

Marker

Pronated R and L

Positioning

1. Female patient stands facing Bucky with feet shoulder-width apart and parallel. She should be as close to the Bucky as possible.
2. Locate the PSIS and the trochanter. Place horizontal central ray between the PSIS and trochanter.
3. The vertical central ray should be aligned down the spinous process of the lumbar spine. Make sure that there is no rotation of the body.
4. Center the film to the horizontal central ray.

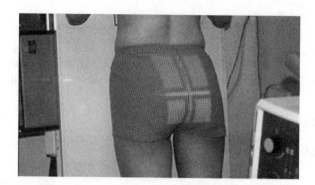

FIGURE 7.46
Coccyx P-A positioning.

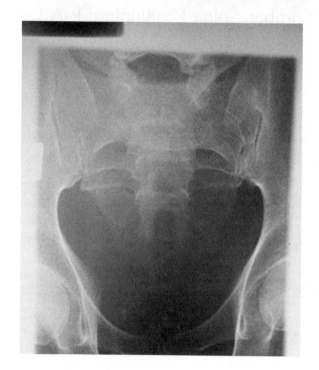

FIGURE 7.47
Coccyx P-A film.

Collimation

Slightly less than film size.

Image Critique

This view is a compromise to reduce radiation exposure on females of child-bearing age. The small focal spot should be used to help compensate for the magnification caused by increased object to film distance. The information on the view will be the same as the A-P sacrum with the exception of the magnification. This view should not be taken on obese patients. Bowel gas will degrade the image more than the A-P view.

Optimum kVp

70–74 kVp

7.18 Lumbar Spine Positioning: Lateral Sacrum and Coccyx View

Measure

Laterally at trochanter

Protection

Lateral gonad shield

SID

40 in. using Bucky

Film

10 in. × 12 in. regular speed rare-earth cassette with I.D. up

Positioning

1. Patient stands with left side to Bucky. If patient has scoliosis with convexity to right, a right lateral is done.
2. Locate the top of the iliac crest and the symphysis pubis. Place horizontal central ray midway between crest and symphysis. Center film to horizontal central ray.

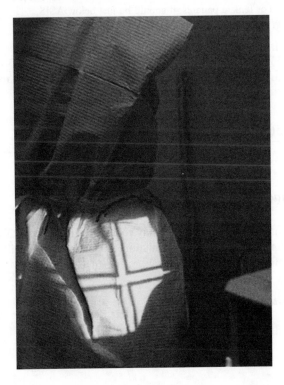

FIGURE 7.48
Sacrum and coccyx lateral positioning.

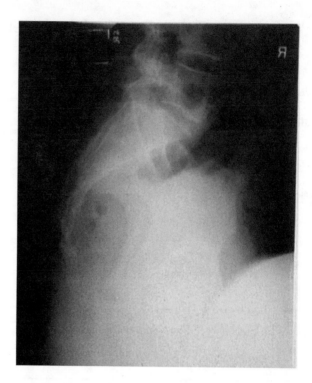

FIGURE 7.49
Sacrum and coccyx lateral film.

3. Find mid-coronal plane by determining the mid-point between the PSIS and ASIS. Center vertical central ray 2 to 3 in. posterior to mid-coronal plane.

4. Collimate and position the lateral gonad shield. For male patients, it should be 2 to 3 in. below ASIS. For female patients, it should be just below ASIS.

Collimation

Top to Bottom: slightly less than film size; Side to Side: to posterior skin, or slightly less than film size.

Breathing Instructions

Full expiration

Image Critique

The image should be free of any rotation of the patient. The view should demonstrate from L-5 to the tip of the coccyx. Collimation to posterior skin will help reduce scatter and provide better visualization of the anatomy.

Optimum kVp

100–110 kVp

7.19 Review of Full Spine, Lumbar Spine, Sacrum, and Coccyx Radiography

1. The key to getting good-quality full spine films is the proper use of filtration, relatively high speed film and cassette, and high-frequency X-ray generators. Without any one of these components, the image will suffer.

2. Subsequent full spine films should be taken P-A on serial scoliosis studies.

3. Some facilities will position the paraspinal lead blockers down to the iliac crest.

4. The only lumbar view that has the horizontal central ray below the iliac crest is the A-P or P-A lumbopelvic view. For the oblique and lateral views, the horizontal central ray is 1 in. above the iliac crest.

5. When palpating the patient to locate the iliac crest, come down from the rib cage. This will help avoid the error of locating the ASIS instead of the crest.

6. All of the lumbar, sacrum, and coccyx views can be taken A-P or P-A. The P-A views will have more magnification but will reduce the exposure for female patients.

7. The patient's lordotic curve will greatly impact the images on erect oblique views. Anterior erect oblique views are less impacted because the divergent rays are in the same plane as the spine.

Chapter 8

Abdominal and Chest Decubitus Radiography

8.1 Abdominal and Chest Decubitus Radiography: Introduction

The basic views taken to evaluate the abdomen are the KUB or supine A-P of the abdomen and an upright view of the abdomen. These views should be somewhat lighter than the views taken of the lumbar spine. The KUB is taken recumbent. A radiographic table with a Bucky or grid is needed to take the KUB. The KUB stands for Kidneys, Ureters, and Bladder, or the anatomy that can be identified on the film. Items or pathologies that can be evaluated with the KUB include gall stones, kidney stones, ileus, or abnormal bowel gas patterns. The positioning is exactly like the A-P lumbopelvic view except it is taken recumbent.

A more detailed evaluation of the abdomen would include a P-A chest view and an erect view of the abdomen. This study is referred to as the *acute abdominal series*. It is important to have the patient upright for at least 10 minutes. The erect views of the abdomen must include the diaphragms. The erect abdomen will demonstrate free air under the diaphragms. One will also see bowel gas and fluid levels. The P-A chest is usually the view of choice to detect free interabdominal air levels under the diaphragms. The patient should be erect for 10 minutes to accurately access the presence of free air. An arrow should be placed on the film to document that the view was taken erect.

A decubitus view is taken to evaluate air and fluid levels. In abdominal radiography, it is used as a substitute for the erect or upright view when the patient cannot stand. The side that the patient lies on is very important. The routine abdominal decubitus is the left lateral decubitus view. The patient lies on the left side. Any free abdominal air will pool above the liver near the right diaphragm. If the patient was on the right side, air in the stomach and colon could be misinterpreted as free air. The patient must remain on the left side for at least 10 minutes to allow the air to pool properly. When marking the decubitus view, mark the side that is up with an arrow and anatomical marker.

Decubitus views are also taken of the chest. They can be very useful when trying to determine the extent of pleural effusions. Both sides of the lung field are very important when taking chest decubitus views. Greater attention is given to the side down because the pleural effusion will pool on the dependent side. Mediastinal or hilar fluid levels can be detected on the side up. Pneumothorax or pneumothorax with effusion can be seen on the side up. The best view for pneumothorax is an erect P-A view with full expiration. It is easier on the patient to do the chest decubitus views A-P. If possible, P-A views will give the most accurate look at the chest. Be careful and lock the gurney or table to avoid the patient rolling off the table and/or falling.

8.2   Abdominal Positioning: KUB or A-P Abdomen View

Measure

A-P at umbilicus

Protection

Bell or apron for males; P-A view may be done on female patients

SID

40 in. using Table Bucky

Tube Angulation

None

Film

14 in. × 17 in. regular speed rare-earth cassette with I.D. up

Positioning

1.   Patient in a supine recumbent position.
2.   Center horizontal central ray 1 in. below iliac crest.
3.   Center film to horizontal central ray.
4.   Align vertical central ray with the mid-sagittal plane of the patient.
5.   Make exposure with full expiration.

Collimation

Top to Bottom: slightly less than film size; Side to Side: skin of abdomen side to side.

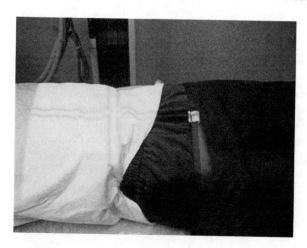

FIGURE 8.1
KUB positioning.

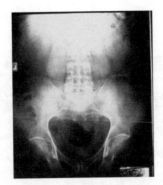

FIGURE 8.2
KUB film.

Breathing Instructions

Full expiration

Image Critique

The view should demonstrate the kidneys, psoas muscles, and the symphysis pubis. There should be no rotation of the patient. Gas patterns in the small and large intestines may be evaluated.

Optimum kVp

70–80 kVp

8.3   Abdominal Positioning: Upright View of Abdomen

Measure

A-P at umbilicus

Protection

Bell for males

SID

40 in. using Bucky

Tube Angulation

None

Film

14 in. × 17 in. regular speed rare-earth cassette with I.D. up

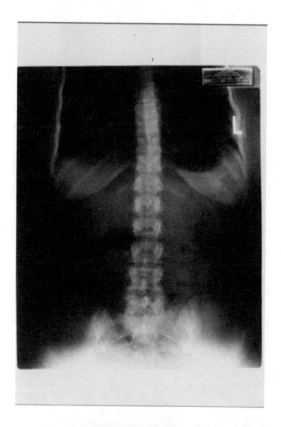

FIGURE 8.3
Erect abdomen film.

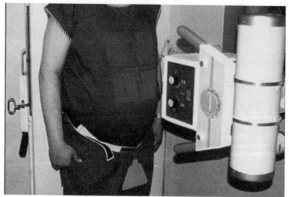

FIGURE 8.4
Erect abdomen positioning.

Positioning

1. Patient stands in front of Bucky, facing the tube.
2. Place top of film 2.5 in. (6.25 cm) above the xiphoid process.
3. Center film to horizontal central ray.
4. Align vertical central ray with the mid-sagittal plane of the patient.
5. Make exposure with full expiration.

Collimation

Top to Bottom: slightly less than film size; Side to Side: skin of abdomen side to side.

Breathing Instructions

Full expiration

Image Critique

The view is usually done to evaluate possible free air in the peritoneal cavity. Therefore, the domes of the diaphragms must be seen at the top of the film. There should be no rotation of the patient. Gas patterns in the small and large intestines may be evaluated.

Optimum kVp

70–80 kVp

8.4   Abdominal Positioning: Left Lateral Decubitus View of Abdomen

Measure

A-P at umbilicus

Protection

Apron draped across lower abdomen

SID

40 in. using Table Bucky

Tube Angulation

None

Film

17 in. × 14 in. regular speed rare-earth cassette with I.D. up

Positioning

1. Patient lies on the left side with table positioned parallel to the upright Bucky. Patient should remain in this position for at least 10 minutes.
2. Center horizontal central ray to mid-sagittal plane of the patient.
3. Center film to horizontal central ray.
4. Align patient so the vertical central ray is 2.5 in. lateral and superior to the iliac crest.
5. Make exposure with full expiration.

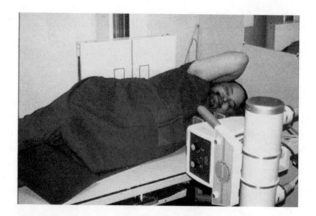

FIGURE 8.5
Left lateral decubitus abdomen positioning.

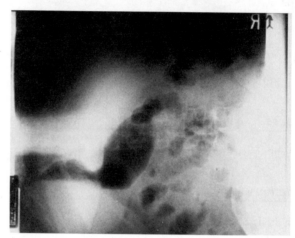

FIGURE 8.6
Left lateral decubitus abdomen film.

Collimation

Top to Bottom: slightly less than film size; Side to Side: skin of abdomen side to side.

Breathing Instructions

Full expiration

Image Critique

The view should demonstrate the presence of free air around the liver under the diaphragm. There should be no rotation of the patient. Gas patterns in the small and large intestines may be evaluated.

Optimum kVp

70–80 kVp

8.5   Chest Positioning: Lateral Decubitus Chest Views

Measure

A-P at mid-chest

Protection

Apron across lower abdomen

SID

72 in. using Table Bucky

Tube Angulation

None

Film

17 in. × 14 in. regular speed rare-earth cassette with I.D. up

Positioning

1. Patient lies on affected side with table positioned parallel to the upright Bucky. Depending on the room layout, view may be done A-P or P-A. For pleural fluid, the affected side should be down. For hilar or pericardial fluid, affected side should be up. Have patient raise arms over head. Patient needs to stay on affected side for 5 to 10 minutes.
2. Center horizontal central ray to mid-sagittal plane of the patient. (Set so bottom of film will be at the level of the film.)
3. Center film to horizontal central ray.
4. Align patient so the top of the film is 2 in. above the shoulder.
5. Make exposure with full inspiration.

Collimation

Top to Bottom: slightly less than film size; Side to Side: skin of chest or film size.

Breathing Instructions

Full inspiration

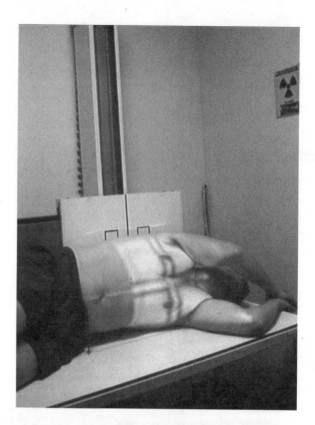

FIGURE 8.7
Decubitus chest positioning.

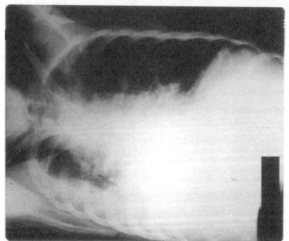

FIGURE 8.8
Decubitus chest film.

Image Critique

The view should demonstrate the presence of free fluid as a layer in the lung field, hilum, or around the heart. Air fluid levels can also be seen on the side up if there is a small pneumothorax with effusion. There should be no rotation of patient.

Optimum kVp

100–125 kVp

Chapter 9

Skull and Facial Radiography

9.1   Skull and Facial Radiography: Introduction

One of the benefits of being very familiar with doing radiography on the wall Bucky or upright radiography is that the skull and facial bones are easier to radiograph erect. For many years, medical facilities spent extra money to purchase head units; they were essentially a wall Bucky. The baselines of the skull discussed in cervical radiography are key to accurate positioning for skull and facial radiography. The routine skull series has generally been replaced by Computed Tomography (CT) or Magnetic Resonance Imaging (MRI) in major hospitals. Because these modalities are not readily available in an office, being able to do routine views is very important. To achieve optimum detail, the small focal spot should always be used for skull or facial films.

Skull films are typically taken with the patient seated in front of the wall Bucky. This allows better visualization of the mid-sagittal plane. Skull radiography should be free of any rotation of the skull. The principal baselines used are the canthomeatal line that runs from the outer canthus of the eye to the external auditory meatus, and the interpupillary line that runs from one eye pupil to the other eye pupil. The canthomeatal line will generally be perpendicular to the film when the nose and forehead are resting on the Bucky. The interpupillary line is used as in the cervical spine to achieve a true lateral view.

Facial bone and sinus studies use the same views. Collimation and the small focal spot are very important. The Waters view is the single most useful view for sinus and facial bone or orbit injuries. Each view will demonstrate a particular area of the sinuses. The Caldwell will give a clear view of the frontal sinuses. The lateral view is good for the sphenoid sinus. The basilar view will demonstrate the sphenoid and ethmoid sinuses.

There are hundreds more views of the skull and spine that are not taught as part of this course. Two very useful views are the Schuller's projection for temporal mandibular joints and the base posterior or basilar view. The Schuller's projection taken with the patient's mouth open and closed will show how the mandibular condyle tracks in the joint. One will see only the osseous portions of the joint. The basilar view is good for evaluation of the upper cervical spine, zygomatic arches, as well as the cranium.

9.2   Skull Positioning: P-A Skull View

Measure

A-P at glabella

Protection

Coat lead apron or half apron draped over back of chair

SID

40 in. using Bucky

Tube Angulation

None

Film

10 in. × 12 in. (24 cm × 30 cm) Lanex regular with I.D. down

Marker

Anatomical

Positioning

1.   Patient seated in chair or on stool P-A in front of wall Bucky or prone on table.
2.   Patient is asked to tuck chin into chest until the canthomeatal line is perpendicular to the film.
3.   Horizontal central ray positioned to exit through the glabella or nasion. Center film to horizontal central ray.

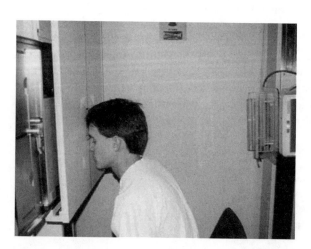

FIGURE 9.1
Skull P-A positioning.

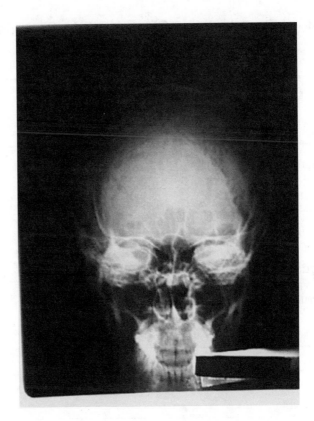

FIGURE 9.2
Skull P-A film.

4. Align the mid-sagittal plane of the patient perpendicular to film. Center vertical central ray to mid-sagittal plane.
5. Check the interpupillary line to make sure it is parallel to the horizontal central ray.
6. Make exposure with suspended respiration.

Collimation

Top to Bottom: skin of skull or film size; Side to Side: skin of skull.

Breathing Instructions

Suspend respiration

Image Critique

The petrous ridges will be in the orbits. There should be no rotation of skull. The skull, frontal sinuses, nasal turbinate, and most of the mandible should be seen.

Optimum kVp

75 kVp

9.3   Skull Positioning: Chamberlain-Town's Skull View

Measure

A-P at glabella

Protection

Coat lead apron

SID

40 in. using Bucky

Tube Angulation

30 to 35° caudal

Film

10 in. × 12 in. (24 cm × 30 cm) Lanex regular with I.D. down

Marker

Anatomical

Positioning

1.   Patient seated in chair or on stool A-P in front of wall Bucky or supine on table.
2.   Patient is asked to tuck chin into chest until the canthomeatal line is perpendicular to the film.

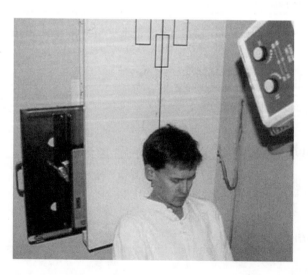

FIGURE 9.3
Chamberlain-Towne's positioning.

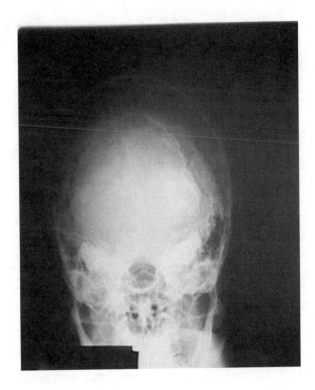

FIGURE 9.4
Chamberlain-Towne's film.

3. Horizontal central ray positioned to exit through the EAM. It should be close to the hairline of the patient. Center film to horizontal central ray.
4. Align the mid-sagittal plane of the patient perpendicular to film. Center vertical central ray to mid-sagittal plane.
5. Check the interpupillary line to make sure it is parallel to film.
6. Make exposure with suspended respiration.

Collimation

Top to Bottom: skin of skull, or film size; Side to Side: skin of skull.

Breathing Instructions

Suspended respiration

Image Critique

The occiput should be clearly seen with no rotation of skull. Both petrous pyramids, foramen magnum, and dorsum sella should be visualized.

Optimum kVp

80 kVp

9.4   Skull Positioning: Lateral View of Skull

Measure

Lateral at external auditory meatus

Protection

Coat lead apron

SID

40 in. using Bucky

Tube Angulation

None; may use angle parallel to interpupillary line

Film

12 in. × 10 in. (30 cm × 24 cm) regular speed rare-earth cassette with I.D. toward mandible.

Positioning

1. Patient seated on stool or chair with affected side of skull lateral to Bucky.
2. Make sure the mid-sagittal plane is parallel to film. Adjust any head tilt to get interpupillary line perpendicular to film.
3. Place horizontal central ray 0.75 in. superior to EAM. Center film to horizontal central ray.
4. Place vertical central ray 0.75 in. superior to the EAM.
5. Ask patient to suspend respiration and hold still.

Collimation

Top to Bottom: skin of skull; Side to Side: skin of skull.

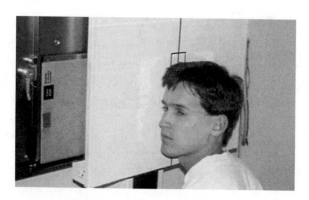

FIGURE 9.5
Lateral skull positioning.

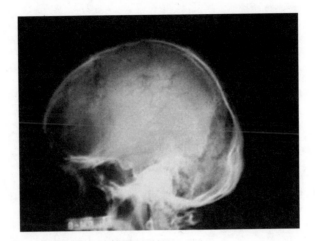

FIGURE 9.6
Lateral skull film.

Breathing Instructions

Hold still and suspend respiration

Image Critique

The EAMs and orbits should be superimposed. The sella should be clearly visualized, with the anterior clinoid processes superimposed. All of the bony structures of the skull should be visualized.

Optimum kVp

65–70 kVp

9.5 Skull Positioning: Base Posterior View of Skull

Measure

A-P at glabella

Protection

Lead apron

SID

40 in. using Bucky

Tube Angulation

None; may angle tube cephalad to get beam perpendicular to inferaorbital-meatal line

Film

10 in. × 12 in. (or 24 cm × 30 cm) Lanex regular cassette with I.D. down

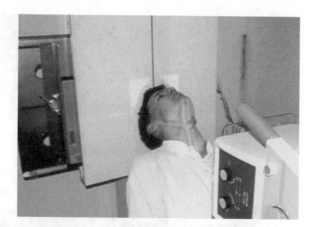

FIGURE 9.7
Skull base posterior positioning.

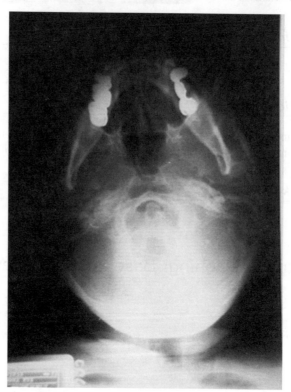

FIGURE 9.8
Skull basilar film.

Positioning

1. Position chair with back about 6 to 10 in. from wall Bucky. Have patient sit in chair.

2. Ask patient to extend head until the inferior orbital meatal line is perpendicular to film. Patient may slouch if necessary.

3. If patient can extend far enough backward, place horizontal central ray at level of EAM or TMJ. Center film to horizontal central ray.

4. If patient is unable to extend far enough, angle tube cephalad until beam is perpendicular to inferior orbital meatal line. Center beam to EAM and film to horizontal central ray.

5. Make sure mid-sagittal plane is perpendicular to film.

6. Ask patient not to breathe, move, or swallow.

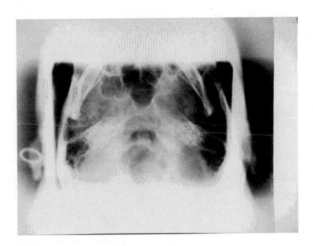

FIGURE 9.9
Skull basilar film.

Collimation

Slightly less than film size

Breathing Instructions

Do not breathe, move, or swallow

Image Critique

There should be no rotation of skull. This is an axial projection of the skull. The foramen magnum will appear round, and C-1 and C-2 will be seen relative to the foramen. The mandible will be superimposed with the frontal bone. With a bright light, the zygomatic arches will appear as teacup handles.

Optimum kVp

80 kVp

9.6 Skull Positioning: Schuller's View of Mastoids and Temporal Mandibular Joints

Measure

Lateral at EAM

Protection

Coat lead apron or apron draped over back of chair

SID

40 in. using Bucky

Tube Angulation

25° caudal

Film

8 in. × 10 in. regular speed rare-earth cassette with I.D. up

Markers

Anatomical and arrow horizontal for closed mouth and pointing down for open mouth, or letters O and C

Positioning

1. Patient seated on stool or in chair with affected side of skull lateral to Bucky.
2. Make sure the mid-sagittal plane is parallel to film. Adjust any head tilt to get interpupillary line perpendicular to film.
3. Center the TMJ next to be Bucky on the center line of the Bucky. Then center the horizontal central ray to the same TMJ. Center the film to the horizontal central ray.
4. Take films with mouth closed and with mouth open.
5. Repeat steps on other TMJ and take films with mouth open and closed.

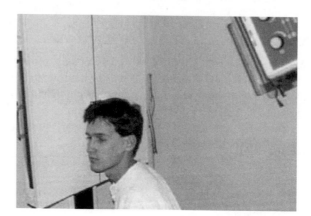

FIGURE 9.10
Schuller's projection, closed mouth.

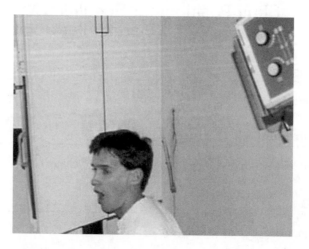

FIGURE 9.11
Schuller's projection, open mouth.

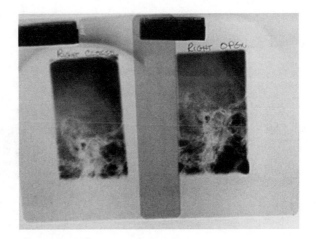

FIGURE 9.12
TMJ films.

Collimation

Top to Bottom: 5 in.; Side to Side: 5 in.

Breathing Instructions

Hold still and suspend respiration

Image Critique

The tube angle will project the TMJ away from the film down, so one should be able to have a clear view of the mandibular condyle and its relationship to the joint at both ends of the range of motion.

Optimum kVp

70 kVp

9.7   Skull Positioning: Caldwell P-A Facial or Sinus View

Measure

A-P at glabella

Protection

Coat lead apron

SID

40 in. Bucky

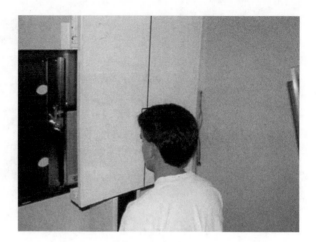

FIGURE 9.13
Sinus Cauldwell positioning.

Tube Angulation

15° caudal

Film

8 in. × 10 in. regular speed rare-earth cassette with I.D. down

Marker

Anatomical

Positioning

1. Patient seated on chair or on stool P-A in front of wall Bucky, or prone on table.
2. Patient is asked to tuck chin into chest until the canthomeatal line is perpendicular to the film.
3. Horizontal central ray positioned to exit through the nasion. Center film to horizontal central ray.
4. Align the mid-sagittal plane of the patient perpendicular to film. Center vertical central ray to mid-sagittal plane.
5. Check the interpupillary line to make sure it is parallel to horizontal central ray.
6. Make exposure with suspended respiration.

Collimation

Top to Bottom: 6–7 in.; Side to Side: 6–7 in.

Breathing Instructions

Suspend respiration

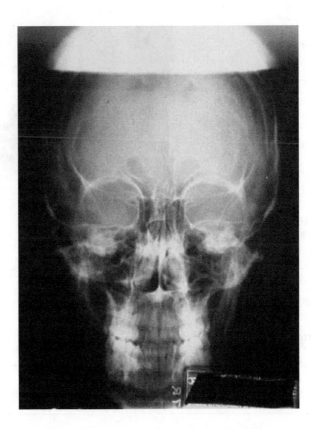

FIGURE 9.14
Sinus Cauldwell film.

Image Critique

The petrous ridges will be below the super orbital rims and above the inferior orbital rims. The frontal sinuses will be clearly identified in the orbits. There should be no rotation of skull. The view may also be done as part of a skull series.

Optimum kVp

75 kVp

9.8   Skull Positioning: Waters View of Facial Bones and Sinuses

Measure

A-P at glabella

Protection

Coat lead apron or apron draped over back of chair

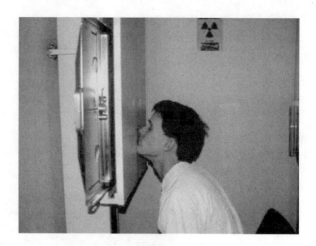

FIGURE 9.15
Sinus Water's positioning.

SID

40 in. using Bucky

Tube Angulation

None

Film

8 in. × 10 in. regular with I.D. down

Marker

Anatomical

Positioning

1. Patient seated in chair or on stool P-A in front of wall Bucky or prone on table.
2. Patient is asked to raise chin until the mentameatal line is perpendicular to the film. The nose should be about 2 cm off the Bucky.
3. Horizontal central ray positioned to exit through the acanthion or tip of nose. To visualize the sphenoid sinus, have patient open mouth. Center film to horizontal central ray.
4. Align the mid-sagittal plane of the patient perpendicular to film. Center vertical central ray to mid-sagittal plane.
5. Check the interpupillary line to make sure it is perpendicular to film.
6. Make exposure with suspended respiration.

Collimation

Top to Bottom: 6–7 in.; Side to side: 6–7 in.

Breathing Instructions

Suspended respiration

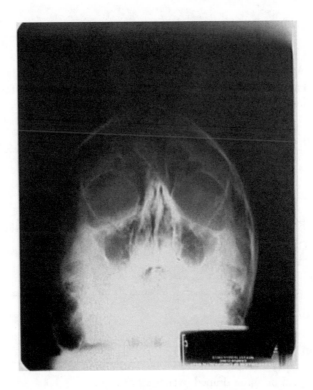

FIGURE 9.16
Sinus Water's film.

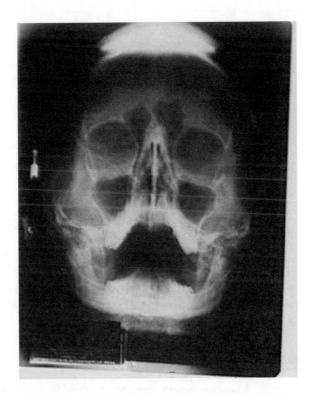

FIGURE 9.17
Sinus Water's film, mouth open.

Image Critique

The petrous ridges will be below the floor of the maxillary sinuses. If done upright, air fluid levels will be identified. The nasal anatomy will also be identified. The zygomas and orbits can be evaluated. Pay attention to the sutures around the orbit and the inferior orbital rim. There should be no rotation of skull.

Optimum kVp

80 kVp

9.9 Skull Positioning: Lateral View of Sinus and Facial Bones

Measure

Lateral at EAM

Protection

Coat lead apron or apron draped over back of chair

SID

40 in. using Bucky

Tube Angulation

None; may use angle parallel to interpupillary line

Film

8 in. × 10 in. regular speed rare-earth cassette with I.D. down

Positioning

1. Patient seated on stool or in chair with affected side of skull lateral to Bucky.
2. Make sure the mid-sagittal plane is parallel to film. Adjust any head tilt to get interpupillary line perpendicular to film.
3. Place horizontal central ray through the outer canthus of the eye. Center film to horizontal central ray.
4. Place vertical central ray through the outer canthus of the eye.
5. Ask patient to suspend respiration and hold still.

Collimation

Top to Bottom: frontal sinuses to mandible; Side to Side: tip of nose to EAM.

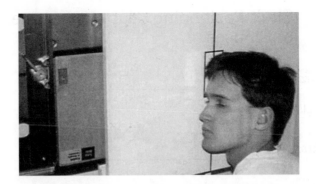

FIGURE 9.18
Sinus lateral positioning.

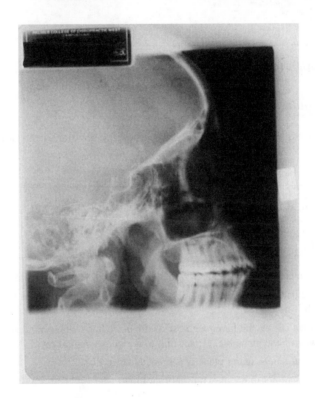

FIGURE 9.19
Sinus lateral film.

Breathing Instructions

Hold still and suspend respiration

Image Critique

The orbits should be superimposed. The sphenoid, frontal, and maxillary sinuses should be clearly visualized. The floor of the maxilla and much of the mandible will be seen. Look for cloudiness or fluid in the sinuses, as well as any air in soft tissues.

Optimum kVp

65–70 kVp

9.10   Skull Positioning: Submentovertex View of Sinuses

Measure

A-P at glabella

Protection

Lead apron

SID

40 in. using Bucky

Tube Angulation

None; may angle tube cephalad to get beam perpendicular to inferior orbital meatal line

Film

8 in. × 10 in. regular speed rare-earth cassette with I.D. down

Positioning

1. Position chair with back about 6 to 10 in. from wall Bucky. Have patient sit in chair.
2. Ask patient to extend head until the inferior orbital meatal line is perpendicular to film. Patient may slouch if necessary.
3. If patient can extend far enough backward, place horizontal central ray 1.5 in. above the EAM or about midway up the mandible. Center film to horizontal central ray.
4. Make sure mid-sagittal plane is perpendicular to film.
5. Ask patient not to breathe, move, or swallow.

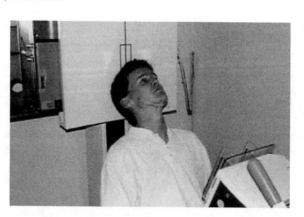

FIGURE 9.20
Sinus basilar view positioning.

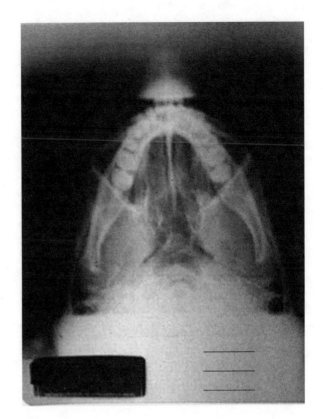

FIGURE 9.21
Sinus basilar view film.

Collimation

Slightly less than film size

Breathing Instructions

Do not breathe, move, or swallow

Image Critique

There should be no rotation of skull. This is an axial projection of the sinuses and skull. The foramen magnum will appear round, and C-1 and C-2 will be seen relative to the foramen. The sphenoid and ethmoid sinuses should be well visualized. The mandible will be superimposed with the frontal bone. With a bright light, the zygomatic arches will appear as teacup handles.

Optimum kVp

80 kVp

Chapter 10

Introduction to Extremity Radiography

Extremity radiography will require some type of table for the patient to place the extremity on. For upper extremities, any table that allows 40 in. focal film or source to image distance is suitable. Any Bucky work can be done with the upright wall Bucky. Most of the extremity views can be taken with the patient standing, seated, or recumbent. Use the method most comfortable for the patient. The small focal spot should always be used for extremity studies to achieve the best possible resolution or geometric detail.

For lower extremity radiography, a recumbent Bucky should be available. This will require a radiographic table or stationary grids. While certainly not recommended, a patient can be positioned on the floor using a stationary grid for recumbent radiography; in such cases, one needs to be able to get the patient down to the floor and back up safely after the exam is completed. This can be the greatest problem with not having a table.

Extremity radiography of the hands, wrists, feet, and ankles requires fine or high detail cassettes. These are typically referred to as "extremity cassettes." Doing extremity radiography on 400 speed rare-earth screen systems is not recommended. The kVp must be dropped so low that the bones may not be penetrated. The resolution is not good enough to see small fractures. Extremity cassettes are used for the smaller body parts. Extremities measuring more than 10 cm are generally taken Bucky. Extremities measuring less than 10 cm are done on extremity cassettes. The extremity cassettes come in both single-screen and two-screen cassette designs. The two-screen cassettes will usually use the same film that is used for spinal work. The single-screen cassettes use a special single-emulsion film. Special care is needed when working with the single-screen cassettes. The emulsion must be placed next to the screen when the cassette is loaded. Single-emulsion film is prone to processing problems and the smallest amount of dirt will be seen on the film. Single-emulsion film is the type of system used for mammography in medical radiography.

Usually, more than one view will be placed on the film when X-rays of the hands, feet, or other small extremities are being studied. This will require the use of lead blockers to protect the exposed section of the film from scatter radiation. Most cassettes have scribed marks or arrows on the border to assist in dividing the cassette into quarters. To do three views on the film, the operator must divide the cassette him/herself. The quarter or four views on the cassette is the most efficient use of the film if the operator accurately positions the extremity.

A full-coat lead apron will provide the best radiation protection for the patient when seated for upper extremity views. The half-apron works fine for lower extremities. For some views of male patients, the bell is the easiest form of gonadal shielding. Never put the patient's lower extremities under the table when taking views of the upper extremity. The radiation will pass through the cassette and provide unnecessary radiation exposure to the legs.

There are some basic principles for extremity radiography. The most important is that the study must include both proximal and distal articulations. Some extremities such as the femur may require more than two views. The minimum study consists of an A-P or P-A and lateral views.

The collimation must be set to include both articulations. This requires a good knowledge of the basic anatomy of the extremity. The collimation should also include the soft tissue around the area of clinical interest. Fat pads and other soft tissue signs are extremely important.

The measurement for the technical factors will generally be where the central ray is placed. This will often be the thickest part of the area of interest. Remember that extremity cassettes are used for extremity studies when the body part usually measures 10 cm or less. The knee can either be done Bucky or with extremity cassettes. The density of the distal femur makes the views of the knee generally Bucky views.

The size of film or cassette used will vary significantly from facility to facility. The greatest variability is in the shoulder and clavicle region. At Palmer-West, 8 in. × 10 in. cassettes are used; other schools use 10 in. × 12 in. Whichever size is used, collimation to less than film size is very important. Wider collimation will result in more scatter radiation, which will reduce contrast and resolution. When opening a practice, one will need to determine what film sizes will be stocked and used.

While extremity views can be taken without positioning aids, radiographic sponges will make it much easier and less painful for the patient. One will also need to have weights or sandbags larger than the 7- to 10-lb bags to be used for the lateral cervical spine.

A stool can be used to provide support for erect lateral views of the knee and hip. Be very careful when having a patient stand on one foot. One patient fall could cost much more than the cost of a radiographic table. The grids in most upright film holders are only 15 in. wide. This can cause problems when taking views of the pelvis or both knees weight-bearing. If the patient leans too hard on the wall Bucky, grid cut-off will result.

The use of the optimum kVp is very important with extremity studies. The use of lower kVp may make the view underpenetrated. This can result in missed fractures. Some screen and film combinations lose speed below 70 kVp. The images may be underexposed when less than 70 kVp is used. It is equally important to not overpenetrate or overexpose extremity views. Calcifications in the bursea can be missed if the views are overexposed. Other soft tissue signs can also be missed when the kVp is set too high and the view lacks contrast.

With precise positioning and the correct equipment, there is no reason why the typical chiropractic office cannot do high-quality extremity radiography. Most views can be done erect or seated. The next few chapters will cover basic extremity radiography as well as some advanced sports medicine type views.

10.1   Basic Concepts of Extremity Radiography

1.   All views must include the proximal and distal articulations of the extremity being radiographed. If the extremity is longer than the film size, additional views will be needed of the missing articulation.

2.   The body part is measured at the point where the central ray will enter the body. The exceptions are the A-P calcaneus and lateral scapula.

3.   Extremities less than 10 cm thick are imaged on the fine or extremity cassettes, except for knees. Years ago, this 10-cm rule was used to determine if films were taken screen or non-screen. If the basic extremity is imaged on these cassettes, larger sized structures may be also done on the extremity cassettes. Examples include ankle views and elbow views.

4. Patient may be seated, recumbent, or standing for extremity views. They may be taken on the wall Bucky, using a tabletop, or a table with a Bucky.

5. When the patient is seated for upper extremity tabletop views, the lower extremities should *never* be under the table.

6. Views that are taken Bucky may also be done recumbent using a stationary grid or table with a Bucky. Watch grid ratio when using stationary grids.

7. When using lead blockers, mask the exposed side of the cassette. Exposed film is more sensitive to fogging. Up to four views may be done on a single cassette.

8. Markers are positioned on the film so the patient cannot read the letter. That is, the letter will be upside down to the patient and right side up to the operator.

9. Collimation is one of the key factors for image quality but it requires the operator to understand the location of the radiographic anatomy that is essential for the view.

10. Typically, when one part of the extremity is in true A-P or lateral position, the rest of the extremity will also be properly positioned for the A-P or lateral type view. This, however, is not true of P-A views.

Chapter 11

Extremity Positioning Quick Reference Charts

11.1 Fingers and Thumbs

View	Measure	Film Size I.D./R or L	FFD	Tube Tilt	Central Ray	Filter/ Shielding	Positioning	Collimation TB = Top to Bottom SS = Side to Side	Essential Anatomy
Fingers P-A	A-P at mid-PIP of finger	Pt. cannot read 10 × 8 Extremity	40 in. Non-Bucky	None 0°	H: proximal interphalangeal joint (PIP). V: long axis of finger.	Lead apron	Pt. seated with affected hand next to the table. Do not put pt. legs under the table. P-A: hand pronated with affected finger extended.	TB: to include entire finger and metacarpal-phalangeal joint. SS: skin of finger	The entire finger and its articulation with the metacarpal must be seen on all three views. The long axis of the finger must remain parallel to film on all three views. If the pt. cannot straighten finger, A-P views may be useful.
Oblique	A-P at mid-PIP of finger				H: to mid film.		Oblique: spread fingers slightly, semi-pronated hand until the involved finger is 45° to film.	Obl. and lateral views *Note:* sponge used to stabilize finger and to keep long axis parallel to film.	
Lateral	Lateral at mid-PIP of finger				H: to mid film.		Lateral: hand in true lateral. Extend affected finger and flex others.		
Thumb P-A	A-P at metacarpal phalangeal joint	Pt. cannot read 10 × 8 Extremity	40 in. Non-Bucky	None 0°	H: through metacarpal-phalangeal joint. H: to mid film. V: long axis of thumb.	Lead apron	Pt. seated with affected hand next to table. P-A: hand lateral on ulnar surface. Thumb is elevated and abducted with sponge for support.	TB: to include trapezium, first metacarpal, and entire thumb. SS: skin of thumb.	Views to see the entire thumb and 1st metacarpal and its articulation with carpal bones. M-P and PIP joint spaces must be open on all views.
A-P							A-P: hand in extreme internal rotation with thumb extended and abducted to touch film.		
Oblique							Obl.: hand pronated with palmar surface flat on film. Thumb extended. Same as P-A hand.		
Lateral							Lat: hand extended with the palmar surface in contact with film. While maintaining contact of thumb and the first metacarpal with film, raise other fingers and palm until the thumb is lateral.		

Basic concepts in extremity radiography:
1. Both joint articulations must be demonstrated on all views of the study.
2. The patient should be seated parallel to the table with the affected extremity next to the table.
3. The lower extremities should never be positioned under the table and the lead apron should protect them and the gonads.
4. The marker is placed on the film in a manner where the letter is upside down to the view of the patient.

11.2 Wrist and Hand Views

View	Measure	Film Size / I.D./R or L	FFD	Tube Tilt	Central Ray	Filter/ Shielding	Positioning	Collimation TB = Top to Bottom / SS = Side to Side	Essential Anatomy
Wrist: P-A	A-P at CR	R or L pt. cannot read. 10 × 12 Extremity	40 in. Non-Bucky	None 0°	H: through mid-carpal bones and distal ulna and radius. V: through third metacarpal.	Lead apron	Pt. seated with affected wrist next to table. Wrist pronated. PA: wrist pronated, fingers flexed or make a fist.	TB: include carpal bones and the articulations with the ulna and radius and metacarpal. SS: skin of wrist.	Wrist series is to evaluate the carpal bones and wrist joint articulation with the distal ulna and radius. It is important to see the area of prime interest. Collimate to include the anatomy that must be seen and the area of interest.
Oblique	A-P at CR				H: through carpal bones and distal ulna and radius. V: through carpal bones and distal ulna and radius.		Oblique: wrist slightly pronated at 45° angle. Thumb to film to support hand.		
Lateral	Lateral at CR						Lateral: Pt. seated. Elbow flexed 90°. Palm is perpendicular to film. Fingers flexed with thumb on index finger.		
Wrist: Ulnar flexion (scaphoid view)	A-P at CR	Pt. cannot read markers 8 × 10 Extremity	40 in. Non-Bucky	15–20° Cephalad	H: mid-carpal bones. V: long axis of ulna and radius. Film center to H.	Lead apron	Pt. seated. Wrist pronated and in maximal ulnar deviation (turned out). Note: Radial flexion can also be used; wrist pronated with maximal radial deviation (turned in). No tube tilt for radial flexion.	TB: include carpal bones and the articulations with the ulna and radius and metacarpal. SS: skin of wrist.	View to see the entire scaphoid bone, usually to rule out fracture.
Wrist: clenched fist A-P view	A-P at CR	R or L pt. cannot read 8 × 10 Extremity	40 in. Non-Bucky	None 0°	H: mid-carpal bones. V: long axis of ulna and radius. Film center to H.	Lead apron	Pt. seated next to table with affected wrist supinated and fist clenched fully.	TB: include carpal bones and the articulations with the ulna and radius and metacarpal. SS: skin of wrist.	A-P view of wrist to evaluate ligaments of wrist.

View	Measure	Film Size I.D./R or L	FFD	Tube Tilt	Central Ray	Filter/ Shielding	Positioning	Collimation TB = Top to Bottom SS = Side to Side	Essential Anatomy
Hand: P-A	A-P at CR	12 × 10 Extremity	40 in. Non-Bucky	None 0°	H: through 3rd metacarpal-phalangeal joint. V: through long axis of hand and 3rd finger. H: Center to film.	Lead apron	PA: Pt. seated next to table. Hand pronated with palm to film. Fingers spread slightly. Oblique: Pt. seated next to table. Hand slightly pronated at 45° angle. Fingers spread slightly but remaining straight. May use a sponge to support hand.	TB: from wrist to fingers. SS: skin of hand.	P-A hand to see the fingers, metacarpals, carpal bones, and the ulna and radius joint. Obl. metacarpals and phalanges or seen in obl. view without superimposition.
Oblique	A-P at CR								
Hand: Lateral view	Lateral at CR	8 × 10 Extremity	40 in. Non-Bucky	None 0°	H: through metacarpal-phalangeal joints. V: through head of 2nd metacarpal joint.	Lead apron	Pt. seated. Hand in true lateral position (elbow flexed 90°). Fingers slightly flexed and spread apart. Thumb and index fingers touching. Sponge may be used to provide support.	TB: from wrist to fingers. SS: to include all fingers and hand.	Lateral view of carpal metacarpals and phalanges.

11.3 — Humerus, Elbow, and Forearm

View	Measure	Film Size I.D./R or L	FFD	Tube Tilt	Central Ray	Filter/ Shielding	Positioning	Collimation TB = Top to Bottom SS = Side to Side	Essential Anatomy
Humerus: A-P	A-P at CR mid-humerus	I.D. down 7 × 17	40 in. Non-Bucky Optional Bucky	None 90°	Top of film 1 in. above shoulder. H: center to film. V: through long axis of humerus.	Lead apron	Pt. standing or recumbent, facing tube. Top of film 1 in. above the humeral head. Hand supinated with arm to side. Must include both joints.	TB: to include shoulder and elbow articulations. SS: skin of arm.	A-P view of entire humerus, including both shoulder and elbow articulations.
Humerus: Lateral	A-P at CR	I.D. down 7 × 17	40 in. Non-Bucky	None 90°	Film 1 in. above humeral head. V: long axis of humerus. H: centered to film or mid-shaft of humerus.	Lead apron	Pt. standing or recumbent, facing tube. Three positions possible: 1. Arm by side and internally rotated. 2. Flex elbow and place on abdomen. 3. Abduct shoulder to 90° and flex elbow. ("Baby Arm") recumbent.	TB: to include shoulder and elbow articulations. SS: skin of arm.	Lateral view of the entire humerus, including shoulder and elbow joints.
Elbow: A-P	A-P at CR	R or L pt. cannot read. 1/2 of 10 × 12 Extremity	40 in. Non-Bucky	None 0°	H: 1 cm distal to epicondyles V: long axis of elbow. Elbow centered on 1/2 of the cassette.	Lead apron	Pt. kneeling next to table with elbow next to table. Arm fully extended and hand supinated. Humeral epicondyles are parallel to film. Sponge may be under the hand for support.	A-P uses 1/2 of the 10 × 12 extremity cassette. TB: distal humerus and proximal forearm. SS: skin of arm.	A-P view of the elbow, including distal humerus and proximal forearm.

View	Measure	Film Size I.D./R or L	FFD	Tube Tilt	Central Ray	Filter/ Shielding	Positioning	Collimation TB = Top to Bottom SS = Side to Side	Essential Anatomy
Elbow: Lateral Oblique	A-P at CR	1/2 of 10 × 12 Extremity	40 in. Bucky	None 0°.	H: 1 cm distal to epicondyles V: long axis of elbow. Elbow centered on 1/2 of the cassette.	Lead apron	Pt. kneeling same position as A-P. Hand supinated and elbow straight. Arm externally rotated 45°. Support hand with sponges.	Oblique view used the remaining half of cassette. Collimation same as A-P.	Oblique elbow view provides an unobstructed view of radial head.
Elbow: Lateral	Lateral at CR	8 × 10 Extremity	40 in. Non-Bucky	None 0°	H: 1 in. distal to epicondyle. V: through long axis of elbow.	Lead apron	Pt. kneeling. Humerus and forearm are parallel to film. Elbow flexed 90° with wrist lateral. Humeral condyles are perpendicular to film.	TB: 6 in. field or to lateral skin. SS: to include proximal forearm.	Lateral view of elbow. Do not collimate off the soft tissue as the fat pad is important.
Elbow: Medial oblique	A-P at CR	8 × 10 Extremity	40 in. Non-Bucky	None 0°	H: 1 cm distal to epicondyles. V: long axis of arm. CR centered to film.	Lead apron	Pt. kneeling with arm straight. Sponge can be used under wrist for comfort. Arm internally rotated until the epicondyles are about 30 to 45° to film.	TB: slightly less than film size. SS: skin of elbow.	View useful for evaluation of the coracoid process of the elbow.
Forearm: A-P and lateral	A-P at CR	I.D. Down 7 × 17 or both views on 14 × 17	40 in. Non-Bucky	None 0°	For both A-P and Lat.: H: mid-shaft of forearm. V: long axis of forearm.	Lead apron	Pt. seated next to table with affected arm extended, with forearm supinated. Lateral position: Pt. seated with the forearm flexed 90°. Ulnar surface on film.	TB: include wrist and elbow joints. SS: to skin of forearm.	Forearm views must include wrist and elbow joints on both views. Both views can be done on a single 14 × 17.

11.4 Clavicle, Acromioclavicular Joints, and Scapula

View	Measure	Film Size I.D./R or L	FFD	Tube Tilt	Central Ray	Filter/Shielding	Positioning	Collimation TB = Top to Bottom SS = Side to Side	Essential Anatomy
Clavicle: P-A Axial or A-P Axial	A-P at mid-clavicle (CR)	Film: Top 1/2 of 8 × 10 or 10 × 12	40 in. Bucky	15–25° Caudal A-P 15–25° cephalad	H: so the beam exits through the clavicle. 4.5 in. × 8 in. field should have a little light above AC joint, beam exits through mid-clavicle P-A. A-P H: 1 in. below clavicle; A-P V: mid-clavicle.	Lead apron	Pt. standing facing Bucky for P-A. Head rotated away from affected side. Pt. standing facing tube for A-P. Head turned away from affected side.	TB: 4.5 in. for top half of film. SS: to film size or to include SC and AC joints.	Axial view of clavicle opens the subacromion area and helps to see angle and displacement of fractures.
P-A or A-P Clavicle	A-P at mid-clavicle (CR)	I.D. down Pronate marker (P-A) 1/2 of 8 × 10 or 10 × 12	40 in. Bucky	None 90°	Film: bottom 1/2 of 8 × 10 Do not use I.D. area. H: mid-clavicle V: mid-clavicle	Lead apron	Same as axial view. Full inspiration.	TB: 4.5 in. centered to bottom half of film. SS: film size or to include SC and AC joints.	P-A or A-P view of clavicle, sternal clavicular, and AC joint.
Acromio-clavicular joints: Bilateral weighted and unweighted	A-P at CR coracoid process	17 × 7 (2) or 17 × 14	72 in. Non-Bucky	Routine no angle. Zanca view. 15° cephalad.	H: mid AC joint. V: mid-sagittal plane. Center top 1/2 of film for non-weighted view. Center bottom 1/2 of film for weighted view with arrow pointing down.	Lead apron	AP: Standing, facing tube, arms to sides and relaxed for non-weighted view. For weighted view, pt. must hold 10–15 lb of weight in each arm. Full inspiration.	Unweighted view: TB: < top 1/2 of film. SS: to include both AC joints Weighted view: TB: < bottom 1/2 of film. SS: to include both AC joints.	Comparison of both AC joints to r/o separation type injury. This method exposed patient to much less radiation than unilateral study.

View	Measure	Film Size I.D./R or L	FFD	Tube Tilt	Central Ray	Filter/ Shielding	Positioning	Collimation TB = Top to Bottom SS = Side to Side	Essential Anatomy
Acromio-clavicular joint: Unilateral weighted and unweighted (Zanca View)	A-P at CR coracoid process	I.D. up 10 × 12	40 in. Bucky	Routine 10–15° cephalad. Optional no angle.	H: mid-AC if no angle, 1 in. below if angle used. Center to top 1/2 film for non-wts. Bottom 1/2 for wts. view. V: through AC joint.	Lead apron	Pt. standing, facing tube. Arms at side. Mid-sagittal plane perpendicular to film. Both unweighted and weighted view with 10–15 lb sandbags are done. Full inspiration.	Unweighted view: TB: to include AC joint to skin. SS: skin of shoulder. Weighted view: TB: include AC joint to skin SS: skin of shoulder.	Unilateral view of the affected AC joint to r/o separation or other pathology.
Scapula: A-P	A-P at CR coracoid process	I.D. to spine 12 × 10	40 in. Bucky	None 90°	H: mid-scapula or 1 in. medial and 1 in. inferior to coracoid process. Pt. rotated to place blade of scapula parallel to film. V: to mid-scapula Film centered to H: CR.	Lead apron	Pt. standing, facing tube. Mid-coronal plane turned 10 to 15° to put scapula parallel to film. Arm at side. Full inspiration.	TB: to include clavicle to inferior blade of scapula SS: to skin of shoulder.	Anterior view of the scapula. Most of the clavicle and head of the humerus will be seen.

11.5   Lateral Scapula, Special Views of AC Joints, Shoulder

View	Measure	Film Size I.D./R or L	FFD	Tube Tilt	Central Ray	Filter/ Shielding	Positioning	Collimation TB = Top to Bottom SS = Side to Side	Essential Anatomy
Scapula: Lateral	A-P at CR coracoid process	I.D. up 10 × 12	40 in. Bucky	0 to 10° Caudal	H: mid-scapula exiting through head of humerus. V: 1 in. medial to spine of scapula (toward spine). Vertical CR is between ribs and scapula.	Lead apron	Pt. in an anterior oblique. Rotate until CR is parallel to blade of scapula. CR passing through the glenoid fossa.	TB: film size or acromion to inferior blade of scapula. SS: film size or skin.	Lateral view of scapula, view of humeral head in glenoid fossa. Good to visualize dislocation.
Acromio-clavicular: Outlet view or anterior oblique shoulder	A-P coracoid process	I.D. up 10 × 12	40 in. Bucky	15 to 40° Caudal; angle depends on body type.	H: mid-scapula exiting through head of humerus. V: 1 in. medial (toward spine) of the scapula blade passing through the glenoid fossa. Film center to H: CR.	Lead apron	Pt. in an anterior oblique. Rotate until CR is parallel to blade of scapula. CR passing through the glenoid fossa. Start with 15° angle.	TB: film size or acromion to inferior blade of scapula. SS: film size or skin.	Clear view of the acromion and underlying acromioclavicular space.
Shoulder: Apical or 30° caudal tilt view	A-P at CR coracoid process	I.D. to spine 12 × 10	40 in. Bucky	30° Caudal	H: 30° caudal angle through acromion process. Film center to H: CR. V: through glenohumeral joint.	Lead apron	A-P: standing facing tube. Arms in neutral position at side. Pt. may need to sit on stool. CR through acromion process.	TB: to include shoulder or film size. SS: to film size or skin of shoulder.	Clear view of the acromion process and superior glenohumeral joint. Useful in trauma shoulder studies.

View	Measure	Film Size I.D./R or L	FFD	Tube Tilt	Central Ray	Filter/ Shielding	Positioning	Collimation TB = Top to Bottom SS = Side to Side	Essential Anatomy
Shoulder internal and external rotation Grashey projection	A-P at CR coracoid process	I.D. to spine 10 × 8 or 12 × 10	40 in. Bucky	None 90°	H: 1 in. inferior to coracoid process. V: through the coracoid process. Film center to H: CR.	Lead apron	Pt. standing, facing tube. Body rotated 15–45° to put scapula parallel to film. 1. Internal rotation of humerus until thumb can touch Bucky. 2. External rotation of humerus until thumb can touch Bucky.	TB: from skin of clavicle to inferior border of shoulder. SS: to skin of shoulder. Arrow points out for ext. Arrow points in for int.	A-P view of shoulder joint in full internal and external rotation. Do not overpenetrate as calcifications in bursa can be missed.
Shoulder Stryker notch	A-P at CR coracoid process	I.D. to spine 8 × 10 or 10 × 12	40 in. Bucky	45° cephalad	H: 2 in. inferior to coracoid process. V: through glenohumeral joint. Film center to H: CR.	Lead apron	Pt. standing, facing tube. Body rotated 15–45° to put scapula parallel to film. Arm abducted with hand behind neck. Arm perpendicular to film.	TB: from skin of clavicle to inferior border of shoulder. SS: to skin of shoulder.	View of inferior glenoid humeral joint and the posterior and inferior humerus. Used to study shoulder instability and Hill-Sachs or Burkart fractures.

11.6 Pelvis, Hip, and Femur

View	Measure	Film Size I.D./R or L	FFD	Tube Tilt	Central Ray	Filter/ Shielding	Positioning	Collimation TB = Top to Bottom / SS = Side to Side	Essential Anatomy
Pelvis A-P	A-P at trochanter	I.D. up 17 × 14	40 in. Bucky	None 0°	H: 1½ in. superior to the pubic symphysis. Center film to H: CR. V: mid-sagittal plane.	Gonadal shield for males only.	Pt. standing or supine, facing the tube. Legs extended with feet internally rotated 15°. (Heels apart and toes together.)	TB: to include from the iliac crests to pubic symphysis and trochanters. SS: to film size or to include trochanters.	A-P of the pelvis and hips. *Note:* if take supine and bilateral hips are needed, the frog leg lateral hips can be done bilaterally.
Hip A-P	A-P at trochanter	I.D. up 10 × 12	40 in. Bucky	None	H: 1.5 in. superior to the pubic symphysis. Film center to H: CR. V: mid-acetabulum or ~2–3 in. lateral to umbilicus.	Gonadal shields: make sure male shield is not over acetabulum	Pt. standing or supine, facing the tube. Mid-coronal plane parallel to film. Lower leg extended with foot internally rotated 15°.	TB: slightly less than film size. SS: slightly less than film size.	A-P of acetabulum and articulation with femur, include below lesser trochanter.
Hip lateral Frog-leg view	A-P at trochanter	I.D. up 10 × 12 or 12 × 10	40 in. Bucky	None 0°	H: 1.5 in. superior to the pubic symphysis. Film center to H: CR. V: mid-acetabulum or ~2–3 in. lateral to umbilicus.	Gonadal shields: make sure male shield is not over acetabulum	Pt. standing or supine, facing tube. Knee of the affected hip is flexed and abducted. For standing: place affected side's foot on stool for support.	TB: slightly less than film size. SS: slightly less than film size.	Apposing view of the head of the femur and articulation of acetabulum
Femur A-P	A-P at CR	I.D. up 7 × 17	40 in. Bucky	None	H: mid-shaft of the femur. Center film to H: CR. V: long axis of femur.	Gonad shields	Pt. standing or supine, facing tube. Affected leg internally rotated 15° or until lower extremity is in true A-P view.	TB: to include from hip to knee. SS: to skin of femur.	A-P of the entire femur to include hip and knee joints. If needed, take A-P hip on separate film to see both articulations.
Femur Lateral	Lateral at CR	I.D. up 7 × 17	40 in. Bucky	None	H: mid-shaft of the femur. Center film to H: CR. V: long axis of femur.	Gonad shield female only	Pt. lying on affected side with other leg abducted out of the way. Standing: Weight supported on non-affected leg. Foot of affected leg resting on stool with knee flexed. Film turned traversely and centered to femur.	TB: to include from hip to knee. SS: to skin of femur.	Lateral view of femur. It is impossible to view hip on lateral. Make sure that the knee joint is included on film.

11.7 Knee and Patella

View	Measure	Film Size I.D./R or L	FFD	Tube Tilt	Central Ray	Filter/ Shielding	Positioning	Collimation TB = Top to Bottom SS = Side to Side	Essential Anatomy
Knee: A-P	A-P at CR	I.D. up Regular 8 × 10	40 in. Bucky	5° Cephalad	H: 1 cm (~1/2 in.) distal to the apex of the patella. Center film to H: CR. V: long axis of knee.	Lead apron	Pt. standing or supine, facing the tube. Knee extended with slight internal rotation to achieve true A-P of leg. Mid-sagittal plane perpendicular to film. Mid-coronal plane parallel to film.	TB: slightly less than film size. SS: to skin of knee.	A-P of knee joint including femoral epicondyles, the patella, and superior tibia and fibula.
Knee: Lateral view	Lateral at CR	I.D. up Regular 8 × 10	40 in. Bucky	5° Cephalad for recumbent; 0° for standing.	H: 1 cm distal to the medial epicondyle. Film center to H: CR. V: center of the medial-epicondyle or mid-coronal plane of femur.	Lead apron	Recumbent: Pt. lying with the affected side to film with grid or Bucky. Knee flexed 45°. Other leg flexed over and out of the way of the affected knee. Standing: Support on the unaffected leg. Put the affected leg on low stool to achieve 45° flexion.	TB: slightly less than film size. SS: slightly less than film size.	Lateral view of the knee, distal femur, patella, and superior tibia and fibula. The epicondyles should be superimposed.

View	Projection	I.D./Film	Distance	CR Angle	Centering	Shielding	Patient Position	TB/SS	Remarks
Knee: Tunnel view Camp-Coventry Intercondylar view P-A	A-P at CR	I.D. up 8 × 10 Regular	40 in. Bucky	40° Caudal	H: through the popliteal fossa. Film center to H: CR. V: long axis of femur.	Lead apron	Pt. recumbent and prone. Knee is flexed 45° and supported with sponge and/or stool. Standing: Pt. standing, facing Bucky with femur on Bucky. Knee bent 45° with foot resting on small stool.	TB: slightly less than film size. SS: skin of knee.	View of the intracondyloid fossa of femur and the medial and lateral condyles.
Patella: P-A View	A-P at CR	I.D. up 8 × 10	40 in. Bucky	5° Cephalad	H: mid-patella. Center film to H: CR. V: long axis of femur.	Lead apron	Pt. standing or recumbent, facing the Bucky. Mid-coronal plane parallel to film. Mid-sagittal plane perpendicular to film.	TB: slightly less than film size. SS: skin of knee.	P-A view improves the detail of the patella as it is next to film.
Patella: Sunrise or Settegast View	AP at CR	I.D. up 8 × 10 Extremity	40 in. Non-Bucky	20° Cephalad	H: through patello-femoral articulation. V: long axis of femur. Film centered to H: CR.	Lead apron	Pt. prone with affected thigh against table with knee flexed back as far as possible or ~140°. The patella should be on the film. Use a strap attached to ankle if needed.	TB: less than 5 in. field or from skin above patella to lateral epicondyle. SS: to skin of knee.	Tangential view of the patella and patellofemoral space.
Patella: Lateral view	Lateral at CR	I.D. up 8 × 10 Extremity	40 in. Non-Bucky	5° Cephalad	H: mid-patella. V: between patella and femoral condyle.	Lead apron	Recumbent: Pt. lying with the affected side to film with grid or Bucky. Knee flexed 15°. Other leg flexed over and out of the way of the affected knee.	TB: less than 5 in. or entire patella. SS: less than 5 in. or include patella and anterior femur.	Lateral view of patella and anterior femur. Patella should be in profile.

11.8 Tibia Fibula and Ankle

View	Measure	Film Size I.D./R or L	FFD	Tube Tilt	Central Ray	Filter/ Shielding	Positioning	Collimation TB = Top to Bottom SS = Side to Side	Essential Anatomy
Tibia-fibula: A-P	A-P at CR	I.D. down 7 × 17	40 in. Non-Bucky	None 0°	Center film to include the ankle and knee joints. H: centered to film. V: long axis of fibula	Lead apron	Pt. sitting or supine. Foot is slightly plantar-flexed to get mid-sagittal plane perpendicular to film.	TB: to include knee and ankle articulations. SS: skin of lower leg.	A-P of lower leg to include knee and ankle joints. For long legs, a 14 × 17 may be turned sideways to get both joints.
Tibia-fibula: Lateral	Lateral at CR	I.D. down 7 × 17	40 in. Non-Bucky	None 0°	Center film to include the ankle and knee joints. H: to center of film. V: long axis of fibula.	Lead apron	Pt. lying on the affected side with mid-coronal plane perpendicular to film. Knee slightly flexed.	TB: to include knee and ankle articulations. SS: to skin of lower leg.	Lateral view of lower leg including both ankle and knee joint. If possible, both A-P and Lat. can be filmed on a 14 × 17 or two 7 × 17s.
Ankle: A-P	A-P at CR	1/2 of 12 × 10 Extremity	40 in. Non-Bucky	None 0°	H: through talo-tibial joint. V: between malleoli Film center to H: CR.	Lead apron	Pt. sitting or supine. Ankle slightly dorsiflexed to get the plantar surface perpendicular to the film. The mid-sagittal plane of ankle is perpendicular to film. Vertical CR should be parallel to 3rd metatarsal.	TB: to include distal tibia and fibula, talus, and calcaneus. SS: skin of ankle on 1/2 of 10 × 12.	A-P view of ankle joint including distal tibia and fibula and talo-tibial space.
Ankle: Oblique or Mortise oblique	A-P at CR	1/2 of 12 × 10	40 in. Non-Bucky	None 0°	H: through talo-tibial joint. V: between malleoli. Film center to H: CR.	Lead apron	Pt. is sitting or supine. Ankle is dorsiflexed to get the plantar surface perpendicular to film. Leg is medially rotated until the mid-sagittal plane is at 45° obliquity. Ankle rolled medially until both malleoli are parallel to film or about 20° of obliquity.	TB: to include distal tibia and fibula, talus, and calcaneus. SS: skin of ankle on 1/2 of 10 × 12.	Oblique view of joint. The lateral malleolar joint space should be open. Slight inversion opens joint space. Used to visualize the mortise joint space.
Ankle: Lateral	Lateral at CR	8 × 10 Extremity	40 in. Non-Bucky	None 0°	H: through talo-tibial joint. Film center to H: CR. V: long axis of tibia and medial malleolus.	Lead apron	Pt. in lateral recumbent position with affected side to film. Ankle dorsi-flexed with lateral side to film. Other leg crossed over and supported.	TB: to include distal tibia and fibula to calcaneus. SS: to include heel and talus bone.	Lateral view of the ankle joint, talus, and calcaneus.

11.9 Calcaneus and Foot

View	Measure	Film Size I.D./R or L	FFD	Tube Tilt	Central Ray	Filter/Shielding	Positioning	Collimation TB = Top to Bottom SS = Side to Side	Essential Anatomy
Calcaneus: Axial	Lateral at CR	1/2 of 10 × 8 Extremity	40 in. Non-Bucky	40° cephalad	H: 2 in. anterior (up) to the calcaneal tuberosity. Center film to H: CR. V: long axis of foot.	Lead apron	Pt. sitting or supine. Foot is slightly dorsi-flexed to get the plantar surface perpendicular to film.	TB: to include entire calcaneus or about 5 in. SS: to skin of foot or less than 1/2 of the 8 × 10.	View of the calcaneus and articulation with other tarsals.
Calcaneus: Lateral	Lateral at CR	1/2 of 10 × 8 Extremity	40 in. Non-Bucky	None 0°	H: mid-calcaneus (1½ in. up front plantar surface of heel). V: long axis of foot.	Lead apron	Pt. lying on the affected side with mid-coronal plane perpendicular to film. Ankle dorsi-flexed.	TB: to include talus and calcaneus. SS: to include entire calcaneus and its articulations on 1/2 of 8 × 10.	Lateral view includes view of subtalar space and entire calcaneus.
Foot: A-P	A-P at CR	1/2 of 10 × 12 Extremity	40 in. Non-Bucky	10° cephalad	H: through base of 3rd metatarsal. Film center to H: CR. V: long axis of foot.	Lead apron	Pt. sitting or supine. Knee flexed to allow pt. to put plantar surface of foot on film.	TB: to film size. SS: skin of foot on 1/2 of a 10 × 12.	A-P view of entire foot.
Foot: Oblique	A-P at CR	1/2 or A-P 10 × 12	40 in. Non-Bucky	None 0°	H: through base of 3rd metatarsal. Film center to H: CR. V: long axis of foot.	Lead apron	From the A-P foot position. Medially rotate the leg and foot 30–45°. The plantar surface of foot should be 30 to 45° to film.	TB: to film size or to include entire foot and toes. SS: skin of foot on 1/2 of a 10 × 12.	Oblique view of foot. The view opens the subtalar space and shows the calcaneus.
Foot: Lateral	Lateral at CR	10 × 12 Extremity	40 in. Non-Bucky	None 0°	H: through long axis of the first metatarsal. V: through navicular bone. Center film to H: CR.	Lead apron	Pt. in lateral recumbent position with affected side to film. Ankle dorsi-flexed with lateral side to film. Other leg crossed over and supported.	TB: to include foot and the ankle joint. SS: to include foot and toes	Lateral view of foot, ankle, and toes.

11.10 Toes and Great Toe

View	Measure	Film Size I.D./R or L	FFD	Tube Tilt	Central Ray	Filter/ Shielding	Positioning	Collimation TB = Top to Bottom SS = Side to Side	Essential Anatomy
Toes: A-P	A-P at CR	1/4 of 12 × 10 Extremity	40 in. Non-Bucky	None	H: through 3rd metatarsal-phalangeal joint. Center film to H: CR. V: long axis of 3rd toe.	Lead apron	Pt. sitting with knee flexed and the plantar surface of affected foot on film.	TB: to include phalanges and metatarsal-phalangeal joints. SS: to skin of toes on 1/4 of 10 × 12.	View of the phalanges of foot and metatarsal joints.
A-P Axial		1/4 of 12 × 10 Extremity		15° cephalid if toes are flat			For axial projection, place toes on a 15° sponge or angle tube 14° cephalad.		Axial view will open joint spaces of toes.
Toes Oblique	A-P at CR	1/4 of 12 × 10 Extremity	40 in. Non-Bucky	None	H: through 3rd metatarsal-phalangeal joint. Center film to H: CR. V: long axis of 3rd toe.	Lead apron	Pt. sitting with knee flexed and the plantar surface on film. Leg rotated medially 45° with plantar surface 45° from film.	TB: to include phalanges and metatarsal-phalangeal joints. SS: to skin of toes or 1/4 of 10 × 2.	Oblique view includes toes and metatarsal-phalangeal joints.
Toes: Lateral	Lateral at CR	1/4 of 12 × 10 Extremity	40 in. Non-Bucky	None	H: through 1st metatarsal-phalangeal joint. Film center to H: CR. V: long axis of toes.	Lead apron	Pt. on lateral recumbent on affected side. Lateral side of foot on film. Tongue depressor may be used to separate the toe of interest.	TB: to include phalanges and metatarsal-phalangeal joints. SS: to skin of toes or 1/4 of 10 × 12.	Lateral view of toes and metatarsal-phalangeal joints.
Great toe: A-P Oblique	A-P at CR	1/3 of 10 × 8 Extremity	40 in. Non-Bucky	None	H: through 1st metatarsal-phalangeal joint. Film center to H: CR. V: long axis of foot.	Lead apron	A-P: same as other toes. Obl.: same as other toes.	TB: to include great toe and metatarsal joint. SS: to skin of great toe on 1/3 of 8 × 10.	Oblique view of foot. The view opens the subtalar space and shows the calcaneus.
Great toe: Lateral	A-P at CR	1/3 of 10 × 8 Extremity	40 in. Non-Bucky	None	H: through 1st M-P joint. V: through 1st M-P joint. Center film to H: CR.	Lead apron	Pt. lies on unaffected side. Leg and ankle turned so the lateral side of the great toe is touching film. Mid-coronal plane of foot is perpendicular to film.	TB: to include great toe and metatarsal joint. SS: to skin of great toe on 1/3 of 8 × 10.	Lateral view of great toe.

11.11   Special Extremity Views

View	Measure	Film Size I.D./R or L	FFD	Tube Tilt	Central Ray	Filter/ Shielding	Positioning	Collimation TB = Top to Bottom SS = Side to Side	Essential Anatomy
Laurin views of the knee: 90° flexion	A-P at patella	17 × 14 Regular	60 in. Non-Bucky	60° Cephalad	H: through patella-femoral space. V: mid-sagittal plane of pt. CR passes inferior-superior to patella.	Lead apron	Pt. seated on table with legs hanging over edge. Knee flexed 90°. Pt. holds film perpendicular to CR on top of thighs. Lower legs tied together to keep femurs parallel to film.	TB: to include patella and femoral condyles. SS: to include both femurs.	Dynamic study of the patellofemoral joint space.
Laurin views of the knee: 60° flexion	A-P at patella	17 × 14 Regular	60 in. Non-Bucky	45° Cephalad	H: through patella-femoral space. V: mid-sagittal plane of pt. CR passes inferior-superior to patella.	Lead apron	Pt. seated on table with legs hanging over edge. Knee flexed 60°. Pt. holds film perpendicular to CR on top of thighs. Lower legs tied together to keep femurs parallel to film.	TB: to include patella and femoral condyles. SS: to include both femurs.	Dynamic study of the patellofemoral joint space.
Laurin views of the knee: 30° flexion	A-P at patella	17 × 14 Regular	60 in. Non-Bucky	30° Cephalad	H: through patella-femoral space. V: mid-sagittal plane of pt. CR passes inferior-superior to patella.	Lead apron	Pt. seated on table with legs hanging over edge. Knee flexed 30°. Pt. holds film perpendicular to CR on top of thighs. Lower legs tied together to keep femurs parallel to film.	TB: to include patella and femoral condyles. SS: to include both femurs.	Dynamic study of the patellofemoral joint space.

Chapter 12

Hand and Wrist Radiography

12.1 Finger, Hand, and Wrist Radiography: Introduction

All views of the fingers, hands, and wrists should be taken using fine detail or extremity cassettes. The small focal spot must also be employed to achieve the best possible resolution. Fractures in this area of the body can be very difficult to see under the best of circumstances.

The patient is seated and any suitable table can be used as long as one can get the 40-in. source to image distance (SID). A full-coat apron will provide better protection than the half-apron. In either case, do not place the patient's legs under the table.

Fingers must be positioned parallel to the film for all views. This will open the joint spaces and make it easier to see fractures. Since multiple views will be done on the same film, lead blockers are used to protect the exposed film from scatter radiation. While the routine view of the second through fifth digits is the P-A view, if the finger is bent and cannot be straightened, A-P views can be helpful. Radiographic sponges will make taking these films much more comfortable for the patient and reduce the possibility of motion on the film.

When positioning fingers and the thumb, use the fingernail as a reference point for positioning. The collimation for fingers must include from the tip of the fingernail to the metacarpal-phalangeal joint. The thumb view should include back to the trapezium. If the palm of the hand blocks the visualization of the full first metacarpal, 10 to 15° of cephalad tube angle can be used.

When taking the hand P-A view, spread the fingers only slightly. This will avoid overlap of the soft tissues and still use just half of the cassette. For all hand views, the fingers should be parallel to the film. The lateral hand view is taken with the fingers fanned so there is no superimposition. The hand views should also include 1 in. of the distal ulna and radius.

When taking views of the wrist, include enough of the distal ulna and radius to rule out a fracture sight. The fingers are cupped but not made into a fist for the P-A view. The entire forearm should be in a lateral position for the lateral wrist view. The ulnar flexion and P-A axial views of the wrist are good views to evaluate the scaphoid. A tube angulation is used to elongate the scaphoid to better visualize the middle of the bone. There will be times when an A-P oblique view of the wrist (Figure 12.1) will be helpful. It may show fractures in the distal radius that are not seen on the other views.

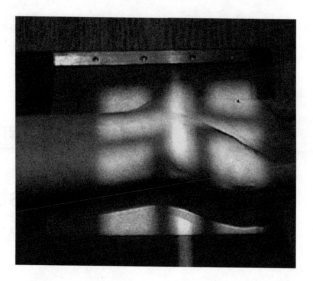

FIGURE 12.1
A-P oblique wrist positioning.

12.2   Thumb Radiography

Measure

A-P at M-P joint

Protection

Coat lead apron

SID

40 in. Non-Bucky using table

Tube Angulation

None; optional 10 to 15° cephalad on A-P if soft tissue of palm obscures view

Film

8 in. × 10 in. Fine (extremity) cassette for all three views

Marker

Anatomical

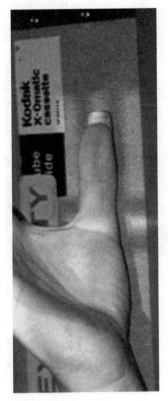

FIGURE 12.2
A-P thumb positioning.

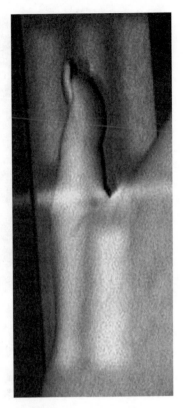

FIGURE 12.3
Oblique thumb positioning.

Positioning

A-P (Figure 12.2):

1. Patient internally rotates arm until thumb is A-P on film.
2. Place horizontal central ray through the M-P joint.
3. Vertical central ray on long axis of thumb. If soft tissue of palm covers metacarpal and trapezium, use tube angulation.

Oblique (Figure 12.3):

1. Hand in P-A position.
2. Center central ray on first M-P joint.

Lateral (Figure 12.4):

1. Hand in P-A position and palm raised until thumb is lateral.
2. Central ray centered on M-P joint.

Collimation

Top to Bottom: from tip of thumb to include trapezium; Side to Side: soft tissue of thumb.

Breathing Instructions

Hold still

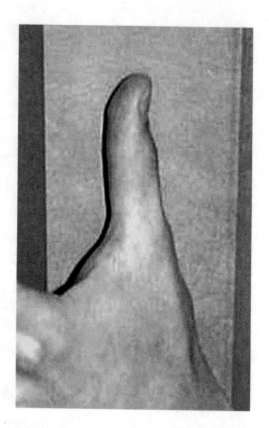

FIGURE 12.4
Lateral thumb positioning.

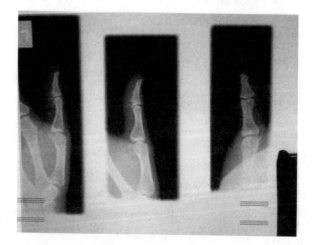

FIGURE 12.5
Thumb series film.

Image Critique

All views must include trapezium to tip of thumb. If palm soft tissue obscures metacarpal and trapezium on A-P view, angle tube or ask patient to pull palm back with other hand.

Optimum kVp

56–65 kVp

12.3   Finger Radiography

Measure

A-P at PIP joint

Protection

Coat lead apron

SID

40 in. Non-Bucky

Tube Angulation

None

Film

8 in. × 10 in. Fine (extremity) cassette

Positioning

P-A (Figure 12.6):

1.   Place pronated hand on film with fingers straight.
2.   Direct central ray through PIP joint of affected finger

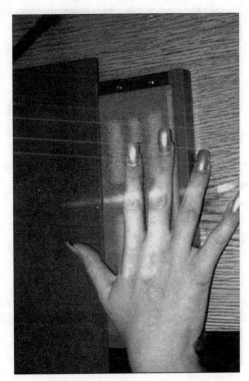

FIGURE 12.6
P-A finger positioning.

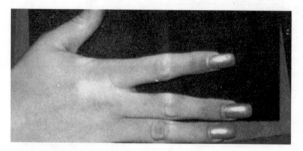

FIGURE 12.7
Oblique finger positioning.

Oblique (Figure 12.7):

1. Hand at 45° angle to film with medial surface on the film.
2. Direct central ray through PIP joint of affected finger. Keep finger parallel to film.

Lateral (Figure 12.8):

1. Hand at 90° angle to film. Have the medial side next to film for 4th and 5th digits. Have lateral side to film for 2nd and 3rd digits.
2. Direct central ray through PIP joint. Keep finger parallel to film.

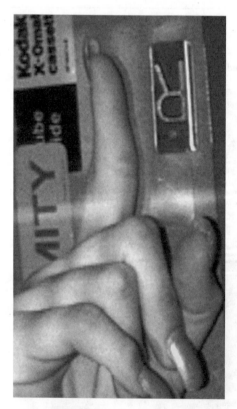

FIGURE 12.8(A)
Lateral index finger.

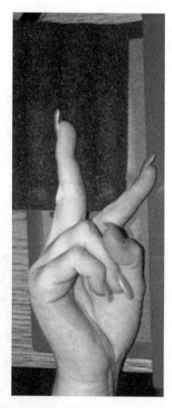

FIGURE 12.8(B)
Lateral 3rd finger.

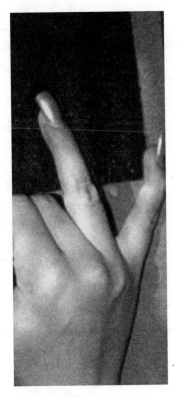

FIGURE 12.8(C)
Lateral 4th finger.

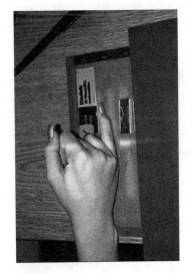

FIGURE 12.8(D)
Lateral 5th finger.

Collimation

Top to Bottom: tuft of finger to M-P joint; Side to Side: skin of finger.

Breathing Instructions

Hold still

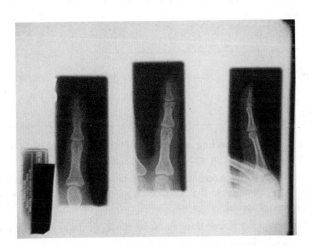

FIGURE 12.9
Finger series film.

Image Critique

The marker must be in the primary beam to be seen on film. All joint spaces of the affected finger should be open on all three projections. If patient cannot straighten finger, the P-A view may be supplemented with the A-P projection. Keep finger as close to film as possible.

Optimum kVp

60 kVp

12.4   Hand Series: P-A View

Measure

P-A at 3rd M-P joint

Protection

Coat lead apron

SID

40 in. using Non-Bucky

Tube Angulation

None

Film

One half of a 10 in. × 12 in. (or 24 cm × 30 cm) Fine (extremity) cassette

Marker

Anatomical

Positioning

1. Patient is seated or kneeling next to table The forearm is placed on the table in the P-A position. The fingers should be straight and resting on cassette.
2. This view may be done on half of the cassette. Cover the other half with a lead blocker. The horizontal central ray is centered to the 3rd metacarpal-phalangeal joint. The hand should be centered with the fingers slightly spread.
3. Vertical central ray placed through the long axis of the hand and wrist.
4. Have patient suspend respiration and hold still.

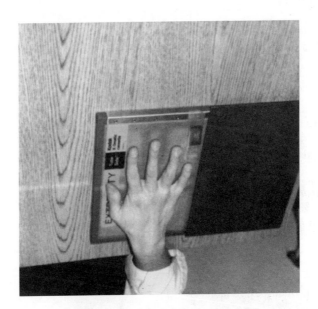

FIGURE 12.10
P-A hand positioning.

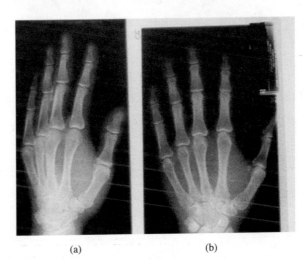

FIGURE 12.11
Hand (a) oblique and (b) P-A films.

(a)   (b)

Collimation

Top to Bottom: to include tips of fingers to distal ulna and radius; Side to Side: soft tissue of hand and fingers.

Breathing Instructions

Hold still

Image Critique

The interphalangeal and metacarpal-phalangeal spaces will be open, and approximately 1 in. of distal radius is seen on the film. There is no overlap of adjacent digits.

Optimum kVp

55–65 kVp

12.5   Hand Series: Oblique View

Measure

A-P at 3rd metacarpal-phalangeal joint

Protection

Coat lead apron

SID

40 in. Non-Bucky using table

Tube Angulation

None

Film

Half of 10 in. × 12 in. (24 cm × 30 cm) Fine (extremity) cassette

Marker

Anatomical

Positioning

1. Patient is seated next to a table with affected hand on the table.
2. The oblique hand sponge is positioned on the unexposed half of the cassette. The exposed portion is protected by a lead blocker.
3. The patient is asked to place hand on sponge with fingers supported by the sponge. This should place hand 45° oblique with the medial surface closest to film. All fingers should be parallel to film.
4. Center horizontal central ray on the 3rd M-P joint.
5. The vertical central ray should be aligned with the long axis of the hand and fingers.

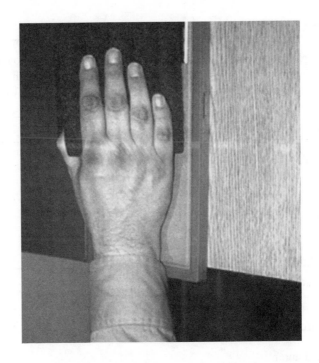

FIGURE 12.12
Hand oblique positioning.

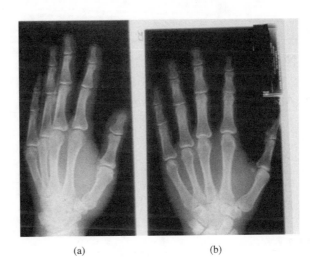

FIGURE 12.13
Hand (a) oblique and (b) P-A films.

(a)   (b)

Collimation

Top to Bottom: soft tissue of hand and phalanges to include 1 in. of distal radius; Side to Side: soft tissue of hand.

Breathing Instructions

Hold still

Image Critique

All intraphalangeal joints should be open. There should be no overlap of the phalanges. The 2nd through 5th metacarpals will appear concave. The 3rd through 5th metacarpal heads will be slightly superimposed. The view must include from the tips of the fingers to include 1 in. of the distal radius.

Optimum kVp

55–65 kVp

12.6   Hand Series: Lateral View

Measure

Lateral across metacarpals

Protection

Coat lead apron

SID

40 in. Non-Bucky using table

Tube Angulation

None

Film

8 in. × 10 in. Fine (extremity) with I.D. toward wrist

Marker

Anatomical

Positioning

1.   Patient is seated next to table with cassette in front of patient. The patient is asked to place hand in lateral position on the cassette.
2.   The patient is then instructed to bend fingers for the "OK" sign, or placed on a special sponge designed for the lateral hand. The fingers should remain parallel to the film.
3.   Center horizontal and vertical central rays on the second M-P joint.
4.   Collimate to include 1 in. of distal radius and the tips of all fingers.
5.   Ask patient to remain still. Make exposure.

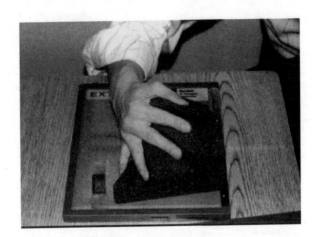

FIGURE 12.14
Hand lateral positioning.

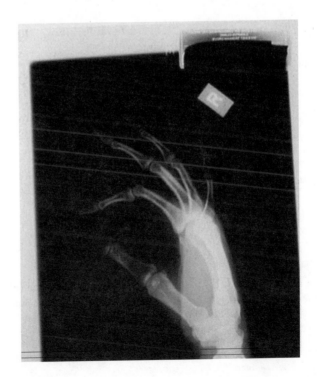

FIGURE 12.15
Hand lateral film.

Collimation

Top to Bottom: distal radius to tips of fingers; Side to Side: soft tissue of hand and fingers.

Breathing Instructions

Hold still

Image Critique

The carpals, metacarpals and distal ulna and radius should be superimposed. The intraphalangeal joints of the 2nd through 5th fingers should be open. The thumb should appear as a P-A view of the digit. All soft tissue of hand should be visualized.

Optimum kVp

60–65 kVp

12.7 Wrist Series: P-A View

Measure

P-A through carpal bones

Protection

Coat lead apron

SID

40 in. using Non-Bucky

Tube Angulation

None

Film

One third or one quarter of a 10 in. × 12 in. (24 cm × 30 cm) Fine (extremity) cassette. If scaphoid view is done, divide cassette in quarters; otherwise, thirds down middle of cassette.

Marker

Anatomical

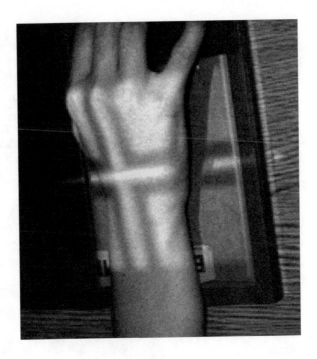

FIGURE 12.16
Wrist P-A positioning.

Positioning

1. Patient is seated or kneeling next to table. The forearm is placed on the table in the P-A position and flexed fingers bent into a loose fist.
2. The film is divided into three or four sections. Lead blockers are positioned to cover the unexposed film. Have patient place wrist in one quarter or one third of the film. The horizontal central ray is centered to the middle of the carpal bones.
3. Vertical central ray placed through the long axis of the carpal bones.
4. Have patient suspend respiration and hold still.

Collimation

Top to Bottom: to include metacarpal articulation to distal ulna and radius; Side to Side: soft tissue of forearm.

Breathing Instructions

Suspend respiration

Image Critique

The articulations of the carpal bones with the metacarpal and distal ulna and radius should be seen. The scaphoid fat stripe should be seen. The radial and ulnar styloid processes will be seen, and metacarpal and radioulnar spaces will be open.

Optimum kVp

60–70 kVp

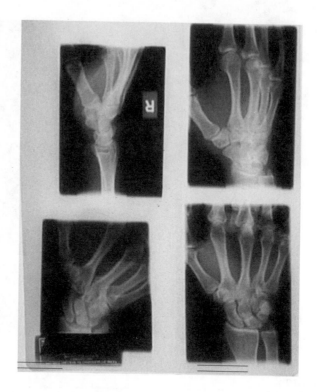

FIGURE 12.17
Wrist P-A series film.

12.8   Wrist Series: Oblique View

Measure

A-P through carpal bones

Protection

Coat lead apron

SID

40 in. using Non-Bucky

Tube Angulation

None

Film

One third or one quarter of a 10 in. × 12 in. (24 cm × 30 cm) Fine (extremity) cassette. If scaphoid view, divide cassette in quarters; otherwise, thirds down middle of cassette.

Marker

Anatomical

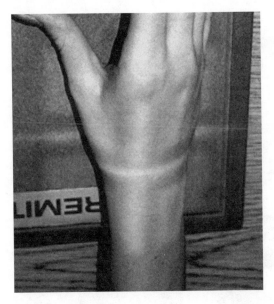

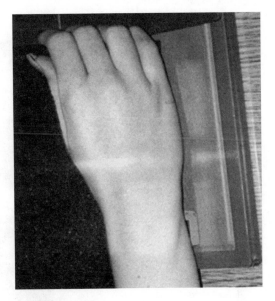

FIGURE 12.18(A)
Wrist oblique positioning.

FIGURE 12.18(B)
Wrist can also rest on sponge with fingers wrapped over top of sponge.

Positioning

1. Patient is seated or kneeling next to table. The forearm is placed on the table in the P-A position and flexed fingers bent into a loose fist.
2. Cover the section of the film that the P-A view has exposed with a lead blocker. Have patient place P-A wrist in the next unexposed section, in one quarter or one third of the film. Ask the patient to roll wrist up 45°, with the ulnar side resting on film. The thumb can be placed in contact with film for support. The horizontal central ray is centered to the first row of carpal bones and distal radius.
3. Vertical central ray placed through the long axis of the 3rd carpa-metacarpal joint and distal radius.
4. Have patient suspend respiration and hold still. Take film.

Collimation

Top to Bottom: to include metacarpal articulation to distal ulna and radius; Side to Side: soft tissue of forearm.

Breathing Instructions

Suspend respiration

Image Critique

The oblique view of the wrist will project the trapezium and trapezoid carpal bones free of any superimposition. The scaphoid tuberosity and wrist will be clearly visualized. The anterior and posterior articular surfaces of the radius should be superimposed.

Optimum kVp

56–65 kVp

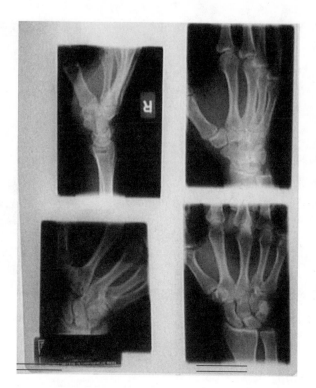

FIGURE 12.19
Wrist oblique series film.

12.9   Wrist Series: Lateral View

Measure

Lateral through carpal bones

Protection

Coat lead apron

SID

40 in. using Non-Bucky

Tube Angulation

None

Film

One third or one quarter of a 10 in. × 12 in. (24 cm × 30 cm) Fine (extremity) cassette. If scaphoid view, divide cassette in quarters; otherwise, thirds down the middle of cassette.

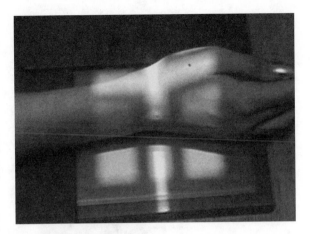

FIGURE 12.20
Wrist lateral positioning.

Marker

Anatomical (best view to place marker)

Positioning

1. Patient is seated or kneeling next to table. The forearm is placed on the table in the lateral position and flexed fingers bent into a loose fist.
2. Cover the exposed area of the film where the P-A and oblique views were taken. Have patient place wrist in one quarter or remaining one third of the film. The horizontal central ray is centered to the middle of the carpal bones.
3. Vertical central ray placed through the long axis of the carpal bones and ulna and radius.
4. Have patient suspend respiration and hold still. Take film.

Collimation

Top to Bottom: to include metacarpal articulation to distal ulna and radius; Side to Side: soft tissue of forearm.

Breathing Instructions

Suspend respiration

Image Critique

The true lateral view will have the distal ulna and radius superimposed. The distal end of the scaphoid and pisiform carpal bones will also be superimposed.

Optimum kVp

56–65 kVp

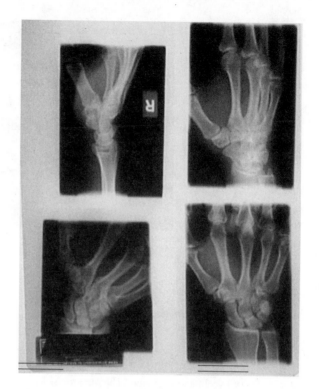

FIGURE 12.21
Wrist lateral series film.

12.10   Wrist Series: P-A View for Scaphoid Injury

Measure

A-P through carpal bones

Protection

Coat lead apron

SID

40 in. using Non-Bucky

Tube Angulation

15 to 20° cephalad

Film

One quarter of a 10 in. × 12 in. (24 cm × 30 cm), or single 8 in. × 10 in. Fine (extremity) cassette

Marker

Anatomical

Positioning

1. Patient is seated or kneeling next to table. The forearm is placed on the table in the P-A position. The fingers should be straight. The patient is unable to ulnar flex wrist. Have patient slightly oblique wrist 10 to 20°.
2. This view may be done in the fourth quarter of the film, or on a separate 8 in. × 10 in. film. Lead blockers are positioned to cover the exposed film. The horizontal central ray is centered to the scaphoid or 0.5 in. distal to the radial styloid process.
3. Vertical central ray placed through the long axis of the carpal bones and radius.
4. Have patient suspend respiration and hold still. Take film.

Collimation

Top to Bottom: to include metacarpal articulation to distal ulna and radius; Side to Side: soft tissue of forearm.

Breathing Instructions

Hold still

Image Critique

The view may open scapholunate, and scapocapitate spaces should be open. If the hand is flat on the film, the trapezium space will be open and the scaphotrapezium space will be closed.

Optimum kVp

55–65 kVp

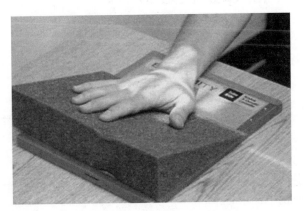

FIGURE 12.22
Wrist P-A axial on sponge.

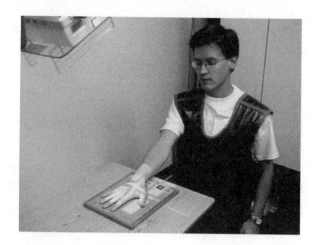

FIGURE 12.23
Wrist P-A axial with tube angle.

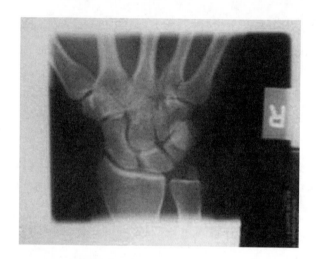

FIGURE 12.24
Wrist P-A axial film.

12.11   Wrist Series: Ulnar Flexion View for Scaphoid Injury

Measure

A-P through carpal bones

Protection

Coat lead apron

SID

40 in. using Non-Bucky

Tube Angulation

15 to 20° cephalad

Film

One quarter of a 10 in. × 12 in. (24 cm × 30 cm), or single 8 in. × 10 in. Fine (extremity cassette)

Marker

Anatomical

Positioning

1. Patient is seated or kneeling next to table. The forearm is placed on the table in the P-A position. The fingers should be straight. The patient is asked to ulnar flex the wrist about 20°.

2. This view may be done in the fourth quarter of the film or on a separate 8 in. × 10 in. film. Lead blockers are positioned to cover the exposed film. The horizontal central ray is centered to the scaphoid, or 0.5 in. distal to the radial styloid process.

3. Vertical central ray placed through the long axis of the carpal bones and radius.

4. Have patient suspend respiration and hold still. Take film.

Collimation

Top to Bottom: to include metacarpal articulation to distal ulna and radius; Side to Side: soft tissue of forearm.

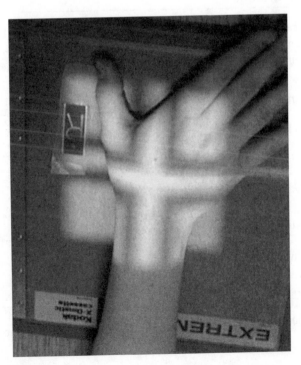

FIGURE 12.25
Wrist ulnar flexion positioning.

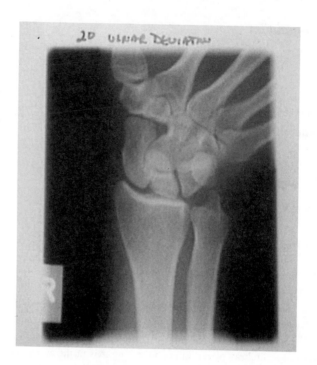

FIGURE 12.26
Wrist ulnar flexion film.

Breathing Instructions

Hold still

Image Critique

The scapholunate and scaphocapitate spaces should be open. If the scaphocapitate space is closed, oblique the wrist about 15°. If the hand is not flat on the film, the second metacarpal base will be superimposed over the trapezium and the scaphotrapezium space will be closed.

Optimum kVp

55–65 kVp

12.12   Wrist Series: A-P Clenched Fist View

Measure

A-P through carpal bones

Protection

Coat lead apron

SID

40 in. Non-Bucky

Tube Angulation

None

Film

One quarter of a 10 in. × 12 in. (24 cm × 30 cm), or single 8 in. × 10 in. Fine (extremity) cassette)

Marker

Anatomical

Positioning

1. Patient is seated or kneeling next to table. The forearm is placed on the table in the A-P position. The fingers should be flexed into a tight fist.
2. This view can be done in the fourth quarter of the film, or on a separate 8 in. × 10 in. film. Lead blockers are positioned to cover the exposed film. The horizontal central ray is centered to the middle of the first row of carpal bones, or 0.5 in. distal to the radial styloid process.
3. Vertical central ray placed through the long axis of the carpal bones and radius.
4. Have patient suspend respiration and hold still. Take film.

Collimation

Top to Bottom: to include metacarpal articulation to distal ulna and radius; Side to Side: soft tissue of forearm.

Breathing Instructions

Hold still

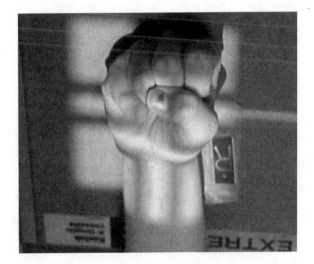

FIGURE 12.27
Wrist A-P stress position.

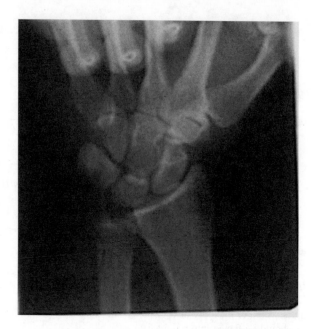

FIGURE 12.28
Wrist A-P stress film.

Image Critique

The view is a stress view of the ligaments in the wrist. There should be no rotation of the wrist or distal ulna and radius.

Optimum kVp

55–65 kVp

Chapter 13

Forearm, Elbow, and Humerus Radiography

13.1 Forearm, Elbow, and Humerus Radiography: Introduction

Forearm Radiography

The forearm views are limited to A-P and lateral views. Sponges can be used under the wrist to get the forearm parallel to the film for both views. Proximal injuries are generally associated with elbow trauma; the ulna and radius can be fractured mid-shaft; and distal injuries are considered as wrist injuries. Distal radius fractures may be difficult to see; they can present just like a scaphoid fracture. Children will often fracture the forearm at the epiphysis. A direct blow to the dorsum of the forearm can fracture the ulna and dislocate the radius. This is called the Monteggia fracture.

Elbow Radiography

Elbow injuries range from soft tissue or muscle and tendon to bone injuries. Many of the soft tissue injuries are a result of micro-trauma or overuse. Radiographically, some hypertrophic changes to the medial or lateral epicondyle can be seen. The bone injuries range from posterior impingement syndrome where repetitive jamming of the olecranon process results in osteophyte formation and hypertrophy of the olecranon process. Hypertrophic changes to the medial aspect of the medial epicondyle and olecranon process can result from repetitive hyperextension of the elbow. Throwing injuries can result in fracture of the lateral aspect of the capitulum or radial head due to impingement of the radial head against the capitulum. This can result in intra-articular fragments of cartilage. Compressive forces to the elbow will also fracture cartilage. These fragments may be seen in the radiocapitellar joint, as the joint has more capacity to accommodate the fragments.

Another throwing injury is osteocondritis dissecans of the capitulum, or Panner's disease. This can be seen radiographically as a subtle flattening of the capitulum.

Fractures may be caused by a fall with outstretched hands, a fall directly on the elbow, or a direct blow to the elbow. The outstretched-hand fall may dislocate the elbow or fracture the radial head or neck. With fractures of the elbow, the anterior fat pad will become angled, and the posterior fat pad will elevate from the olecranon fossa. Displacement of the posterior fat pad is referred to as a "positive fat pad sign" and is a reliable indication of a fracture. A fall with outstretched hands with the elbow in flexion can result in an avulsion fracture of the olecranon.

Knowing the method of injury can help tailor what view will be taken of the elbow. The routine views are A-P, lateral oblique, and lateral. On the lateral view, it may be very important to use sponges under the distal forearm; this is a common mistake that results in the epicondyles not being superimposed on the lateral view.

Supplementary views are the axial and medial oblique views. The Coyle Trauma, or Radial Head and Capitulum view, and a lateral view are used for acute trauma when the patient cannot straighten the arm. The medial oblique view will demonstrate the medial trochlear-coronoid process articulation. The radial head will be superimposed over the ulna; this view can also be used to see avulsion fracture of the olecranon process.

The axial view of the elbow will provide a more detailed look at the soft tissues immediately around the olecranon and olecranon fossa. This area is a site for calcium deposits and frequent inflammatory processes. A 15° medial rotation of the arm will demonstrate the cubital tunnel.

Humerus Radiography

The humerus views are generally taken Non-Bucky using the Non-Bucky film holder. The film is centered to the humerus, and the central ray is centered to the film. Proximal humerus injuries are often seen as part of the shoulder series (Hill-Sachs lesions as an example). It is very important to demonstrate both articulations on both views of the humerus.

The A-P view is very straightforward. The arm is externally rotated until the epicondyles are parallel to the film. There are numerous methods to take the lateral view of the humerus. For the non-trauma case, the A-P internal rotation method is easier for the patient. The "baby arm" lateral is also taken on the non-acute trauma patient. A modification of the "baby arm" view can be used to evaluate the cartilage in the glenohumeral joint. The patient abducts the humerus 90° and holds a light weight (a 12-oz. filled soda can will work) in the hand; this provides full-weighted stress on the shoulder.

The patient who may have fractured his/her humerus presents a challenge for positioning. The P-A lateral with the arm across the chest can be taken with the patient in a sling. It will involve no movement of the injured humerus. An A-P view in the sling can be taken by rotating the patient toward the affected side. The elbow area will be foreshortened.

There is one Bucky view of the humerus when a fracture is very likely. A reverse swimmer's view or trans-thoracic lateral can be taken by leaving the affected humerus to the side and aligned next to the Bucky. The unaffected arm (i.e., the arm toward the tube) is raised over the head. A swimmer's technique is used.

13.2   A-P Forearm View

Measure

A-P at middle of forearm

Protection

Coat lead apron

SID

40 in. Non-Bucky

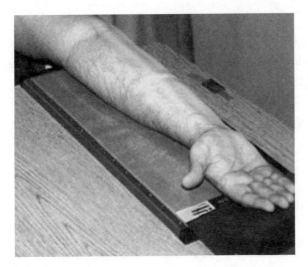

FIGURE 13.1
Forearm A-P positioning.

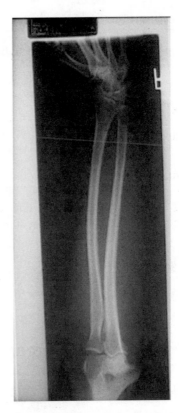

FIGURE 13.2
Forearm A-P film.

Tube Angulation

None

Film

7 in. × 17 in. Regular rare-earth cassette

Marker

Anatomical

Positioning

1. Patient is seated or kneeling next to table. The forearm is placed on the table in the A-P position with palm up.
2. The film is positioned to include the elbow and wrist joint spaces. The horizontal central ray is centered to the film.
3. Vertical central ray is placed through the long axis of the forearm.
4. A sponge can be placed under the hand for comfort. Make sure the entire arm is as straight as possible. The epicondyles should be parallel to the film.
5. Have patient suspend respiration and hold still. Take film.

Collimation

Top to Bottom: slightly less than film size, or to include elbow and wrist; Side to Side: soft tissue of forearm.

Breathing Instructions

Hold still

Image Critique

The view should include the ulna and radius, free of significant superimposition. The epicondyles should be equidistant from the film. The soft tissue should be seen. Film must not be overexposed.

Optimum kVp

65–70 kVp

13.3   Lateral Forearm View

Measure

Lateral at middle of the forearm

Protection

Coat lead apron

SID

40 in. using Non-Bucky

Tube Angulation

None

Film

7 in. × 17 in. regular speed rare-earth cassette

Marker

Anatomical

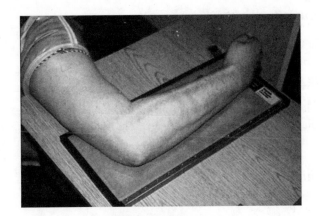

FIGURE 13.3
Forearm lateral positioning.

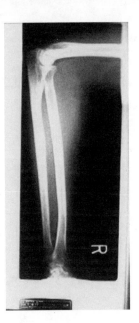

FIGURE 13.4
Forearm lateral film.

Positioning

1. Patient is seated or kneeling next to table. The forearm is placed on the table in the lateral position and flexed 90°. Make sure that the humerus and forearm are parallel to the film.

2. The film is positioned to include both elbow and wrist joints. The horizontal central ray is centered to the film.

3. Vertical central ray is placed through the long axis of the forearm.

4. The epicondyles and the carpal bones should be perpendicular to the film.

5. Have patient suspend respiration and hold still. Take film.

Collimation

Top to Bottom: slightly less than film size, or to include elbow and wrist; Side to Side: soft tissue of forearm.

Breathing Instructions

Hold still

Image Critique

The epicondyles should be superimposed and olecranon process and fossa will be seen. Most of the radial head will be clear of the ulna. The wrist should also be in a true lateral position with the distal ulna and radius superimposed.

Optimum kVp

65–70 kVp

13.4 A-P Elbow View

Measure

A-P at 1 cm distal to epicondyles

Protection

Coat lead apron

SID

40 in. using Non-Bucky

Tube Angulation

None

Film

One half of 10 in. × 12 in. Fine (extremity) cassette

Marker

Anatomical

Positioning

1. Patient is seated or kneeling next to table. The elbow is placed on the table in the A-P position with palm up.
2. The horizontal central ray is placed 1 cm distal to the epicondyles. One half of the extremity cassette is centered to the horizontal central ray.
3. Vertical central ray is placed through the long axis of the elbow.
4. A sponge can be placed under the hand for comfort. Make sure the entire arm is as straight as possible. The epicondyles should be parallel to the film.
5. Have patient suspend respiration and hold still. Take film.

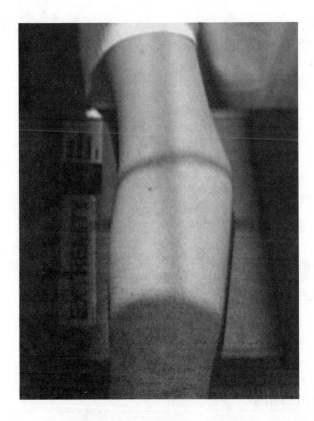

FIGURE 13.5
Elbow A-P positioning.

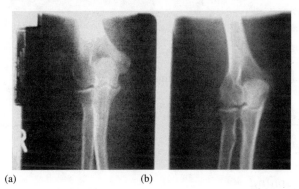

FIGURE 13.6
Elbow (a) A-P and (b) oblique film.

(a)   (b)

Collimation

Top to Bottom: slightly less than film size; Side to Side: soft tissue of elbow.

Breathing Instructions

Hold still

Image Critique

The view should demonstrate the elbow joints. The epicondyles should be equidistant from the film. The soft tissue should be seen. If the patient is not able to straighten arm fully, a view with the humerus parallel to film and one with the forearm parallel to film should be taken. Film must not be overexposed.

Optimum kVp

70 kVp

13.5   Lateral Oblique Elbow View

Measure

A-P at 1 cm distal to epicondyles

Protection

Coat lead apron

SID

40 in. using Non-Bucky

Tube Angulation

None

Film

One half of 10 in. × 12 in. Fine (extremity) cassette

Marker

Anatomical

Positioning

1. Patient is seated or kneeling next to table. The elbow is placed on the table in the A-P position with palm up. The patient is asked to externally or laterally rotate the arm about 40°.
2. The horizontal central ray is placed 1 cm distal to the epicondyles. One half of the extremity cassette is centered to the horizontal central ray.
3. Vertical central ray is placed through the long axis of the elbow.
4. A sponge can be placed under the hand for comfort. Make sure the entire arm is as straight as possible. The epicondyles should be 40° to the film.
5. Have patient suspend respiration and hold still. Take film.

Collimation

Top to Bottom: slightly less than film size; Side to Side: soft tissue of elbow.

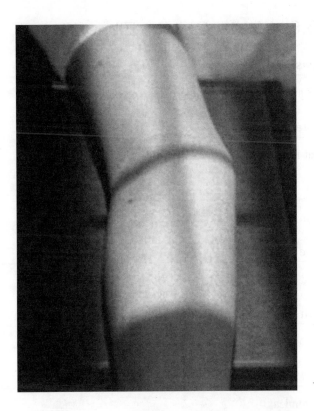

FIGURE 13.7
Elbow lateral oblique positioning.

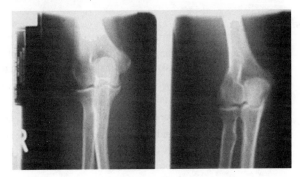

FIGURE 13.8
Elbow (a) A-P and (b) oblique films.

Breathing Instructions

Suspend respiration

Image Critique

The view should demonstrate the radial head clear of the ulna. The olecranon process and fossa will be seen. The soft tissue should be seen. If the patient is not able to straighten arm fully, take view with the arm as straight as possible. Opening the joint space depends on the arm being straight.

Optimum kVp

70 kVp

13.6   Medial Oblique Elbow View

Measure

A-P at 1 cm distal to epicondyles

Protection

Coat lead apron

SID

40 in. using Non-Bucky

Tube Angulation

None

Film

8 in. × 10 in. Fine (extremity) cassette

Marker

Anatomical

Positioning

1.   Patient is seated or kneeling next to table. The elbow is placed on the table in the A-P position with palm up. The patient is asked to internally or medially rotate the arm about 40°.
2.   The horizontal central ray is placed 1 cm distal to the epicondyles. One half of the extremity cassette is centered to the horizontal central ray.
3.   Vertical central ray is placed through the long axis of the elbow.
4.   A sponge can be placed under the hand for comfort. Make sure the entire arm is as straight as possible. The epicondyles should be 40° to the film.
5.   Have patient suspend respiration and hold still. Take film.

Collimation

Top to Bottom: slightly less than film size; Side to Side: soft tissue of elbow.

Breathing Instructions

Suspend respiration

Image Critique

The olecranon process and fossa will be seen. The coracoid process will also be seen. The radial head will be superimposed on the ulna. The soft tissue should be seen. If the patient is not able to straighten arm fully, take view with the arm as straight as possible. Opening the joint space depends on the arm being straight.

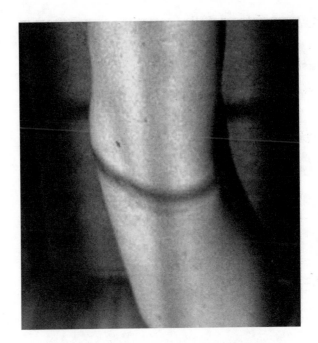

FIGURE 13.9
Elbow medial oblique positioning.

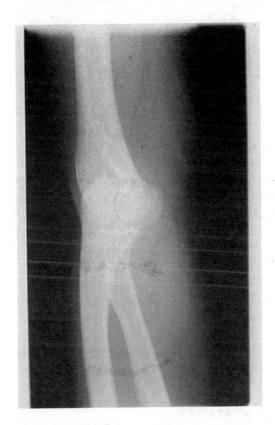

FIGURE 13.10
Elbow medial oblique film.

Optimum kVp

70 kVp

13.7   Lateral Elbow View

Measure

A-P at 1 in. distal to epicondyles

Protection

Lead apron

SID

40 in. using Non-Bucky

Tube Angulation

None

Film

8 in. × 10 in. Fine or Detail (extremity) cassette

Marker

Anatomical

Positioning

1. Patient is seated or kneeling next to table. The elbow is placed on the table in the lateral position and flexed 90°. Make sure that the humerus and forearm are parallel to the film.
2. The horizontal central ray is placed 1 in. distal to the epicondyles. The horizontal central ray is centered to the long axis of the forearm. The extremity cassette is centered to the horizontal central ray.
3. Vertical central ray is placed through the long axis of the forearm.
4. A sponge can be placed under the hand for comfort. Make sure the entire arm is true lateral. The epicondyles should be perpendicular to the film.
5. Have patient suspend respiration and hold still. Take film.

Collimation

Top to Bottom: slightly less than film size; Side to Side: soft tissue of elbow.

Breathing Instructions

Suspend respiration

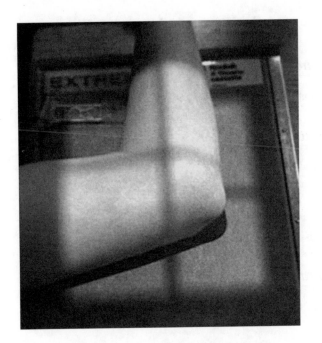

FIGURE 13.11
Elbow lateral positioning.

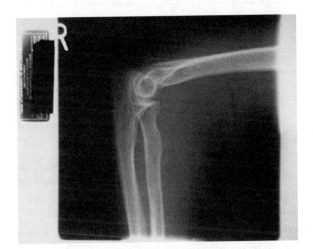

FIGURE 13.12
Elbow lateral film.

Image Critique

The epicondyles should be superimposed, and olecranon process and fossa will be seen. Most of the radial head will be clear of the ulna. Pay very close attention to the exposure factors, as soft tissue detail is important. If the film is overexposed, the fat pad signs cannot be evaluated.

Optimum kVp

65–70 kVp

13.8   Coyle Trauma View of Elbow

Measure

Lateral at the epicondyles

Protection

Coat lead apron

SID

40 in. using Non-Bucky

Tube Angulation

45° toward shoulder

Film

8 in. × 10 in. Fine (extremity) cassette

Marker

Anatomical

Positioning

1. Patient is seated or kneeling next to table. The elbow is placed on the table in the lateral position and flexed 90°. Make sure that the humerus and forearm are parallel to the film.
2. The horizontal central ray is placed 1 in. distal to the epicondyles along the long axis of the forearm. The extremity cassette is centered to the horizontal central ray.
3. Vertical central ray is placed through the long axis of the humerus.
4. A sponge can be placed under the hand for comfort. Make sure the entire arm is true lateral. The epicondyles should be perpendicular to the film.
5. Have patient suspend respiration and hold still. Take film.

Collimation

Top to Bottom: slightly less than film size; Side to Side: soft tissue of elbow.

Breathing Instructions

Hold Still

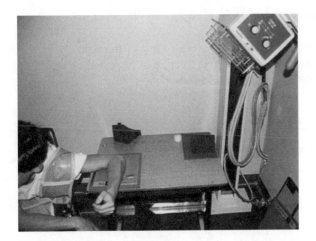

FIGURE 13.13
Elbow trauma view: positioning 1.

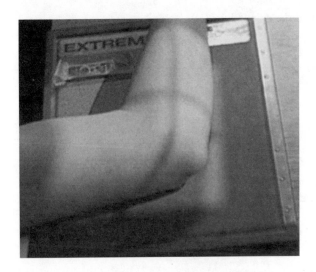

FIGURE 13.14
Elbow trauma view: positioning 2.

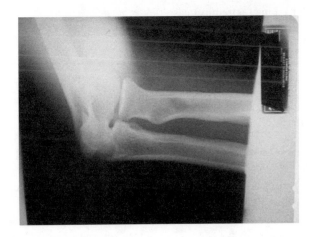

FIGURE 13.15
Elbow trauma view film.

Image Critique

The view will provide a clear view of the radial head and capitellum. It should be the first view taken when a radial head fracture is suspected. A view for the coronoid process can be taken with the tube angled toward the brachial crease and the elbow flexed less than 80°.

Optimum kVp

70 kVp

13.9   Axial View of Elbow

Measure

A-P at the epicondyles

Protection

Coat lead apron

SID

40 in. using Non-Bucky

Tube Angulation

None

Film

8 in. × 10 in. Fine (extremity) cassette

Marker

Anatomical

Positioning

1. Patient is seated or kneeling next to table. The elbow is placed on the table in the A-P position and flexed 45°. Make sure that the humerus is parallel to the film.
2. The horizontal central ray is placed through the epicondyles along the long axis of the forearm. The extremity cassette is centered to the horizontal central ray.
3. Vertical central ray placed through the long axis of the humerus.
4. Have patient suspend respiration and hold still. Take film.
5. To view the cubital tunnel, medially rotate the arm 15°.

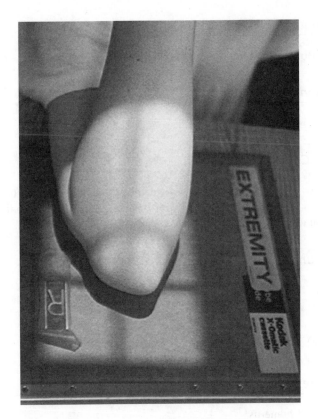

FIGURE 13.16
Elbow axial positioning.

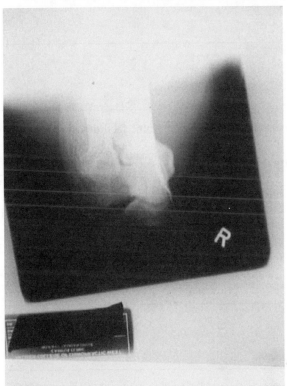

FIGURE 13.17
Elbow axial film.

Collimation

Top to Bottom: soft tissue around elbow, or 5 in.; Side to Side: soft tissue of elbow, or 5 in.

Breathing Instructions

Suspend respiration and hold still

Image Critique

The view will provide a clear view of the soft tissue adjacent to the olecranon process and the olecranon process. It is very good for detecting loose bodies in this area. The modified view for the cubital tunnel and the axial view should not be overexposed.

Optimum kVp

70 kVp

13.10   A-P Humerus View

Measure

A-P at mid-humerus

Protection

Lead apron

SID

40 in. using Non-Bucky film holder (some facilities may use Bucky technique)

Tube Angulation

None

Film

7 in. × 17 in. regular speed rare-earth with I.D. down

Marker

Anatomical

Positioning

1.   Patient stands in front of Bucky, facing tube. The shoulder and humerus should be touching the film.
2.   Center film by placing top of film 2 in. above shoulder. Center horizontal central ray to film.

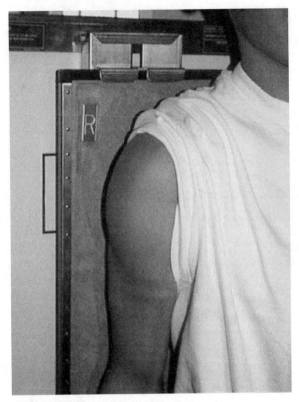

FIGURE 13.18
Humerus A-P positioning.

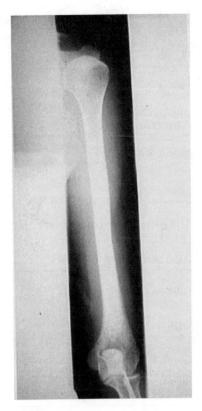

FIGURE 13.19
Humerus A-P film.

3. Vertical central ray is placed through the long axis of the humerus.
4. Patient is instructed to externally rotate arm until the epicondyles are parallel to film.
5. Have patient suspend respiration and hold still. Take film.

Collimation

Top to Bottom: shoulder to elbow; Side to Side: soft tissue of arm.

Breathing Instructions

Suspend respiration and hold

Image Critique

The view should demonstrate both the shoulder and elbow joints. The epicondyles should be equidistant from the film. The soft tissue should be seen. Film must not be overexposed.

Optimium kVp

70 kVp

13.11   Lateral Humerus with Arm Across Chest View

Measure

A-P at mid-humerus

Protection

Lead apron

SID

40 in. using Non-Bucky film holder (some facilities take this film Bucky)

Tube Angulation

None

Film

7 in. × 17 in. regular speed rare-earth cassette with I.D. down

Marker

Anatomical marker pronated

Positioning

1. Patient stands in front of Bucky facing Bucky. The shoulder and humerus should be touching the film.
2. Center film by placing top of film 2 in. above shoulder. Center horizontal central ray to film.
3. Vertical central ray is placed through the long axis of the humerus.
4. Patient is instructed to flex elbow 90° with arm across chest or until the epicondyles are perpendicular to film. May be done with arm in sling. Patient may need to lean into Bucky to keep humerus parallel to film.
5. Have patient suspend respiration. Take film

Collimation

Top to Bottom: shoulder to elbow; Side to Side: soft tissue of arm.

Breathing Instructions

Suspend respiration

Image Critique

The view should demonstrate both the shoulder and elbow joint space. The epicondyles should be equally superimposed on the film. The soft tissue should be seen. Film must not be overexposed.

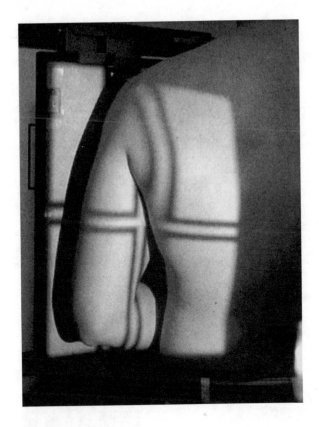

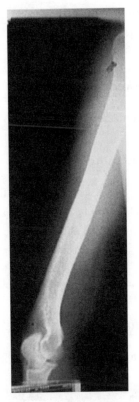

FIGURE 13.21
Humerus lateral with arm
across chest film.

FIGURE 13.20
Humerus lateral with arm across chest positioning.

Optimum kVp

70 kVp

13.12   Lateral Humerus with Internal Rotation

Measure

A-P at mid-humerus

Protection

Lead apron

SID

40 in. using Non-Bucky

Tube Angulation

None

Film

7 in. × 17 in. regular speed rare-earth cassette with I.D. down

Marker

Anatomical

Positioning

1. Patient stands in front of Bucky, facing tube. The shoulder and humerus should be touching the film.
2. Center film by placing top of film 2 in. above shoulder. Center horizontal central ray to film.
3. Vertical central ray is placed through the long axis of the humerus.
4. Patient is instructed to internally rotate arm until the epicondyles are perpendicular to film (may be done with arm in sling).
5. Have patient suspend respiration and hold still. Take film.

Collimation

Top to Bottom: shoulder to elbow; Side to Side: soft tissue of arm.

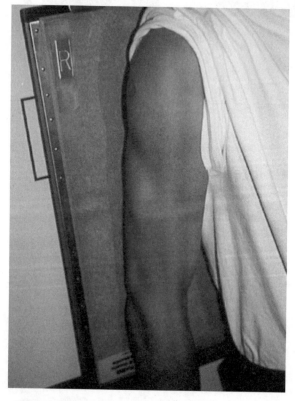

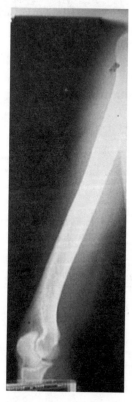

FIGURE 13.22
Humerus lateral with internal rotation positioning.

FIGURE 13.23
Humerus lateral with internal rotation film.

Breathing Instructions

Suspend respiration

Image Critique

The view should demonstrate both the shoulder and elbow joint space. The epicondyles should be equal-superimposed on the film. The soft tissue should be seen. Film must not be overexposed.

Optimium kVp

70 kVp

13.13   Lateral Humerus (Baby Arm) View

Measure

A-P at mid-humerus

Protection

Lead apron

SID

40 in. using Non-Bucky (Some facilities take this view Bucky.)

Tube Angulation

None

Film

7 in. × 17 in. regular speed rare-earth cassette with I.D. down .

Marker

Anatomical

Positioning

1.   Patient stands in front of Bucky, facing tube. The arm is abducted 90° with elbow flexed.
2.   Center film by placing to the long axis of the humerus. Center horizontal central ray to film.
3.   Vertical central ray is placed through the long axis of the humerus to include both shoulder and elbow joints.

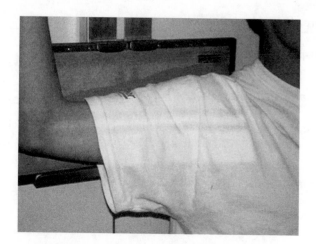

FIGURE 13.24
Humerus baby arm lateral positioning.

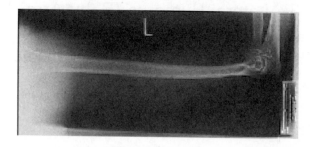

FIGURE 13.25
Humerus baby arm lateral film.

4. Patient instructed to externally rotate arm until the epicondyles are perpendicular to film. The forearm will be parallel to Bucky. The patient may be in a slight oblique position to have the humerus parallel to the film.

5. Have patient suspend rspiration. Take film.

Collimation

Top to Bottom: shoulder to elbow; Side to Side: soft tissue of arm.

Breathing Instructions

Suspend respiration

Image Critique

The view should demonstrate both the shoulder and elbow joint space. The humerus epicondyles should be superimposed on the film. The soft tissue should be seen. Film must not be overexposed.

Optimum kVp

70 kVp

14

Shoulder, Scapula, and Clavicle Radiography

14.1 Shoulder, Scapula and Clavicle Radiography: Introduction

The shoulder, scapula, and clavicle are common areas of upper extremity pain and injury. The shoulder and scapula can be radiographically evaluated at the same time. The clavicle and acromioclavicular joints require different patient positioning. Therefore, a study to rule out fracture of the shoulder may not demonstrate clavicle or acromioclavicular joint pathology as well as dedicated views. All views of the clavicle or shoulder should be taken erect; this will provide some weight-bearing effect and generally less discomfort for the patient.

Shoulder Radiography

The shoulder is a very complex joint. Many muscle groups are used in its function. The shoulder can be easily injured in contact sports or during work involving lifting, pulling, and pushing heavy objects. The shoulder is prone to arthritic changes, bursitis and other nontraumatic injuries. Besides radiography, computed tomography and magnetic resonance are used to evaluate injuries. None of the present imaging modalities will demonstrate all causes for pain and discomfort.

The radiographic study of the shoulder requires precise and accurate positioning. The glenohumeral joint should always be open on frontal views of the shoulder. The patient should be turned toward the shoulder of interest until the scapula is parallel to the film. This generally requires the patient to be turned from 15 to 45°; this is referred to as the true A-P or Grashey shoulder projection. Accurate positioning also requires that attention be paid to the position of the humerus. The external rotation shoulder views should have the humerus epicondyle parallel to the film. This will have the humerus in an A-P position. The internal rotation view will have the epicondyle perpendicular to the film, or the humerus in a lateral position.

The internal and external rotation views are routinely taken on nontraumatic injury shoulder studies. When concerned about supraspinatus muscle impingement, the outlet view is very important. An A-P view with the arm abducted to 90° can be very useful in evaluating the joint space. Placing a full soda can in the hand of the affected arm will provide adequate stress to evaluate the cartilage in the glenohumeral joint space. The full soda can will provide 95% of full weight-bearing stress.

Post-traumatic shoulder studies should not involve movement of the humerus. It is relatively easy to provide a complete evaluation of the shoulder with the arm in a sling or never moved. Post-trauma views are definitely better tolerated by the patient when taken upright or erect. One of the best views to evaluate a dislocation is the "Y", Outlet view or lateral scapula. By taking A-P, apical, Stryker Notch, and "Y" views, the shoulder can be comprehensively evaluated for fractures or dislocation. Bankart and Hill-Sachs defects will be seen on the apical or Stryker Notch views. These trauma views are also used to study the unstable shoulder. (We have experimented with doing internal and external rotational views with weights to further study the unstable shoulder.)

Radiographic equipment generally found in chiropractic offices is not designed to easily image the shoulder in the axial plane. Ceiling-suspended X-ray tubes are able to provide the compound angles needed to take the routine A-P axillary view. The West Point, or military axillary, view can be done with chiropractic equipment if a suitable small table is available. The patient is asked to lean over the table in a prone position. The shoulder and anterior chest are placed on radiographic sponges. This is a rather cumbersome position. The other trauma view can be used to replace the axillary view for most patients.

Clavicle and Acromioclavicular Joint Studies

The clavicle can be imaged P-A or A-P. Recumbent views should never be taken P-A. When taking clavicle X-rays, the P-A view will provide less magnification but better detail; it is also more difficult to position. If the operator does not feel comfortable taking the films P-A, the exam can be taken A-P. The other advantage of the A-P clavicle view is that greater tube angulation can be used for the axial view. With tall patients, the chiropractor may be limited to 10° or less caudal tube angulation. It is much easier to get up to 25° of cephalad tube angulation on A-P axial views of the clavicle. The axial view is very important when evaluating fracture direction, degree of reduction, and healing progress of clavicle fractures.

For clavicle or acromioclavicular joints, the patient should not be rotated. The mid-sagittal plane should be perpendicular to the film. On P-A views, the shoulders can be rolled forward — similar to chest radiography. This will get the long axis of the clavicle running more parallel to the film.

The Zanca view of the acromioclavicular joint is the view of choice for evaluation of separation or resorption from steroid use. The tube angulation and deep inspiration will open the subacromion space much better than the straight A-P view. This view can be taken as a unilateral study at 40 in. SID using the Bucky or at 72 in. SID using Non-Bucky. The 72 in. SID Non-Bucky view will reduce exposure by about 75%.

Weighted and non-weighted views of the acromioclavicular (AC) joints are taken to evaluate a potential acromioclavicular joint separation. The bilateral view allows easier comparison if the shoulders are not too wide. The amount of weight needs to exceed 15 lb. The weights should be strapped around both wrists so that arm muscles are not used to support the weight. This is key for accurate diagnostic value.

Scapula

The arm position for views of the scapula may be different from the routine shoulder position. The rotation of the humerus is not important. (This author routinely leaves the arm in a neutral position.) The arm can be raised to pull the body of the scapula clear of the ribs for the frontal view. The arm can be placed behind the patient's back, raised over the patient's head, or pulled across the patient's chest on the lateral view. If shoulder dislocation is not a concern, sometimes placing the arm behind the patient's back will pull the scapula clear of the ribs.

14.2 Shoulder: A-P Shoulder with Internal Rotation

Measure

A-P at coracoid process

Protection

Lead apron

SID

40 in. using Bucky

Tube Angulation

None

Film

10 in. × 8 in. regular speed rare-earth cassettes with I.D. toward spine (some facilities use 10 in. × 12 in. film size)

Marker

Anatomical plus INT or arrow pointing in

Positioning

1. Patient stands in front of Bucky, facing tube.
2. Patient rotated about 15 to 45° until the scapula is parallel to film.
3. Horizontal central ray placed 1 in. below coracoid process. Film centered to horizontal central ray.

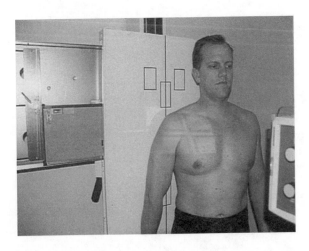

FIGURE 14.1
Shoulder internal rotation positioning.

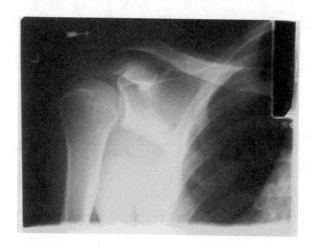

FIGURE 14.2
Shoulder internal rotation film.

4.   Vertical central ray placed on coracoid process.
5.   Patient internally rotates humerus until the humeral condyles are perpendicular to film.
6.   Patient is instructed to hold breath and stand still. Exposure made.

Collimation

Soft tissue of shoulder or slightly less than film size

Breathing Instructions

Suspend respiration

Image Critique

Glenohumeral joint space must be open. The soft tissue around shoulder should be seen. The lesser tubericle will be in profile medially with the humeral head and greater tubericle superimposed.

Optimum kVp

70 kVp

14.3   Shoulder: A-P Shoulder with External Rotation

Measure

A-P at coracoid process

Protection

Lead apron

SID

40 in. using Bucky

Tube Angulation

None

Film

8 in. × 10 in. regular speed rare-earth cassette with I.D. to spine (some facilities use 10 in. × 12 in. cassettes)

Markers

Anatomical plus EXT or arrow pointing out.

Positioning

1. Patient stands in front of Bucky, facing tube.
2. Patient rotated about 15° until the scapula is parallel to film.
3. Horizontal central ray placed 1 in. below coracoid process. Film centered to horizontal central ray.
4. Vertical central ray placed on coracoid process.
5. Patient internally rotates humerus until the humeral condyles are parallel to film.
6. Patient is instructed to hold breath and stand still. Exposure made.

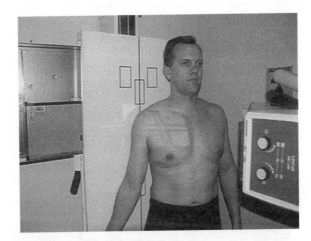

FIGURE 14.3
Shoulder external rotation positioning.

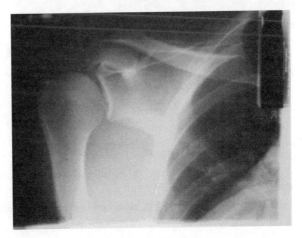

FIGURE 14.4
Shoulder external rotation film.

Collimation

Soft tissue of shoulder, or slightly less than film size

Breathing Instructions

Suspend respiration

Image Critique

Glenohumeral joint space must be open. Soft tissue of shoulder should be seen. Distal clavicle should also be well visualized. The greater tubercle and humeral head will be seen in profile.

Optimum kVp

70–75 kVp

14.4   Shoulder: Apical Oblique View

Measure

A-P at coracoid process

Protection

Lead apron

SID

40 in. using Bucky

Tube Angulation

30° caudal

Film

10 in. × 12 in. regular speed rare-earth cassette with I.D. to spine

Marker

Anatomical

Positioning

1.   Patient stands in front of Bucky, facing tube. The patient is rotated about 15° to position the scapula parallel to the film. The patient's arm is in an internal rotation.
2.   Horizontal central ray placed 2 in. superior to the coracoid process. Film centered to horizontal central ray.

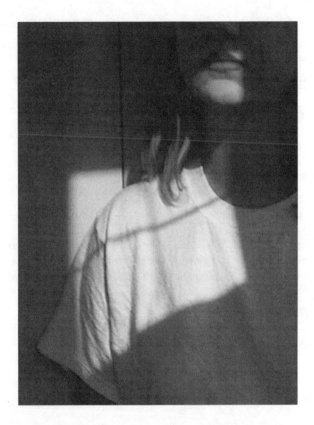

FIGURE 14.5
Shoulder apical oblique positioning.

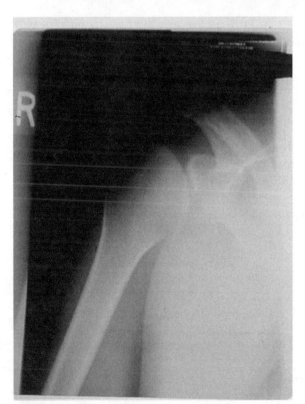

FIGURE 14.6
Shoulder apical film.

3. The vertical central ray is positioned through the glenohumeral joint space.

4. Patient is instructed to suspend respiration. Exposure made.

Collimation

Soft tissue around shoulder to include scapula, or slightly less than film size

Breathing Instructions

Suspended respiration

Image Critique

This view provides a tangential view of head of the humerus in the glenohumeral joint space and the glenoid fossa. The view provides minimal superimposition of adjacent structures. This view is used to detect dislocations and Hill-Sachs and Burkhart defects.

Optimum kVp

70 kVp

14.5 Shoulder: Prone Axillary or West Point View

Measure

A-P at coracoid process

Protection

Lead apron

SID

40 in. using Bucky

Tube Angulation

15 to 25° caudal

Film

8 in. × 10 in. regular speed rare-earth cassette with I.D. to spine

Marker

Anatomical

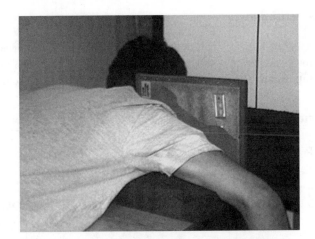

FIGURE 14.7
Shoulder axial positioning.

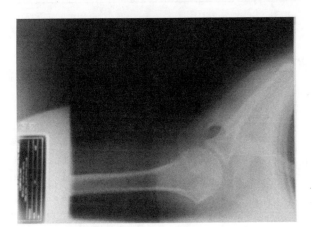

FIGURE 14.8
Shoulder axial film.

Positioning

1. Patient prone, leaning over table. The mid-sagittal plane of the patient is rotated 10 to 25° medially. The humerus is abducted 90°. The shoulder is resting on radiographic sponges. The film is placed above or superior to the shoulder.

2. If the tube angle is used, the horizontal central ray is placed 2 in. above the glenoid fossa. If no tube angle is used, the horizontal central ray is placed through the glenoid fossa.

3. The vertical central ray is positioned through the glenohumeral joint space. The film is centered to the vertical central ray.

4. Patient is instructed to take full inspiration. Exposure is made.

Collimation

Soft tissue around shoulder and proximal humerus

Breathing Instructions

Suspended respiration

Image Critique

Clear view of head of the humerus in the glenohumeral joint space and the glenoid fossa. The posterior and anterior aspects of the humeral head will be seen in profile with the least amount of superimposition. This view is used to detect dislocation or fracture in the joint space.

Optimum kVp

70 kVp

14.6   Shoulder: Outlet or Lateral Scapula View

Measure

A-P at coracoid process

Protection

Lead apron

SID

40 in. using Bucky

Tube Angulation

15 to 30° caudal for outlet; 0 to 10° caudal for lateral scapula

Film

10 in. × 12 in. regular speed rare-earth cassette with I.D. up

Marker

Anatomical

Positioning

1. Patient stands in front of Bucky, facing Bucky. Align the humeral head of the affected shoulder with the center line of the Bucky.
2. Horizontal central ray is placed through the head of the humerus. Film is centered to horizontal central ray.
3. Position patient in a 60° anterior oblique or align the scapula perpendicular to film. Vertical central ray should be 1 in. medial to the body of the scapula.
4. Patient is instructed to take full inspiration. Exposure made.

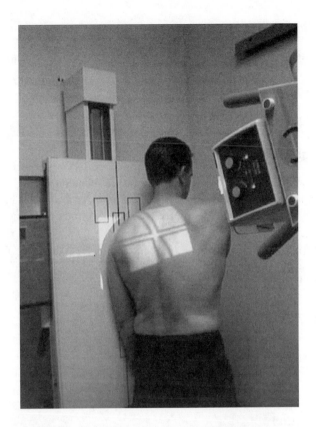

FIGURE 14.9
Shoulder outlet view positioning.

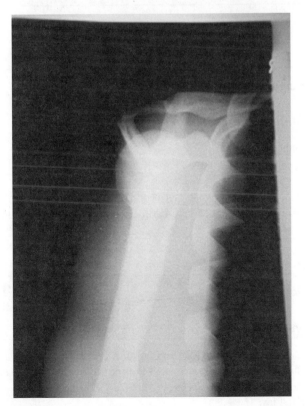

FIGURE 14.10
Shoulder outlet view film.

Collimation

Soft tissue around distal clavicle and shoulder to include scapula, or slightly less than film size

Breathing Instructions

Full inspiration

Image Critique

Clear view of head of the humerus in the glenohumeral joint space or position of humerus in relation to the joint if dislocated. Subacromion space should be open and well visualized. Scapula should be in true lateral position. Film must not be overexposed.

Optimum kVp

70 kVp

14.7   Shoulder: Stryker Notch View

Measure

A-P at coracoid process

Protection

Lead apron

SID

40 in. using Bucky

Tube Angulation

45° cephalad

Film

8 in. × 10 in. regular speed rare-earth cassette with I.D. to spine (some facilities use a 10 in. × 12 in. cassette)

Marker

Anatomical

Positioning

1. Patient stands in front of Bucky, facing tube. The patient is rotated about 15° to position the scapula parallel to the film. The patient abducts arm with hand behind neck. The humerus should be perpendicular to the film.
2. Horizontal central ray is placed 2 in. inferior to the coracoid process. Film is centered to horizontal central ray.

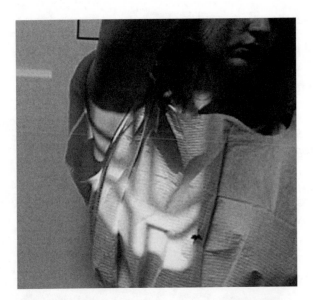

FIGURE 14.11
Shoulder Stryker notch positioning.

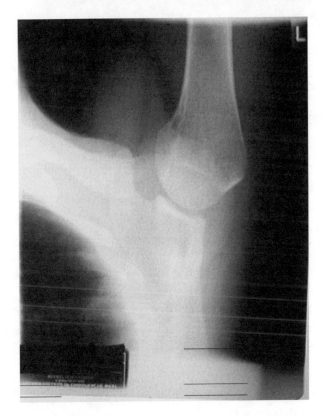

FIGURE 14.12
Shoulder Stryker notch film.

3. The vertical central ray is positioned through the glenohumeral joint space.
4. Patient instructed to take full inspiration. Exposure made.

Collimation

Soft tissue around shoulder to include scapula, or slightly less than film size

Breathing Instructions

Full inspiration

Image Critique

Clear view of head of the humerus in the glenohumeral joint space and the glenoid fossa. The posterior and superior aspects of the humeral head will be seen in profile. This view is used to detect anterior instability and Hill-Sachs defects.

Optimum kVp

70 kVp

14.8   Clavicle: P-A Clavicle View

Measure

A-P at mid-clavicle

Protection

Lead apron

SID

40 in. using Bucky

Tube Angulation

None

Film

8 in. × 10 in. regular speed rare-earth cassette with I.D. down (some facilities use a 10 in. × 12 in. cassette)

Marker

Anatomical (pronated)

Positioning

1.   Patient stands in front of Bucky, facing Bucky.
2.   The mid-sagittal plane should be perpendicular to film.

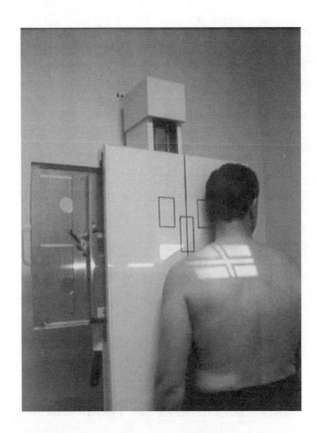

FIGURE 14.13
Clavicle P-A positioning.

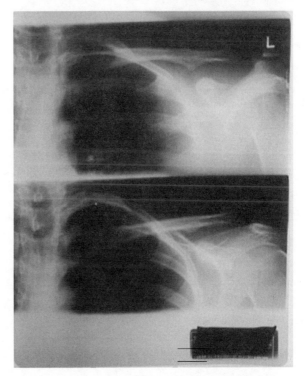

FIGURE 14.14
Clavicle series film.

3. Horizontal central ray through the long axis of the clavicle. The AC joint can be used as a reference. Top half of film is centered to horizontal central ray.

4. Vertical central ray is placed at the middle of the clavicle.

5. Patient is instructed to hold breath and stand still. Exposure made.

Collimation

Top to Bottom: soft tissue of clavicle; Side to Side: to include AC joint and sternoclavicular joints.

Breathing Instructions

Suspend respiration

Image Critique

The entire clavicle should be seen. The AC joint will be open. There should be no rotation, as demonstrated by visualization of the sternoclavicular joint.

Optimum kVp

70 kVp

14.9   Clavicle Views: P-A Axial Clavicle

Measure

A-P at mid-clavicle

Protection

Lead apron

SID

40 in. using Bucky

Tube Angulation

10 to 15° caudal

Film

8 in. × 10 in. (or 10 in. × 12 in.) regular speed rare-earth cassette with I.D. down. Use bottom of film used for P-A clavicle view.

Marker

Anatomical

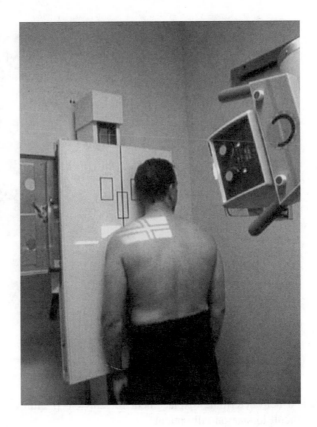

FIGURE 14.15
Clavicle P-A axial positioning.

Positioning

1. Patient stands in front of Bucky, facing Bucky.
2. The mid-sagittal plane will be perpendicular to film.
3. Horizontal central ray 1 in. above the long axis of the clavicle. The AC joint can be used as a reference. Bottom half of film centered to horizontal central ray.
4. Vertical central ray is placed at the middle of the clavicle.
5. Patient is instructed to hold breath and stand still. Exposure made.

Collimation

Top to Bottom: soft tissue of clavicle; Side to Side: to include AC joint and sternoclavicular joints.

Breathing Instructions

Suspend respiration

Image Critique

The entire clavicle should be seen. The AC joint will be open. There should be no rotation, as demonstrated by visualization of the sternoclavicular joint. The axial view will open the acromion

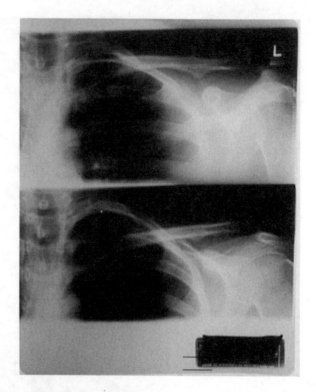

FIGURE 14.16
Clavicle series film.

space and help determine displacement for clavicle fractures. Tube height limits will make this view difficult to take on tall patients.

Optimum kVp

70 kVp

14.10   Clavicle: A-P Clavicle View

Measure

A-P at mid-clavicle

Protection

Lead apron

SID

40 in. using Bucky

Tube Angulation

None

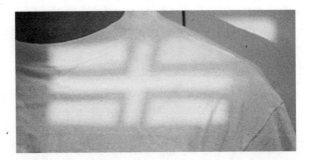

FIGURE 14.17
Clavicle A-P positioning.

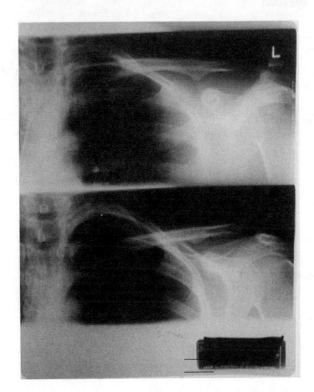

FIGURE 14.18
Clavicle series film.

Film

8 in. × 10 in. (or 10 in. × 12 in.) regular speed rare-earth cassette with I.D. down. Use top half of cassette.

Marker

Anatomical

Positioning

1. Patient stands in front of Bucky, facing tube.
2. Patient has back to film with no rotation.
3. Horizontal central ray through the long axis of the clavicle. Top half of film is centered to horizontal central ray.

4. Vertical central ray is placed at the middle of the clavicle.
5. Patient is instructed to hold breath and stand still. Exposure made.

Collimation

Top to Bottom: soft tissue of clavicle; Side to Side: to include AC joint and sternoclavicular joints.

Breathing Instructions

Suspend respiration

Image Critique

The entire clavicle should be seen. The AC joint will be open. There should be no rotation, as demonstrated by visualization of the sternoclavicular joint.

Optimum kVp

70 kVp

14.11 Clavicle: A-P Axial Clavicle View

Measure

A-P at mid-clavicle

Protection

Lead apron

SID

40 in. using Bucky

Tube Angulation

15 to 25° cephalad

Film

8 in. × 10 in. (or 10 in. × 12 in.) regular speed rare-earth cassette with I.D. down. Done on bottom half of A-P clavicle film.

Marker

Anatomical

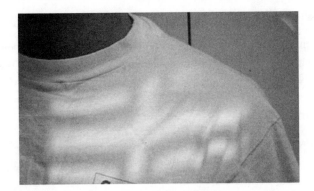

FIGURE 14.19
Clavicle A-P axial positioning.

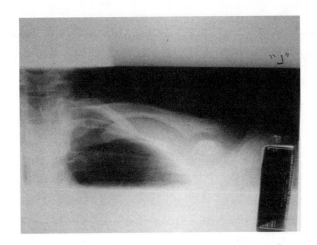

FIGURE 14.20
Clavicle A-P axial film.

Positioning

1. Patient stands in front of Bucky, facing tube.
2. Patient has back to film with no rotation.
3. Horizontal central ray 1 in. below the long axis of the clavicle. Bottom half of film centered to horizontal central ray.
4. Vertical central ray is placed at the middle of the clavicle.
5. Patient is instructed to hold breath and stand still. Exposure made.

Collimation

Top to Bottom: soft tissue of clavicle; Side to Side: to include AC joint and sternoclavicular joints.

Breathing Instructions

Suspend respiration

Image Critique

The entire clavicle should be seen. The AC joint will be open. There should be no rotation, as demonstrated by visualization of the sternoclavicular joint. The axial view will open the acromion space and help determine displacement for clavicle fractures.

Optimum kVp

70 kVp

14.12   Shoulder: A-P Acromioclavicular Joint Unilateral

Measure

A-P at coracoid process

Protection

Lead apron

SID

40 in. using Bucky

Tube Angulation

None. 15° cephalad for Zanca modification

Film

10 in. × 12 in. regular speed rare-earth cassette with I.D. toward spine; 8 in. × 10 in. for view not needing weights

Marker

Anatomical plus arrow pointing down for weighted view

Positioning

1. Patient stands in front of Bucky, facing tube. Both shoulders should be touching Bucky.
2. Horizontal central ray is placed through the AC joints. Film is centered to horizontal central ray. Have patient take full inspiration to determine centering.
3. Vertical central ray is placed on AC joint.
4. Patient is instructed to take full inspiration. Exposure made.
5. If weighted view is needed, strap 15 to 20 lb of weight around both wrists and repeat steps 1 through 4.

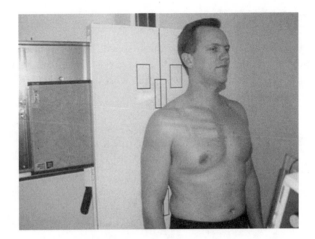

FIGURE 14.21
AC joint unilateral positioning.

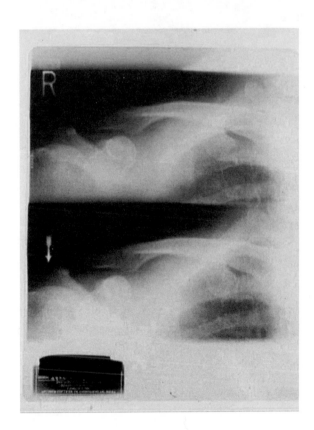

FIGURE 14.22
Unilateral AC joint film (Zanca).

Collimation

Soft tissue around distal clavicle and shoulder

Breathing Instructions

Full inspiration

Image Critique

Clear view of AC joint and acromion space. Must not be overexposed. For a clearer view of the acromion space, the Zanca modification is recommended. Make sure the patient does not move the AC joint out of the area of exposure (with the deep inspiration). Full inspiration will provide a clearer view of the acromion space.

Optimum kVp

70 kVp

14.13   Shoulder: A-P Acromioclavicular Joints Bilateral

Measure

A-P at coracoid process

Protection

Lead apron

SID

72 in. using Non-Bucky

Tube Angulation

None; optional 15° cephalad (Zanca)

Film

17 in. × 14 in. (or 7 in. × 17 in.) regular speed rare-earth cassette with I.D. toward unaffected side

Marker

Anatomical plus arrow pointing down on weighted view

Positioning

1.   Patient stands in front of Bucky, facing tube.
2.   Patient places both shoulders on film with no rotation.
3.   Horizontal central ray is placed at coracoid process. Top half of film is centered to horizontal central ray.
4.   Vertical central ray is placed at mid-sternum.
5.   Patient takes deep breath, and image is taken.
6.   15 to 20 lb of weight are strapped to both wrists. Horizontal central ray is centered to bottom half of film.
7.   Patient is instructed to take deep breath and stand still. Exposure made.

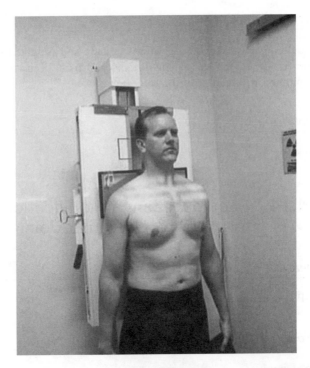

FIGURE 14.23
AC joint bilateral weighted positioning.

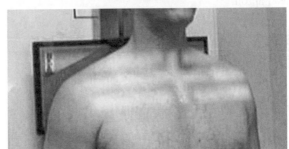

FIGURE 14.24
AC joint bilateral without weights positioning.

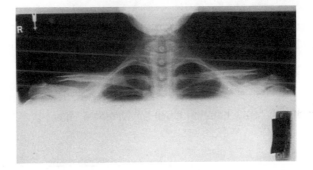

FIGURE 14.25
AC joint bilateral film.

Collimation

Both AC joints and soft tissue above the shoulders

Breathing Instructions

Deep inspiration

Image Critique

Should demonstrate both AC joints in static and weighted position. Important not to overexpose film. Make sure that the patient does not move out of the field of view with deep inspiration. Deep inspiration will help open the acromion space.

Optimum kVp

70 kVp

14.14   Shoulder: Zanca Modification for Acromioclavicular Joint

Measure

A-P at coracoid process

Protection

Lead apron

SID

40 in. using Bucky

Tube Angulation

15° cephalad

Film

10 in. × 12 in. Lanex regular with I.D. toward spine; 8 in. × 10 in. for view not needing weights

Marker

Anatomical plus arrow pointing down for weighted view

Positioning

1. Patient stands in front of Bucky, facing tube. Both shoulders should be touching Bucky.
2. Horizontal central ray is placed 1 in. below AC joints. Film is centered to horizontal central ray. Have patient take full inspiration to determine centering.
3. Vertical central ray is placed on AC joint.
4. Patient is instructed to take full inspiration. Exposure made.
5. If weighted view is needed, strap weight around both wrists and repeat steps 1 through 4.

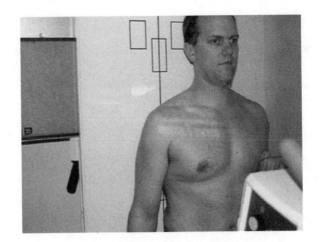

FIGURE 14.26
AC joint Zanca positioning.

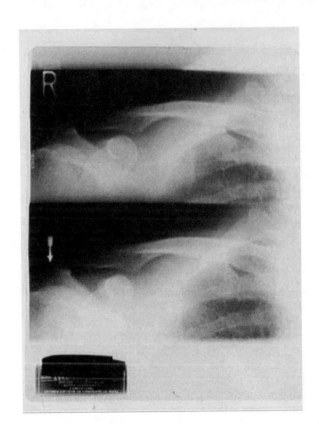

FIGURE 14.27
AC joint Zanca film.

Collimation

Soft tissue around distal clavicle and shoulder

Breathing Instructions

Full inspiration

Image Critique

Clear view of AC joint and acromion space. Must not be overexposed.

Optimium kVp

70 kVp

14.15   Shoulder: A-P Scapula

Measure

A-P at coracoid process

Protection

Lead apron

SID

40 in. using Bucky

Tube Angulation

None

Film

12 in. × 10 in. regular speed rare-earth cassette with I.D. toward spine

Marker

Anatomical

Positioning

1. Patient stands in front of Bucky, facing tube.
2. Patient rotated about 15° until the scapula is parallel to film.
3. Horizontal central ray is placed 1 in. below and 1 in. medial to the coracoid process. Film is centered to horizontal central ray.
4. Vertical central ray is placed 1 in. inferior to coracoid process.
5. Patient may leave arm in neutral position.
6. Patient is instructed to hold breath and stand still. Exposure made.

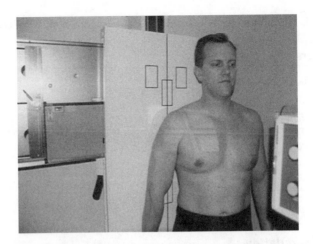

FIGURE 14.28
Scapula A-P positioning.

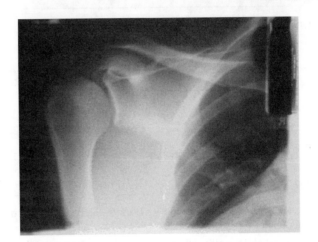

FIGURE 14.29
Scapula A-P film.

Collimation

Soft tissue of shoulder, or slightly less than film size

Breathing Instructions

Suspend respiration

Image Critique

Glenohumeral joint space and the entire scapula should be seen on the film. The soft tissue around shoulder should be seen. Variations of this view include raising the arm over the patient's head to get the scapula clear of the ribs.

Optimum kVp

70 kVp

14.16   Shoulder: Lateral Scapula or Outlet

Measure

A-P at coracoid process

Protection

Lead apron

SID

40 in. using Bucky

Tube Angulation

15 to 30° caudal for outlet; 0 to 10° caudal for lateral scapula

Film

10 in. × 12 in. regular speed rare-earth cassette with I.D. up

Marker

Anatomical

Positioning

1. Patient stands in front of Bucky, facing Bucky. Align the humeral head of the affected shoulder with the center line of the Bucky.
2. Horizontal central ray is placed through the head of the humerus. Film is centered to horizontal central ray.
3. Position patient in a 60° anterior oblique or align the scapula perpendicular to film. Vertical central ray should be 1 in. medial to the body of the scapula.
4. Patient is instructed to take full inspiration. Exposure made.

Collimation

Soft tissue around distal clavicle and shoulder to include scapula, or slightly less than film size

Breathing Instructions

Full inspiration

Image Critique

Clear view of head of the humerus in the glenohumeral joint space or position of humerus in relation to the joint if dislocated. Subacromion space should be open and well visualized. Scapula should be in true lateral position. Film must not be overexposed.

Optimum kVp

70 kVp

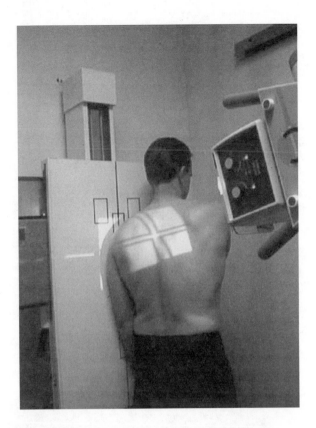

FIGURE 14.30
Lateral scapula/outlet positioning.

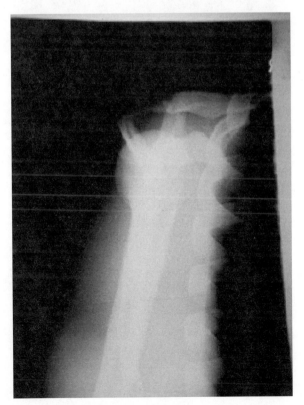

FIGURE 14.31
Lateral scapula/outlet film.

Chapter 15

Pelvis, Hip, and Femur Radiography

15.1 Pelvis, Hip, and Femur Radiography: Introduction

A-P Pelvis and Bilateral Hips View

The A-P view of the hips and pelvis is generally taken recumbent. Most modern wall Bucky units are only 14 in. wide. In order to see the pelvis, both hips, and the soft tissue of the hips, the film is placed 17 in. × 14 in. This can be done only on a table Bucky or with a stationary grid. The legs are internally rotated until the heels and toes touch. This will generally be about 15°.

Particularly with cases of recent trauma, it is important to have a clear view of the pubis. Hip pain after a fall may be the result of a fracture in the ischium or pubis. If gonad shields obscure the demonstration of this area, the view should be repeated. Great care must be taken in placement of the bell shield on male patients.

When the routine A-P pelvis demonstrates a potential for a pubic region fracture, a 30 to 35° cephalad tube angle can be used to better demonstrate the pubic bone, sacroiliac joints, sacrum, and ischial rami. This is referred to as Ferguson's view. Another modification of the A-P pelvis would be a 20° caudal tube angle. This will give a superior to inferior view of the ischium and pubic area. This is useful in determining the displacement of a fracture. Oblique views of the pelvis are also special pelvic views that may better evaluate the acetabulum. These specialized views are rarely taken and therefore mentioned only in this introduction.

A bilateral frog leg oblique view can also be taken. This is the routine lateral view for nontraumatic pain. The patient places the plantar surfaces of the feet together and knees are bent. The patient is then asked to laterally rotate both femurs as far as possible. The patient's pelvis and the film are not moved from the A-P view.

Unilateral Hip View

The unilateral hip can be taken recumbent or erect. The A-P view is centered in the same way, except the vertical central ray is moved to the acetabulum. The lower leg is internally rotated until the leg is in a true A-P position. The unilateral view must include the pubis and ischium of the affected side.

The positioning is exactly the same for the erect and recumbent A-P unilateral hip.

The lateral view should have the femur parallel to the film. The pelvis can be rotated to achieve the true lateral of the upper femur. Extra care must be taken with bell shield placement on the lateral hip with a rotated pelvis. The patient can place the foot of the affected side on a stool when taking this view erect.

Femur View

The femur is too long to get both proximal and distal joints on a single 7 in. × 17 in. or 14 in. × 17 in. film. The complete study must include both articulations. This author generally takes A-P and lateral hip views. The femur will be taken from the knee joint up.

The alternative is to take a film from the hip down and then take knee views to complete the study. The top of the film would be placed at the level of the ASIS for the A-P and lateral views from the hip down. The leg should not be bent for the lateral hip, but the pelvis should be rotated into a posterior oblique of the affected side.

15.2   A-P Pelvis and Hips

Measure

A-P at trochanter

Protection

Males, bell below symphysis; female, none

SID

40 in. using Table Bucky

Tube Angulation

None

Film

17 in. × 14 in. (or 43 cm × 35 cm) Lanex regular with I.D. up

Marker

Anatomical

Positioning

1. Have patient lie on back on table. Put bell belt on male patient before having patient lie down. Make sure tube is centered to Bucky after patient is on table.
2. Have patient internally rotate legs until toes touch.

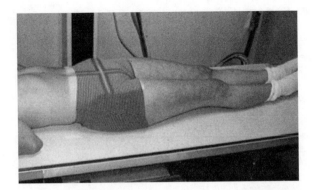

FIGURE 15.1
Pelvis A-P positioning.

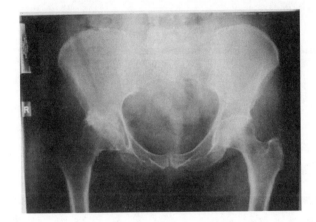

FIGURE 15.2
Pelvis A-P film.

3. Place horizontal central ray 1½ in. above the symphysis pubis. Center film to horizontal central ray.
4. Adjust patient position so the vertical central ray will be down the mid-sagittal plane.
5. Ask patient to suspend respiration. Take film.

Collimation

Top to Bottom: iliac crests to lesser trochanter, or slightly less than film size; Side to Side: film size.

Breathing Instructions

Full expiration

Image Critique

There should be no rotation of the pelvis. The hips will be in true A-P position. Must see all of the pelvis, including both iliac crests.

Optimum kVp

70–76 kVp

15.3   A-P Pelvis with Bilateral Frog Leg Hips

Measure

A-P at trochanter

Protection

Males, bell below symphysis; female, none

SID

40 in. using Table Bucky

Tube Angulation

None

Film

17 in. × 14 in. (or 43 cm × 35 cm) Lanex regular with I.D. up

Marker

Anatomical

Positioning

1.   Have patient lie on back on table. Put bell belt on male patient before having patient lie down. Make sure tube is centered to Bucky after patient is on table.
2.   Have patient bend knees and place heels together. Then externally rotate legs as far as possible.
3.   Place horizontal central ray 1½ in. above the symphysis pubis. Center film to horizontal central ray.
4.   Adjust patient position so the vertical central ray will be down the mid-sagittal plane.
5.   Ask patient to suspend respiration. Take film.

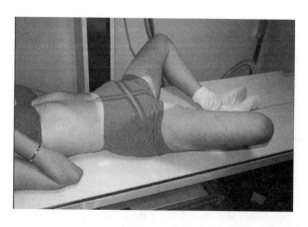

FIGURE 15.3
Pelvis A-P with bilateral frog leg hips positioning.

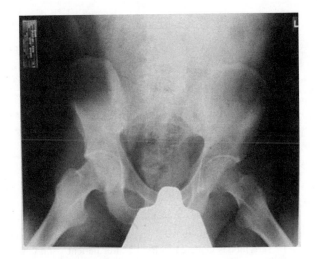

FIGURE 15.4
Pelvis A-P with frog leg hps film (Note poor placement of bell shield).

Collimation

Top to Bottom: iliac crests to lesser trochanter, or slightly less than film size; Side to Side: film size

Breathing Instruction

Full expiration

Image Critique

There should be no rotation of the pelvis. The hips will be in lateral position. There will be some foreshortening of the proximal femurs. Must see all of the pelvis, including both iliac crests.

Optimum kVp

70–76 kVp

15.4   A-P Hips

Measure

A-P at trochanter

Protection

Males, bell below symphysis; female, none

SID

40 in. using Table Bucky

Tube Angulation

None

Film

10 in. × 12 in. (or 24 cm × 30 cm) regular speed rare-earth cassette with I.D. up

Marker

Anatomical

Positioning

1. Have patient lie on back on table. Put bell belt on male patient before having patient lie down. Make sure tube is centered to Bucky after patient is on table.
2. Have patient internally rotate legs until toes touch.
3. Place horizontal central ray 1½ in. above the symphysis pubis. Center film to horizontal central ray.
4. Adjust patient position so the vertical central ray is 2 to 3 in. lateral to the mid-sagittal plane or through the acetabulum.
5. Ask patient to suspend respiration. Take film.

Collimation

Top to Bottom: iliac crests to lesser trochanter, or slightly less than film size; Side to Side: to include soft tissue of hip.

Breathing Instructions

Full expiration

Image Critique

There should be no rotation of the pelvis. The hip will be in true A-P position. The gonad shielding must not obscure the symphysis pubis. The pubis of the affected side must be on the film.

Optimum kVp

70–76 kVp

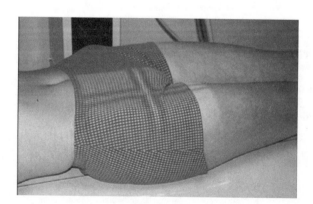

FIGURE 15.5
Hip A-P positioning.

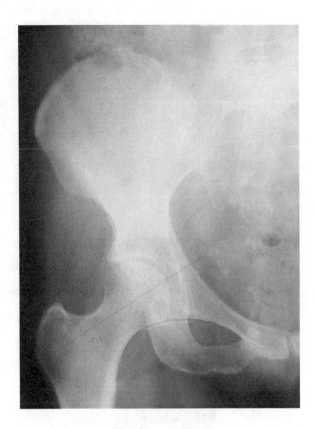

FIGURE 15.6
Hip A-P film.

15.5 Frog Leg Lateral Hip

Measure

A-P at trochanter

Protection

Males, bell below symphysis; female, none

SID

40 in. using Table Bucky

Tube Angulation

None

Film

10 in. × 12 in. (or 24 cm × 30 cm) regular speed rare-earth cassette with I.D. up

Marker

Anatomical

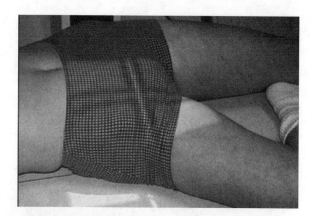

FIGURE 15.7
Hip lateral positioning.

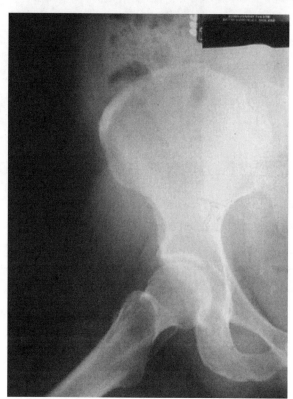

FIGURE 15.8
Hip lateral film.

Positioning

1. Have patient lie on back on table. Put bell belt on male patient before having patient lie down. Make sure tube is centered to Bucky after patient is on table.

2. Have patient externally rotate leg and put foot behind knee of unaffected leg. This will look like a figure "4." Oblique patient if necessary to get the femur parallel to the film.

3. Place horizontal central ray 1½ in. above the symphysis pubis. Center film to horizontal central ray.

4. Adjust patient position so the vertical central ray is 2 to 3 in. lateral to the mid-sagittal plane or through the acetabulum.

5. Ask patient to suspend respiration. Take film.

Collimation

Top to Bottom: iliac crests to lesser trochanter, or slightly less than film size; Side to Side: to include soft tissue of hip.

Breathing Instructions

Full expiration

Image Critique

The hip should be in true lateral position and the acetabulum will be clearly demonstrated. Obliquity of the pelvis is preferred to foreshortening of the proximal femur.

Optimum kVp

70–76 kVp

15.6   A-P Lower Femur

Measure

A-P at mid-thigh

Protection

Males, Bell below symphysis; females, apron on abdomen

SID

40 in. using Table Bucky

Tube Angulation

None

Film

7 in. × 17 in. regular speed rare-earth cassette with I.D. up

Marker

Anatomical

Positioning

1. Have patient lie on back on table. Put bell belt on male patient before having patient lie down. Make sure tube is centered to Bucky after patient is on table.

2. Align the long axis of the femur with the center line of the table. Have patient internally rotate leg until the condyles are parallel to film. This is usually about 15°.

3. Place bottom of film 2 in. below the condyles. Center the horizontal central ray to the film.

4. Ask patient to suspend respiration. Take film.

5. If hip joint is not on film, take A-P hip view.

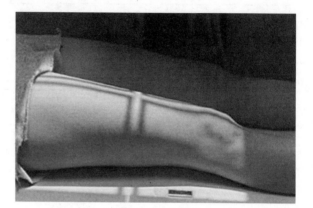

FIGURE 15.9
Femur A-P positioning.

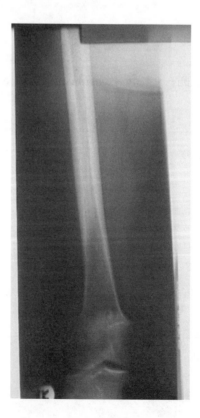

FIGURE 15.10
Femur A-P film.

Collimation

Top to Bottom: knee articulation to hip; Side to Side: to include soft tissue of femur.

Breathing Instructions

Suspend respiration and hold still

Image Critique

The exam must include both articulations. If hip is not seen, take A-P hip view. There should be no rotation of femur. For most patients, a separate hip film will be needed. A film can be taken from hip down with top of film placed at level of ASIS.

Optimum kVp

70–76 kVp

15.7   Lateral Lower Femur

Measure

A-P at mid-thigh

Protection

Males, bell below symphysis; female, apron on abdomen

SID

40 in. using Table Bucky

Tube Angulation

None

Film

7 in. × 17 in. regular speed rare-earth cassette with I.D. up

Marker

Anatomical

Positioning

1. Have patient lie on affected side on table. Have patient bend unaffected leg 90° to get it clear of the affected femur. Make sure tube is centered to Bucky after patient is on table.
2. Align the long axis of the femur with the center line of the table. Have patient internally rotate leg until the condyles are perpendicular to film. Have patient bend knee 45°.

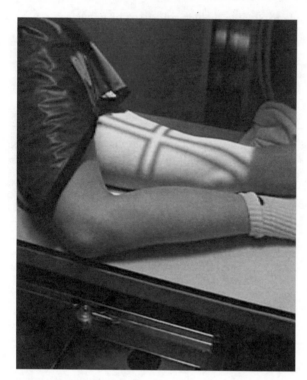

FIGURE 15.11
Femur lateral positioning.

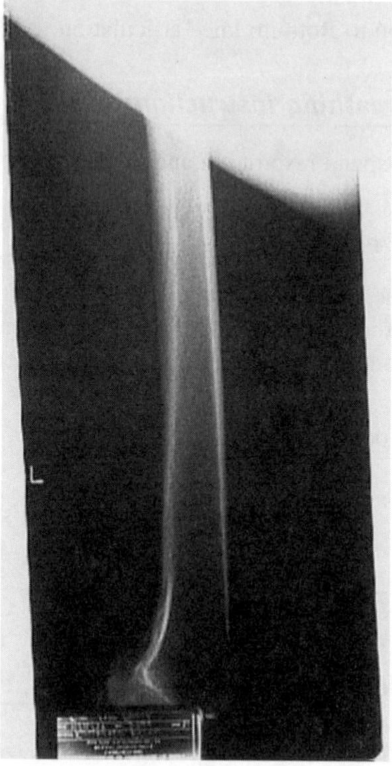

FIGURE 15.12
Femur lateral film.

3. Place bottom of film 2 in. below the condyles. Center the horizontal central ray to the film.
4. Ask patient to suspend respiration. Take film.

Collimation

Top to Bottom: knee articulation to hip, or slightly less than film size; Side to Side: to include soft tissue of femur.

Breathing Instructions

Full expiration

Image Critique

The exam must include knee articulation. Femur condyles should be superimposed. The hip will not be seen. If the hip is the joint closest to the pathology, put top of film at ASIS and do not cross unaffected leg over femur. Have patient in a slightly oblique position to make it more comfortable for the patient to have the femur in lateral position. If film is taken from hip down, gonad shielding should be omitted.

Optimum kVp

70–76 kVp

Chapter 16

Knee and Patella Radiography

16.1 Knee and Patella Radiography: Introduction

Knee Radiography

Adult knee films are generally taken using the Bucky. The bone density of the distal femur generally makes too much scatter radiation for non-grid films. The A-P, oblique, and lateral views can be easily taken upright or recumbent. A 5° cephalad tube angulation is used for all A-P and oblique views. This tube angulation helps to open the joint space. The A-P and oblique views will demonstrate the distal femur and femoral condyles, proximal tibia and tibia plateaus, tibial spines, medial and lateral joint compartments, and the fibular head. The oblique views are less frequently taken. The lateral oblique will demonstrate the medial condyle in profile. The medial oblique will demonstrate the lateral condyle in profile and provide a clear view of the head of the fibula.

The recumbent lateral view of the knee is improved by using a 5° cephalad tube angulation. For this to work, the long axis of the femur should be centered to the table. The tube angle compensates for the taper of the thigh. The knee should be bent 45°. The tube angle will generally not help improve the view on erect views because the only way to get the long axis of the femur aligned vertically with the Bucky is to have the patient stand with no flexion and place all weight on the injured knee. Generally, a stepstool is used as a platform for the patient to rest the foot on the affected side. The flexion of the knee may approach 90°. The long axis of the lower leg should be parallel to the wall Bucky to get the knee in a true lateral position.

The advantage of erect radiography of the knee is the visualization of the joint space weight-bearing. The effects of weight-bearing will help determine the loss of cartilage in the knee. The typical study for this purpose is a limited A-P and lateral view. The A-P view can be taken bilateral using a 7 in. × 17 in. cassette.

The tunnel or Camp Coventry view can also be taken upright or recumbent. This view is useful when looking for loose bodies in the knee. The intercondylar notch and intercondylar eminences of the tibia are demonstrated with the tunnel view. It is much easier to take the view recumbent. To do the view erect, the affected foot would be placed on a stool or stack of books to achieve more than 30° of flexion with the patient standing P-A. The lower leg would be positioned as close to the Bucky as possible. Try to picture the patient on their hands and knees recumbent. This would be the basic position erect.

Patella Radiography

When the body part is as close to the film as possible, one obtains better detail. This is very true with the patella. The frontal projection of the patella is taken P-A. The Bucky is used to reduce scatter radiation. The patella will be much less magnified using the P-A view.

The lateral views are taken non-grid using detail or extremity cassettes. The lateral patella view is different from the lateral knee view. The knee flexion is limited to only 10 to 15°. The central ray is centered to the patella.

The Settegast or sunrise view is an axial view of the patella. The success of this view is limited by the amount of flexion the patient can tolerate. A belt or strap placed around the ankle and held by the patient will help the patient hold the flexion that he/she can tolerate. Because the knee flexion is usually greater than 100°, the sunrise view cannot be used to evaluate subluxation or patella tracking problems.

Patella Subluxation Views

Anterior knee pain and the potential for patellofemoral joint instability are common complaints from patients with knee pain. The routine sunrise or Settegast view will reduce any subluxation of the patella resulting in a false negative X-ray.

Merchant's axial or Lauren axial views are used to demonstrate subluxation of the patella. The Lauren views can be taken with a table or chair for the patient to sit on and hang the knees off the edge. The central ray is directed inferior to superior, perpendicular to the long axis of the patella. The tube direction significantly increases the level of radiation exposure. This view requires the patient to be relatively slender. The knee is flexed 30°, 60°, and occasionally 90°, with bilateral views taken at each position. The Lauren view will yield an accurate and undistorted view of the patellofemoral joint with varied degrees of knee flexion. This allows evaluation of the joint as the patella travels through the range of motion. The Merchant view requires the use of a special film holder. The holder will help produce accurate undistorted images with varied knee flexion. The central ray is directed superior to inferior. This significantly reduces the radiation exposure. The Merchant view will generally be more accurate as it is easier to position, but the film holder/jig should be purchased from Dr. Merchant.

16.2   A-P Knee

Measure

A-P at patella

Protection

Recumbent: apron; upright: bell for males, apron held high for females

SID

40 in. using Bucky

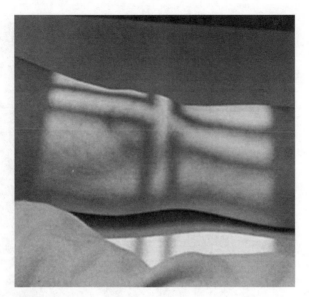

FIGURE 16.1
Knee A-P positioning.

Tube Angulation

5° cephalad

Film

8 in. × 10 in. regular speed rare-earth cassette with I.D. up

Positioning

1. Patient standing, facing tube; or supine on table. Center the long axis of femur with the center line of the Bucky.
2. Have patient internally rotate leg 15° or until the condyles are parallel to film.
3. Place horizontal central ray 1 cm distal to the apex of the patella. Center film to horizontal central ray.
4. Vertical central ray will be centered to mid-sagittal plane or long axis of femur.
5. Have patient remain still. Make exposure.

Collimation

Top to Bottom: slightly less than film size; Side to Side: soft tissue of distal femur.

Breathing Instructions

Remain still

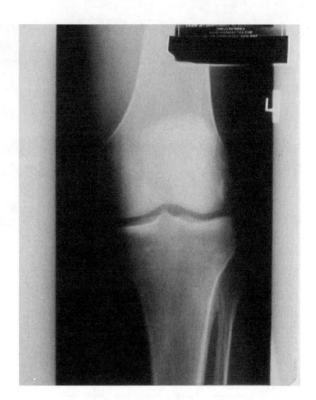

FIGURE 16.2
Knee A-P film.

Image Critique

The joint space should be open. The patella should be mid-line to the distal femur. The soft tissue structures adjacent to the knee will be seen.

Optimum kVp

70 kVp

16.3   Medial Oblique Knee

Measure

A-P at patella

Protection

Recumbent: apron. Upright: bell for males, apron high for females.

SID

40 in. using Bucky

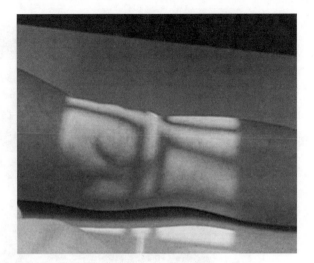

FIGURE 16.3
Knee medial oblique positioning.

Tube Angulation

5° cephalad

Film

8 in. × 10 in. Lanex regular with I.D. up

Positioning

1. Patient standing, facing tube; or supine on table. Center the long axis of femur with the center line of the Bucky.
2. Have patient internally rotate leg until the condyles are 40 to 45° to the film.
3. Place horizontal central ray 2 cm distal to the medial condyle. Center film to horizontal central ray.
4. Vertical central ray will be centered to the long axis of femur.
5. Have patient remain still. Make exposure.

Collimation

Top to Bottom: Slightly less than film size; Side to Side: soft tissue of distal femur.

Breathing Instructions

Remain still

Image Critique

The fibular head will be seen clear of the tibia. The lateral femoral condyle will be seen in profile. The femoral-fibular joint space will be open. The soft tissue structures adjacent to the knee will

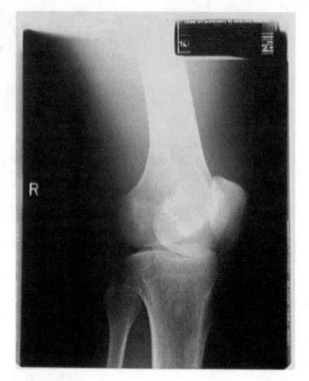

FIGURE 16.4
Knee medial oblique film (phantom).

be seen. Be careful and watch the object to film distance. It will almost always be less of a problem with the patient recumbent.

Optimum kVp

70 kVp

16.4   Lateral Oblique Knee

Measure

A-P at patella

Protection

Recumbent: apron. Upright: bell for males, apron high for females.

SID

40 in. using Bucky

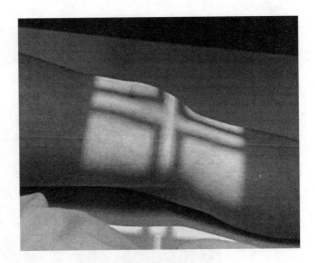

FIGURE 16.5
Knee lateral oblique positioning.

Tube Angulation

5° cephalad

Film

8 in. × 10 in. Lanex regular with I.D. up

Positioning

1. Patient standing, facing tube; or supine on table. Center the long axis of femur with the center line of the Bucky.
2. Have patient externally rotate leg until the condyles are 40 to 45° to the film.
3. Place horizontal central ray 2 cm distal to the medial condyle. Center film to horizontal central ray.
4. Vertical central ray will be centered to the long axis of femur.
5. Have patient remain still. Make exposure.

Collimation

Top to Bottom: slightly less than film size; Side to Side: soft tissue of distal femur.

Breathing Instructions

Remain still

Image Critique

The medial femoral condyle will be seen in profile. The femoral-fibular joint space will be open. The fibular head, neck, and shaft will be superimposed by the tibia. The fibular head will align with the anterior edge of the tibia. The soft tissue structures adjacent to the knee will be seen. Be

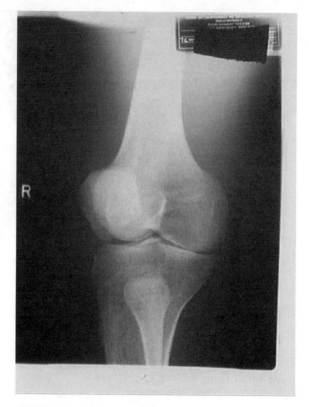

FIGURE 16.6
Knee lateral oblique film (phantom).

careful and watch the object to film distance. It will almost always be less of a problem with the patient recumbent.

Optimum kVp

70 kVp

16.5   Lateral Knee

Measure

Lateral through condyles

Protection

Recumbent: apron. Upright: bell for males, apron high for females.

SID

40 in. using Bucky

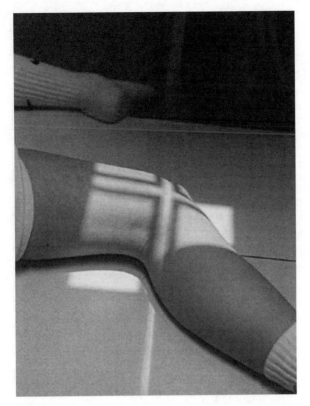

FIGURE 16.7
Knee lateral positioning.

Tube Angulation

5° cephalad

Film

8 in. × 10 in. regular speed rare-earth cassette I.D. up

Positioning

1. Patient standing with affected knee next to Bucky and foot resting on stool; or recumbent on table lying on affected side. Center the long axis of femur with the center line of the Bucky on the table.

2. The unaffected leg is brought over and in front of the affected knee with the patient recumbent. Align the long axis of femur parallel to vertical central ray. For erect film, have patient rest affected foot on stool.

3. Have patient bend knee 45° and place horizontal central ray 1 cm distal to the medial condyle. Center film to horizontal central ray.

4. Vertical central ray will be centered to the long axis of the tibia erect and long axis of femur recumbent.

5. Have patient remain still. Make exposure.

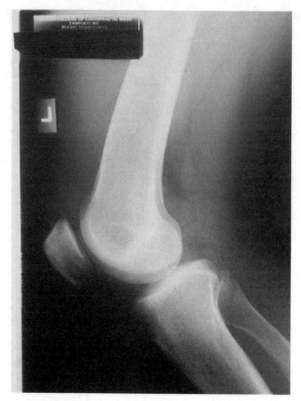

FIGURE 16.8
Knee lateral film.

Collimation

Top to Bottom: to include distal femur, patella, and proximal tibia, or slightly less than film size; Side to Side: soft tissue of distal femur and patella.

Breathing Instructions

Remain still

Image Critique

The joint space should be open. The condyles should be superimposed. The soft tissue structures adjacent to the knee will be seen.

Optimum kVp

70 kVp

16.6   Camp-Coventry or Tunnel View of Knee

Measure

A-P at patella

Protection

Lead apron

SID

40 in. using Bucky

Tube Angulation

30 to 40° caudal

Film

8 in. × 10 in. Lanex regular with I.D. up

Marker

Anatomical pronated

Positioning

1.   Patient standing, facing Bucky; or prone on table. Center the long axis of femur with the center line of the Bucky.
2.   Have patient internally rotate leg 15° or until the condyles are parallel to film.
3.   Patient bends knee until the long axis of the tibia and fibula is perpendicular to central ray. A sponge or stool can be used for support.
4.   Place horizontal central ray through the intercondylar fossa. Center film to horizontal central ray.
5.   Vertical central ray will be centered to mid-sagittal plane or long axis of femur.
6.   Have patient remain still. Make exposure.

Collimation

Top to Bottom: slightly less than film size; Side to Side: soft tissue of distal femur.

Breathing Instructions

Remain still

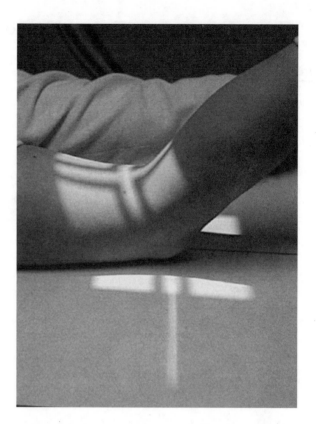

FIGURE 16.9
Knee tunnel positioning.

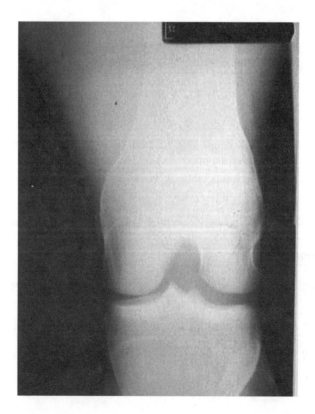

FIGURE 16.10
Knee tunnel film.

Image Critique

The joint space should be open. The intercondylar fossa will be open and its proximal and lateral surfaces demonstrated free of rotation. The intercondylar eminence will be seen. The soft tissue structures adjacent to the knee will be seen.

Optimum kVp

70 kVp

16.7   Bilateral A-P Knees Weight-Bearing

Measure

A-P at patella

Protection

Upright: bell for males, apron high for females

SID

40 in. using Bucky

Tube Angulation

5° cephalad

Film

17 in. × 14 in. or 17 in. × 7 in. regular speed rare-earth cassette with I.D. up or away from the affected knee

Positioning

1. Patient standing, facing tube. Center the long axis of femurs equidistant from the center line of the Bucky.
2. Have patient internally rotate legs 15° or until the condyles are parallel to film. The heels and toes should be touching.
3. Place horizontal central ray 1 cm distal to the apex of the patella. Center film to horizontal central ray.
4. Vertical central ray will be centered to mid-sagittal plane or long axis of femur.
5. Have patient remain still. Make exposure.

Collimation

Top to Bottom: slightly less than film size; Side to Side: soft tissue of both distal femurs.

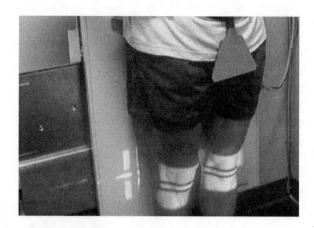

FIGURE 16.11
Knees bilateral A-P positioning.

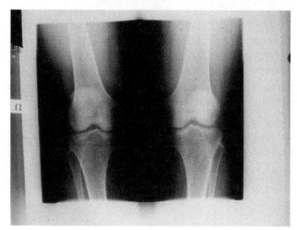

FIGURE 16.12
Knees bilateral A-P film.

Breathing Instructions

Remain still

Image Critique

The joint space should be open. The patellas should be mid-line to the distal femurs. The soft tissue structures adjacent to the knee will be seen. Make sure the patient does not lean on Bucky or grid cut-off will result. If Bucky is not perfectly aligned to tube, grid cut-off will be seen as one knee being more dense than the other. This can be noted on the example comparing the right knee density to that of the left knee.

Optimum kVp

70 kVp

16.8   P-A Patella

Measure

A-P at patella

Protection

Lead apron

SID

40 in. using Bucky

Tube Angulation

5° cephalad

Film

8 in. × 10 in. regular speed rare-earth cassette with I.D. up

Positioning

1. Patient stands facing Bucky, or prone on table. Center long axis of femur with center line of Bucky.
2. Have patient internally rotate leg 15° or until the condyles are parallel to film.
3. Center the horizontal central ray to the patella. Center film to horizontal central ray.
4. Vertical central ray will be centered to the mid-sagittal plane or long axis of femur.
5. Have patient remain still. Make exposure.

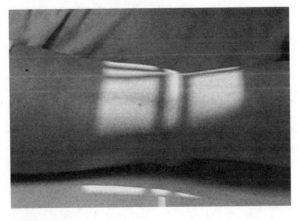

FIGURE 16.13
Patella P-A positioning.

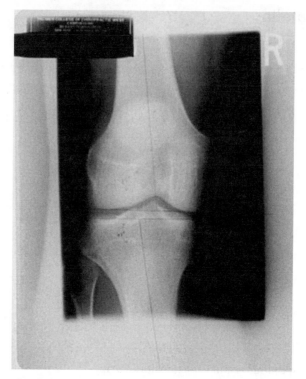

FIGURE 16.14
Patella P-A film.

Collimation

Top to Bottom: 5 in., or to include patella; Side to Side: soft tissue of patellal femur.

Breathing Instructions

Remain still

Image Critique

The joint space should be open. The patella should be mid-line to the distal femur. The soft tissue structures adjacent to the knee will be seen.

Optimum kVp

70 kVp

16.9   Lateral Patella

Measure

Lateral at condyles

Protection

Lead apron

SID

40 in. using Non-Bucky

Tube Angulation

5° cephalad

Film

8 in. × 10 in. Fine (extremity) cassette with I.D. up

Positioning

1.   Patient lies on the affected side. The knee is flexed about 10 to 15°. Center the long axis of femur with the center line of the Bucky.
2.   Slide the film under the affected knee. Center the horizontal central ray to the patella.

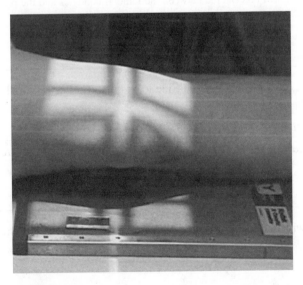

FIGURE 16.15
Patella lateral positioning.

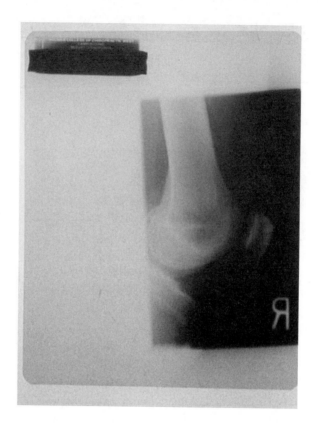

FIGURE 16.16
Patella lateral film.

3. Center film to horizontal central ray.
4. Vertical central ray will be centered between the femoral condyles and the patella.
5. Have patient remain still. Make exposure.

Collimation

Top to Bottom: 5 in., or to include patella; Side to Side: soft tissue of patellal femur.

Breathing Instructions

Remain still

Image Critique

The lateral patella will provide a true lateral view of the patella. The distal femur will appear underexposed.

Optimum kVp

60 kVp

16.10   Settegast or Sunrise View of Patella

Measure

A-P at patella

Protection

Lead apron

SID

40 in. using Non-Bucky

Tube Angulation

20° cephalad

Film

8 in. × 10 in. Lanex Fine (extremity) cassette with I.D. up

Marker

Anatomical pronated

Positioning

1.   Patient lies face-down on table. Center the long axis of femur with the center line of the Bucky.
2.   Have patient internally rotate leg 15° or until the condyles are parallel to film.

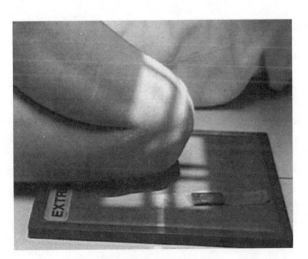

FIGURE 16.17
Patella sunrise positioning.

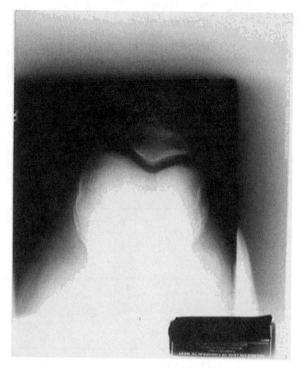

FIGURE 16.18
Patella sunrise film.

3.　Patient bends knee back 110° or as far as possible. Place extremity cassette under knee.
4.　Place horizontal central ray through the patella-femoral joint space. Center film to horizontal central ray.
5.　Vertical central ray will be centered to mid-sagittal plane or long axis of femur.
6.　Have patient remain still. Make exposure.

Collimation

Top to Bottom: slightly less than film size; Side to Side: soft tissue of distal femur.

Breathing Instructions

Remain still

Image Critique

The ability of the patient to hold knee in maximum flexion is key to the view. A strap placed around the lower leg and given to the patient to hold may help patient hold the position for a longer period of time. The patella will be projected superior to the femoral condyles. The joint space should be open. The soft tissue structures adjacent to the knee will be seen.

Optimum kVp

70 kVp

16.11   Lauren Views of Interpatella Fossa

Measure

A-P at patella

Protection

None

SID

60 in. using Non-Bucky

Tube Anglulation

1.   Knee flexed 30°; tube angle is 30° cephalad;
2.   Knee flexed 60°; tube angle is 45° cephalad;
3.   Knee flexed 90°; tube angle is 45° cephalad.

Film

17 in. × 7 in. regular speed rare-earth cassette with I.D. toward the unaffected side.

Positioning

1.   Patient is seated on a table with legs hanging over the edge of the table.
2.   Patient's thighs and lower legs are strapped together to prevent external rotation of the limbs.
3.   Have patient flex limbs until the knee forms a 30° angle. The tube is angled 30° cephalad or 120°. The patient will hold the film perpendicular to the beam.
4.   The horizontal central ray is directed through patellofemoral joints. The vertical central ray is through the mid-sagittal plane. The patient holds the film perpendicular to the horizontal central ray.
5.   Repeat view at 45° and 60° of knee flexion.

Collimation

Slightly less than film size

Image Critique

Both patellofemoral joints should be seen on the films at all three levels of knee flexion. It is very important that the femurs and lower legs be strapped together to avoid external femur rotation, which can lead to a misdiagnosis of a low lateral condyle. Knee flexion greater than 60° will reduce an otherwise subluxed patella and distort the actual depth of the sulcus. The Settegast view is of little use in the evaluation of the extensor mechanics of the knee or anterior knee pain.

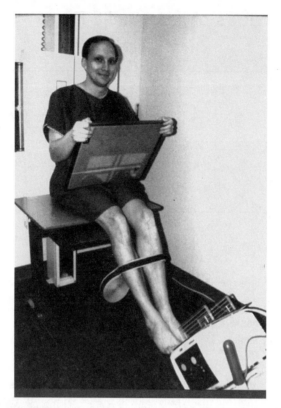

FIGURE 16.19
Laurin view positioning.

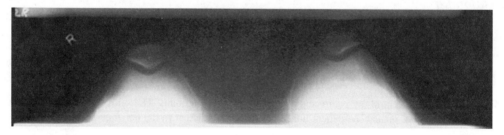

FIGURE 16.20
Laurin view film.

Chapter 17

Lower Leg and Ankle Radiography

17.1 Lower Leg and Ankle Radiography: Introduction

Tibia/Fibula Radiography

The tibia/fibula or lower leg views are generally limited to A-P and lateral views. These views are taken on a regular speed rare-earth cassette. The views are taken tabletop. The lower leg can be a challenge to fit both proximal and distal articulations on the same film. With tall patients, the lower leg is positioned diagonally on a 14 in. × 17 in. regular speed rare-earth cassette. For a shorter person, the study can be done on 7 in. × 17 in. cassettes, or both the A-P and lateral on a single 14 in. × 17 in. cassette.

Tibial fractures are generally caused by rotational or torsional forces common in skiing. These forces will generally produce a spiral fracture. Better binding release systems have reduced the number of spiral fractures. Bending forces can produce transverse or oblique fractures, referred to as "boot-top" fractures. In skiing, a fall forward with the ski fixed can cause a transverse fracture. Football can also produce lower leg fractures.

Ankle Radiography

The ankle is the most commonly injured weight-bearing joint in the athlete who engages in running, skiing, basketball, and/or gymnastics. Most (85%) injuries are inversion sprains. The less-frequent eversion sprain can also result in an avulsion of the medial malleolus. The Achilles tendon rupture results from a sudden contraction of the gastrocnemius and soleus muscles; for example, in pushing off with the knee extended or forced dorsi flexion as in landing from a jump. Ankle fractures are classified by anatomical location: unimalleolar, bimalleolar, or trimalleolar. They result from inversion, eversion, or a combination of both. A common nonathletic source of severe ankle fractures are platform shoes.

The routine study of the ankle consists of the A-P view, an oblique view, and a lateral view. All views need to be taken with plantar flexion sufficient to have the plantar surface of the foot perpendicular to the lower leg. This will help open the talotibial joint space.

Two basic oblique views are routinely taken. Both are internal oblique views. One is more a variant of the A-P projection; it uses only 10 to 15° of internal rotation. The ankle will be in the proper position when the medial and lateral malleoli are parallel to the film. It is called the Mortise view because it opens the mortise joint of the ankle and eliminates any overlap of the medial aspect of the distal fibula and the lateral aspect of the talus.

The other routine oblique view is the 30 to 45° of internal oblique view. This view will demonstrate the tibiofibular and talofibular joints. This view is more difficult because the patient must internally rotate the affected leg to a significant extent. The external rotation oblique view is rarely taken to evaluate the lateral malleolus or the anterior tibial tubercle.

The lateral view must be taken with the entire lower leg in a lateral position. The properly positioned lateral view will clearly demonstrate the anterior aspect of the distal tibia and the posterior lip of the tibia, the third malleolus. The view also shows the talotibial joint space and the calcaneus.

17.2   A-P Lower Leg

Measure

A-P at mid-lower leg

Protection

Lead apron

SID

40 in. using Non-Bucky

Tube Angulation

None

Film

7 in. × 17 in. regular with I.D. down

Marker

Anatomical

Positioning

1. Have patient lie on back on table.
2. Align the long axis of the lower leg with the center line of the table. Have patient internally rotate leg until the condyles are parallel to film. This is usually about 15°.
3. Place top of film 2 in. above the condyles. Make sure that the ankle joint is also on the film. Center the horizontal central ray to the film.
4. The vertical central ray should align with the long axis of the lower leg.
5. Ask patient to hold still. Take film.

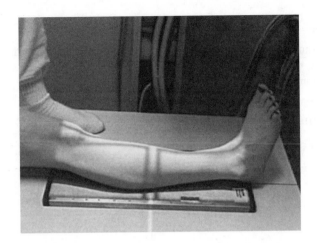

FIGURE 17.1
Lower leg A-P positioning.

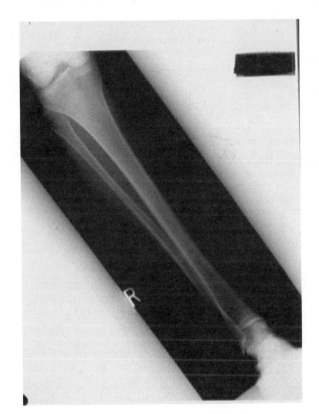

FIGURE 17.2
Lower leg A-P film.

Collimation

Top to Bottom: knee articulation to ankle; Side to Side: to include soft tissue of lower leg.

Breathing Instructions

Hold still

Image Critique

The exam must include both articulations. Since the film is done Non-Bucky, a 14 in. × 17 in. cassette can be turned diagonally to get both joints on the film for tall patients. Both knee and ankle joints should be open and free of rotation.

Optimum kVp

60–70 kVp

17.3   Lateral Lower Leg

Measure

A-P at mid-lower leg

Protection

Lead apron

SID

40 in. using Non-Bucky

Tube Angulation

None

Film

7 in. × 17 in. regular speed rare-earth with I.D. down, or 14 in. × 17 in. cassette with I.D. up

Marker

Anatomical

Positioning

1. Have patient lie on affected side on table.
2. Align the long axis of the lower leg with the center line of the table, with the knee slightly flexed. Rotate leg until the condyles are perpendicular to film. The ankle should also be in a true lateral position.
3. Place top of film 2 in. above the condyles. Make sure that the ankle joint is also on the film. Center the horizontal central ray to the film.
4. The vertical central ray should align with the long axis of the lower leg.
5. Ask patient to hold still. Take film.

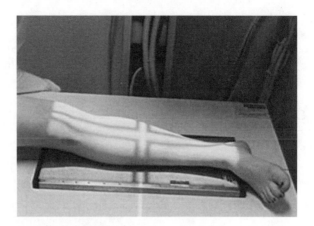

FIGURE 17.3
Lower leg lateral positioning.

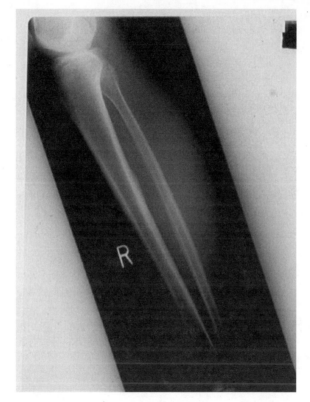

FIGURE 17.4
Lower leg lateral film.

Collimation

Top to Bottom: knee articulation to ankle; Side to Side: to include soft tissue of lower leg.

Breathing Instructions

Hold still

Image Critique

The exam must include both articulations. Since the film is done Non-Bucky, a 14 in. × 17 in. cassette can be turned diagonally to get both joints on the film for tall patients. Both knee and ankle joints should be open and free of rotation.

Optimum kVp

60–70 kVp

17.4   A-P Ankle

Measure

A-P at malleoli

Protection

Lead apron

SID

40 in. using Non-Bucky

Tube Angulation

None

Film

One half of 30 cm × 24 cm or 12 in. × 10 in. Fine (extremity) cassette with I.D. up

Marker

Anatomical

Positioning

1. Have patient lie on back on table.
2. Align the long axis of the lower leg with the center line of the table. Have patient internally rotate leg until the condyles are parallel to film. This is usually about 15°. Have patient dorsiflex the ankle until the plantar surface is perpendicular to the film.
3. Place the horizontal central ray at the level of the malleoli. Center the film to the horizontal central ray.
4. The vertical central ray should align with the long axis of the lower leg.
5. Ask patient to hold still. Take film.

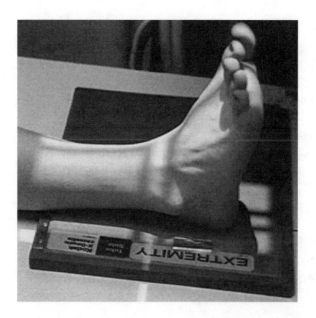

FIGURE 17.5
Ankle A-P positioning.

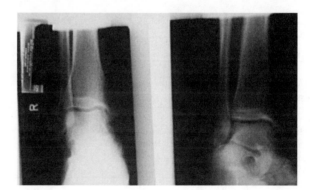

FIGURE 17.6
Ankle A-P and oblique films.

Collimation

Top to Bottom: distal fibula to soft tissue below calcaneus; Side to Side: to include soft tissue of lower leg.

Breathing Instruction

Hold still

Image Critique

The ankle should be seen with no rotation, as evidenced by the medial mortise joint being open. The foot should be perpendicular to the fibula. The talotibular joint must be open.

Optimum kVp

70–76 kVp

17.5   Oblique Ankle

Measure

A-P at malleoli

Protection

Lead apron

SID

40 in. using Non-Bucky

Tube Angulation

None

Film

One half of 30 cm × 24 cm or 12 in. × 10 in. Fine (extremity) cassette with I.D. up

Marker

Anatomical

Positioning

1.   Have patient lie on back on table.
2.   Align the long axis of the lower leg with the center line of the table. Have patient internally rotate leg until the long axis of the foot is 45° to film. Have patient dorsiflex the ankle until the plantar surface is perpendicular to the film. The vertical axis of the foot is 90° to the lower leg and film.
3.   Place the horizontal central ray at the level of the malleoli. Center the film to the horizontal central ray.
4.   The vertical central ray should align with the long axis of the lower leg.
5.   Ask patient to hold still. Take film.

Collimation

Top to Bottom: distal fibula to soft tissue below calcaneus; Side to Side: to include soft tissue of lower leg.

Breathing Instructions

Hold still

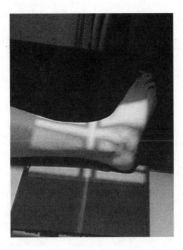

FIGURE 17.7
Ankle oblique positioning. (Image 45° oblique usually taken on same film as the A-P)

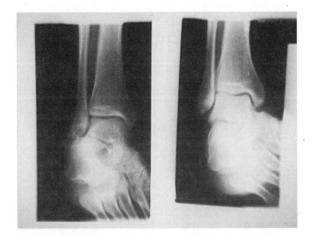

FIGURE 17.8
Ankle oblique and mortise films.

Image Critique

The lateral malleolus ankle should be seen clear of the talus. The medial mortise joint may be open. The foot should be perpendicular to the fibula. The talotibular joint must be open. The tarsal sinus will be open. The calcaneus will be seen in the collimated field.

Optimum kVp

70–76 kVp

17.6   Mortise View of Ankle

Measure

A-P at malleoli

Protection

Lead apron

SID

40 in. using Non-Bucky

Tube Angulation

None

Film

One half of 30 cm × 24 cm or 12 in. × 10 in. Fine (extremity) cassette with I.D. up

Marker

Anatomical

Positioning

1. Have patient lie on back on table.
2. Align the long axis of the lower leg with the center line of the table. Have patient internally rotate leg until the medial and lateral malleoli are parallel to the film. Have patient dorsiflex the ankle until the plantar surface is perpendicular to the film. The angle of the ankle will be about 15 to 20° medial from A-P. The vertical axis of the foot is 90° to the lower leg and film.
3. Place the horizontal central ray at the level of the malleoli. Center the film to the horizontal central ray.
4. The vertical central ray should align with the long axis of the lower leg.
5. Ask patient to hold still. Take film.

Collimation

Top to Bottom: distal fibula to soft tissue below calcaneus; Side to Side: to include soft tissue of lower leg.

Breathing Instructions

Hold still

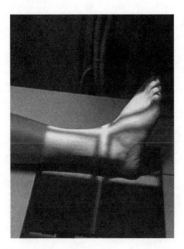

FIGURE 17.9
Ankle mortise positioning.

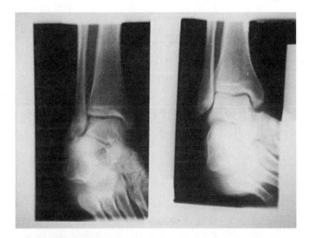

FIGURE 17.10
Ankle oblique and mortise films.

Image Critique

The lateral malleolus ankle should be seen clear of the talus. The medial mortise joint will be open. The foot should be perpendicular to the fibula. The talotibular joint must be open. The calcaneus will be seen in the collimated field.

Optimum kVp

70–76 kVp

17.7   Lateral Ankle

Measure

Lateral at malleoli

Protection

Lead apron

SID

40 in. using Non-Bucky

Tube Angulation

None

Film

8 in. × 10 in. Fine (extremity) cassette with I.D. up

Marker

Anatomical

Positioning

1. Have patient lie on affected side on table.
2. Align the long axis of the lower leg with the center line of the table, with the knee slightly flexed. Rotate leg until the malleoli are perpendicular to the film. The foot should also be in a true lateral position.

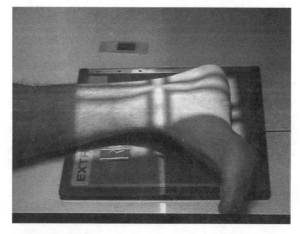

FIGURE 17.11
Ankle lateral positioning.

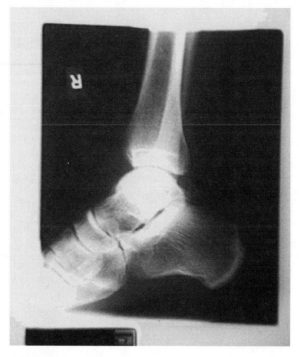

FIGURE 17.12
Ankle lateral film.

3. Place horizontal central ray on the medial malleolus. Center the film to the horizontal central ray.
4. The vertical central ray should align with the long axis of the lower leg.
5. Ask patient to hold still. Take film.

Collimation

Top to Bottom: distal tibia to soft tissue below calcaneus; Side to Side: to include soft tissue of calcaneus.

Breathing Instructions

Hold still

Image Critique

The exam must include the distal tibia, talus, and calcaneus. The talus domes will be superimposed. The distal fibula will overlie the posterior fibula. The talotibial joint space will be open.

Optimum kVp

60–66 kVp

18

Calcaneus, Foot, and Toe Radiography

18.1 Calcaneus, Foot, and Toe Radiography: Introduction

Calcaneus Radiography

Calcaneus fractures are generally the result of falls from heights that result in compressive force to the calcaneus. Parachuting and pole vaulting can cause these fractures. About 60% of tarsal bone injuries are calcaneus fractures. The fractures are categorized by involvement of the subtalar joint (75%) and not involving the subtalar joint. Patients with calcaneus fractures should also be evaluated for compression fractures in the thoracolumbar region. Stress fractures are common in runners and typically are not seen on radiographs. While not a traumatic fracture, plantar fascitis or heel spurs are common overuse injuries.

The views of the calcaneus are totally different from foot radiographs. If a heel injury or condition is suspected, heel or calcaneal views should be taken. The routine views of the calcaneus are an axial view and a lateral view. The properly positioned axial view will have the plantar surface of the foot perpendicular to the film. The lateral view is positioned just like the lateral ankle, with the exception of lowering the horizontal central ray to about 1 in. above the plantar surface of the foot. Another view that can be very useful is a 30° medial oblique view. The lateral and oblique views will demonstrate the subtalar joint.

Foot Radiography

The routine foot views will include the tarsal bone, metatarsals, and phalanges. A tube angle is used to open the tarsal bone on the A-P view of the foot; the greater the arch of the foot, the greater the angle required. A flat foot will not need the tube angulation. The tube angle is not needed on the medial oblique and lateral views. The medial oblique view is particularly useful; it demonstrates a clear view of the tarsal bones, the 4th and 5th metatarsals, the intertarsal joints, and detail of the 5th metatarsal.

The "basketball foot" is a traumatic medial subtalar dislocation that results from landing on an inverted foot. The talocalcaneal and talonavicular joints dislocate with the navicular, calcaneus, and distal bone displaced medially. Another basketball injury is the Jones' fracture or an avulsion fracture off the base of the 5th metatarsal. Any of the metatarsals can be fractured when the foot is trodden upon. Ballet dancers can fracture the sesamoid bones. Stress fractures of the metatarsals are generally transverse fractures. They can result from marching in the military or jumping in figure skating.

Toe Radiography

Toes can present significant challenges in positioning. The natural curve of the toes toward the plantar surface of the foot makes the evaluation of the joint spaces and phalanx difficult due to foreshortening. Along with the A-P, oblique, and lateral views, an axial view is added to the toe routine views. A tube angle or the film and toe position is altered to open the PIP joints and demonstrate a more accurate view of the phalanx. Many toe fractures will involve the joint space; others are spiral in nature. Perhaps the most challenging toe view is the lateral view. Tongue depressors and tape may be needed to obtain a true lateral view clear of the other toes.

The turf toe is caused by the patient's shoe gripping an artificial surface during a sudden stop. The foot moves forward in the shoe, resulting in severe dorsi flexion of the toe. The ligaments are usually stretched and the capsule torn. Radiographically, soft tissue swelling will be evident.

18.2   Axial View of the Calcaneus

Measure

Lateral at calcaneus

Protection

Lead apron

SID

40 in. using Non-Bucky

Tube Angulation

40° cephalad

Film

One half of 10 in. × 8 in. Fine (extremity) cassette with I.D. up

Marker

Anatomical

Positioning

1. Have patient lie on back on table.

2. Align the long axis of the lower leg with the center line of the table. Have patient internally rotate leg until the condyles are parallel to the film; this is usually about 15°. Have patient dorsiflex the ankle until the plantar surface is perpendicular to the film. A strap can be placed around the foot to help the patient hold this position.

3. Place the horizontal central ray 1.5 to 2 in. up the calcaneal tuberosity. Center the film to the horizontal central ray.

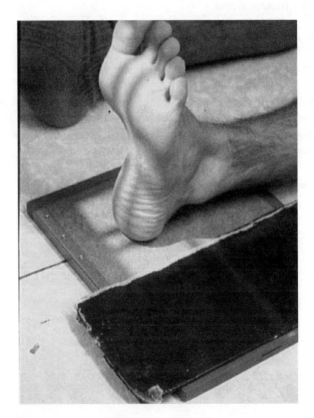

FIGURE 18.1
Heel axial positioning.

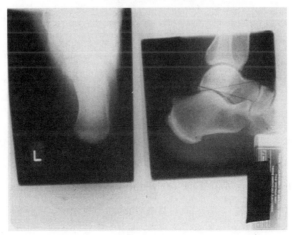

FIGURE 18.2
Heel series film.

4.   The vertical central ray should align with the long axis of the lower leg and the 3rd metatarsal.

5.   Ask patient to hold still. Take film.

Collimation

Top to Bottom: to include entire calcaneus and soft tissue below calcaneus; Side to Side: to include soft tissue of the calcaneus.

Breathing Instructions

Hold still

Image Critique

The axial view will demonstrate the calcaneal tuberosity without distortion and have the talocalcaneal joint space open. If the plantar surface of the foot was not perpendicular to the film, the tuberosity will be foreshortened and the talocalcaneal joint will not be seen. If the dorsiflexion is greater than 90°, reduce the tube angle.

Optimum kVp

70–76 kVp

18.3   Lateral Calcaneus

Measure

Lateral at calcaneus

Protection

Lead apron

SID

40 in. using Non-Bucky

Tube Angulation

None

Film

One half of the 10 in. × 8 in. Fine (extremity) cassette used for the axial view

Marker

Anatomical

Positioning

1. Have patient lie on affected side on table.
2. Align the long axis of the lower leg with the center line of the table, with the knee slightly flexed. Rotate leg until the lateral side of the foot is flat on the film. The malleoli are perpendicular to film.
3. Place horizontal central ray 2 in. above the heel and aligned with the medial malleolus. Center the film to the horizontal central ray.

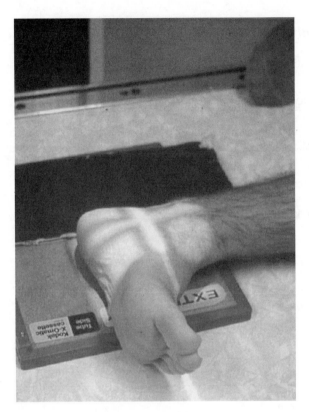

FIGURE 18.3
Calcaneus lateral positioning.

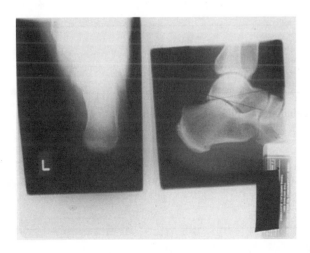

FIGURE 18.4
Heel series film.

4.   The vertical central ray should align with the medial malleoli.

5.   Ask patient to hold still. Take film.

Collimation

Top to Bottom: distal tibia to soft tissue below calcaneus; Side to Side: to include soft tissue of calcaneus.

Breathing Instructions

Hold still

Image Critique

The exam must include the distal tibia, talus, and calcaneus. The talus domes will be superimposed. The distal fibula will overlie the posterior fibula. The talotibial joint space will be open.

Optimum kVp

60–66 kVp

18.4   A-P Foot

Measure

A-P at base of 3rd metatarsal

Protection

Lead apron

SID

40 in. using Non-Bucky

Tube Angulation

A-P: 10° cephalad; oblique: no angulation.

Film

One half of 10 in. × 12 in. or 24 cm × 30 cm Fine (extremity) cassette with I.D. up

Marker

Anatomical

Positioning

1. Have patient lie on table, with knee bent and plantar surface of foot on table.
2. Align the long axis of the foot with the center line of the table. Place foot on cassette with I.D. toward heel.
3. Place horizontal central ray on the base of the 3rd metatarsal. Center the film to the horizontal central ray.
4. The vertical central ray should align with the long axis of the foot.
5. Ask patient to hold still. Take film.

Collimation

Top to Bottom: distal tibia to tips of toes or slightly less than film size; Side to Side: to include soft tissue of foot.

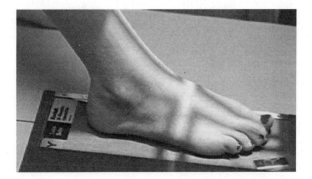

FIGURE 18.5
Foot A-P positioning.

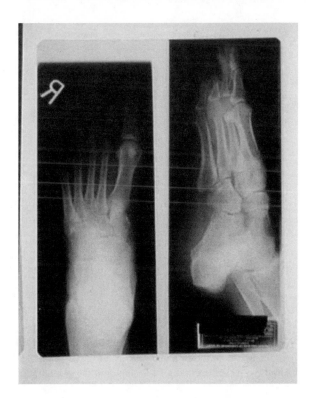

FIGURE 18.6
Foot A-P and oblique film.

Breathing Instructions

Hold still

Image Critique

The exam must include from the distal tibia to the tips of the toes. The tarsal bone joint spaces will be open. Principally, the joint spaces between the first and second cuneiform will be open. The tarsal-metatarsal joint spaces will be open. Part of the calcaneus will be seen without the talus being superimposed.

Optimum kVp

60–66 kVp

18.5   Medial Oblique Foot

Measure

A-P at base of 3rd metatarsal

Protection

Lead apron

SID

40 in. using Non-Bucky

Tube Angulation

None

Film

One half of 10 in. × 12 in. or 24 cm × 30 cm Fine (extremity) cassette with I.D. up

Marker

Anatomical

Positioning

1.   Have patient lie on table, with knee bent and plantar surface of foot on table.
2.   Align the long axis of the foot with the center line of the table. Place foot on cassette with I.D. toward heel. Have the patient medially rotate leg until the plantar surface of the foot is 30 to 40° to the film.

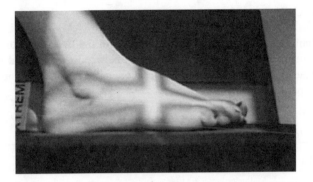

FIGURE 18.7
Foot oblique positioning.

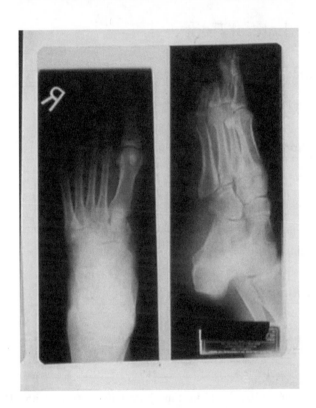

FIGURE 18.8
Foot A-P and oblique films.

3. Place horizontal central ray on the base of the 3rd metatarsal. Center the film to the horizontal central ray.
4. The vertical central ray should align with the long axis of the foot.
5. Ask patient to hold still. Take film.

Collimation

Top to Bottom: distal tibia to tips of toes; Side to Side: to include soft tissue of foot.

Breathing Instructions

Hold still

Image Critique

The exam must include from the distal tibia to the tips of the toes. The tarsal bones joint spaces will be open. Principally, the joint spaces between the first and second cuneiform will be open. The tarsal-metatarsal joint spaces will be open. Part of the calcaneus will be seen without the talus being superimposed.

Optimum kVp

60–66 kVp

18.6 Lateral Foot

Measure

Lateral at base of 1st metatarsal

Protection

Lead apro

SID

40 in. using Non-Bucky

Tube Angulation

None

Film

8 in. × 10 in. or 10 in. × 12 in. Fine (extremity) cassette with I.D. up

Marker

Anatomicaln

Positioning

1. Have patient lie on affected side on table.
2. Align the long axis of the lower leg with the center line of the table, with the knee slightly flexed. Rotate leg until the malleoli are perpendicular to film. The long axis of the foot should be at 90° to the lower leg. The lower leg should be parallel to the film. The plantar surface of the foot will be perpendicular to film.
3. Place horizontal central ray on the base of the 1st metatarsal. Center the film to the horizontal central ray.

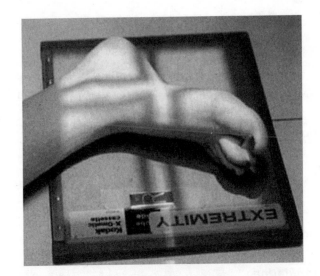

FIGURE 18.9
Foot lateral positioning.

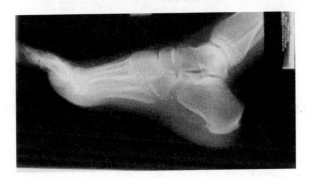

FIGURE 18.10
Foot lateral film.

4. The vertical central ray should align with the long axis of the foot.
5. Ask patient to hold still. Take film.

Collimation

Top to Bottom: distal tibia to soft tissue below calcaneus; Side to Side: to include soft tissue of calcaneus to toes.

Breathing Instructions

Hold still

Image Critique

The exam must include from the distal tibia to the tips of the toes. The talus domes will be superimposed. The distal fibula will overlie the posterior fibula. The talotibial joint space will be open.

Optimum kVp

60–66 kVp

18.7   A-P Toes and Axial A-P Toes

Measure

A-P at base of 3rd metatarsal-phalangeal (M-P) joint or affected toe

Protection

Lead apron

SID

40 in. using Non-Bucky

Tube Angulation

A-P: None
Axial: 15° cephalad

Film

One quarter of 10 in. × 12 in. Lanex Fine (extremity) cassette with I.D. up

Marker

Anatomical

Positioning

A-P (Figure 18.11)

1.   Have patient lie on table, with knee bent and plantar surface of foot on table.
2.   Align the long axis of the foot with the center line of the table. Place foot on cassette with I.D. toward heel.
3.   Place horizontal central ray at the 3rd M-P joint. Center one quarter of the film to horizontal central ray.
4.   The vertical central ray should align with the long axis of the foot.
5.   Ask patient to hold still. Take film.

Axial (Figure 18.12)

1.   Same as A-P, except 15° cephalad tube angulation.

Collimation

Top to Bottom: metatarsal-phalangeal joints to tips of toes; Side to Side: to include soft tissue of foot or affected toe.

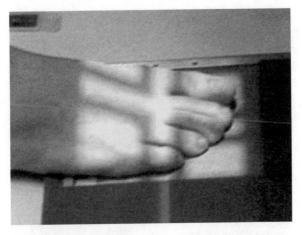

FIGURE 18.11
Toes A-P positioning.

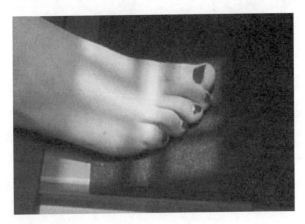

FIGURE 18.12
Toes A-P axial positioning.

Breathing Instructions

Hold still

Image Critique

The exam must include from the metatarsal-phalangeal joint to the tips of the toes. The axial view will open the PIP joints better than the A-P view.

Optimum kVp

56–60 kVp

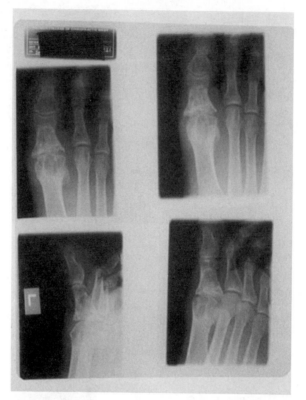

FIGURE 18.13
Toes series film.

18.8   Oblique and Lateral Views of Toes

Measure

A-P at base of 3rd metatarsal-phalangeal (M-P) joint or affected toe

Protection

Lead apron

SID

40 in. using Non-Bucky

Tube Angulation

None

Film

One quarter of 10 in. × 12 in. Fine (extremity) cassette with I.D. up

Marker

Anatomical

Positioning

A-P (Figure 18.14)

1. Have patient lie on table, with knee bent and plantar surface of affected foot on table.
2. Align the long axis of the foot with the center line of the table. Have patient medially rotate leg until the plantar surface is 30 to 45° to film.
3. Place horizontal and vertical central ray at the 3rd M-P joint. Center one quarter of the film to horizontal central ray.
4. Ask patient to hold still. Take film.

Lateral (Figure 18.5)

1. Have patient rotate leg medially for 1st and 2nd toes lateral until the foot is in profile.
2. Have patient rotate leg laterally for 3rd to 5th toes until the foot is lateral.
3. Tape unaffected toes away from toe of interest. Center on M-P joint. Take film.

Collimation

Top to Bottom: M-P joints to tips of toes; distal tibia to tips of toes; Side to Side: to include soft tissue of foot or affected toe.

Breathing Instructions

Hold still

Image Critique

The exam must include from the metatarsal-phalangeal joint to the tips of the toes. The axial view will open the PIP joints better than the A-P view.

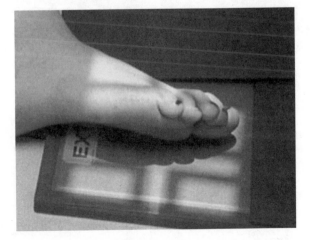

FIGURE 18.14
Toes oblique positioning.

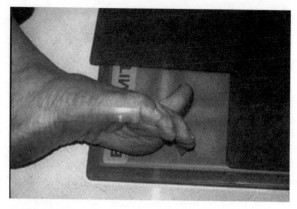

FIGURE 18.15
Toes lateral positioning.

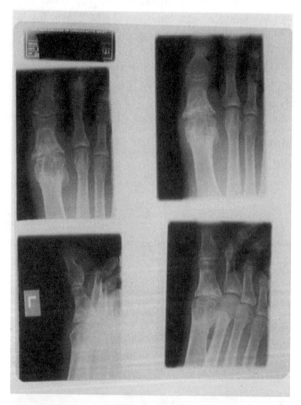

FIGURE 18.16
Toe series film.

Optimum kVp

56–60 kVp

Individual Lateral Toes (Figure 18.17)

Positioning of lateral toe views will require tape and a tongue depressor or hobby stick. It is very important to get a lateral view clear of the other toes. Keep the toe parallel to film and as close to the film as possible..

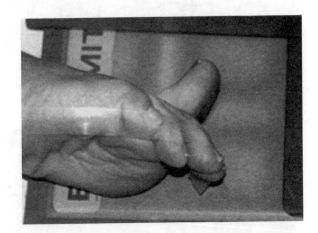

(a)

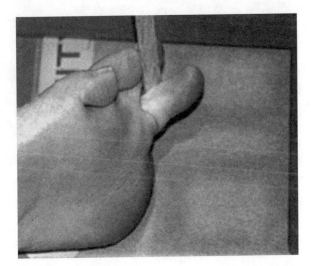

(b)

FIGURE 18.17
Individual lateral toes: (a) lateral great toe; (b) lateral 2nd toe; (c) lateral 3rd toe; (d) lateral 4th toe; and (e) lateral 5th toe.

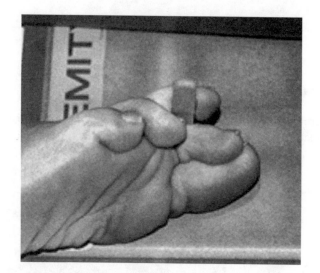

(c)

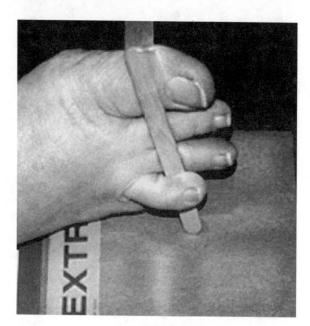

(d)

FIGURE 18.17 (continued)

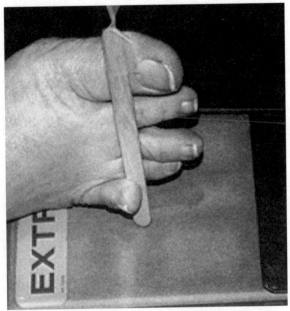

(e)

FIGURE 18.17 (continued)

Chapter **19**

Introduction to Quality Assurance and Radiographic Quality Control*

19.1 Introduction to Quality Assurance and Quality Control

Quality Assurance and Quality Control have been practiced in hospital radiology departments for years. These programs are designed to remove as many of the variables as possible and to correct problems before they degrade image quality.

There are so many things that can go wrong during the performance of a radiographic examination. Without a quality control program, the equipment will be in control and one will wonder if any study will come out properly. Patients expect and demand good-quality X-ray studies. The ability to make the diagnosis depends on obtaining films with the proper density, contrast, and resolution.

The Quality Assurance program in this book was formulated by a committee working with the California Department of Health Services, Department of Radiologic Health. It is very extensive. In many cases, more cost-effective methods are demonstrated in each section.

Quality Assurance is a management tool used to optimize the performance of X-ray facility personnel and radiographic and ancillary equipment operations. The purpose is to optimize the diagnostic quality of the radiograph.

Quality Assurance includes:

1. Policies and procedures that establish standards for training, performance, and competence of staff
2. Quality control of radiographic and ancillary equipment
3. Preventive and corrective maintenance of the equipment
4. Repeat or retake analysis to quantify that staff is appropriately trained and the variables of radiography are under control
5. Defined administrative accountability and standards

---

* The format for this chapter was adapted from *Syllabus on Radiography Radiation Protection*, State of California Department of Health Services, Sacramento, 1995. With permission from Edgar D. Bailey.

Quality Control is the performance of standardized tests that, when performed with care at prescribed intervals, will detect slowly evolving problems before they cause significant deterioration of image quality. The equipment is divided into three groups:

1. Accessories that include cassettes, grids, lead aprons, and gonadal shields
2. Radiographic equipment and calibration
3. Darkroom and automatic processing equipment

Costs Associated with Startup of a Quality Assurance Program

Because the main reason for Quality Assurance (QA) is to optimize the diagnostic quality of the radiograph, quantified benefits can be realized. If multiple repeat films are taken, the patient receives unnecessary exposure to radiation. If pathology that is present is missed due to poor quality, the clinician may misdiagnose the patient and could be subject to legal action by the patient. For these reasons, the expenditure for a QA program is warranted. The costs include:

- Training of personnel to perform the tests and continued costs of time to perform the tests
- Costs of the quality control equipment (less than $2000), which is relatively small when compared to operational and X-ray equipment costs
- Decreased patient flow if testing is done during patient visit time
- Cost of physicist or specialist to test the equipment

Cost Savings and Benefits of the Quality Assurance Program

The primary savings will be in reduced numbers of repeated films and avoidance of unnecessary radiation to the patient. Other associated cost savings include:

- Cost of film, which varies from $1.50 to $7.00 per sheet of film
- Cost of processing chemicals and hazardous waste removal
- Wear and tear on the equipment
- Less downtime of the equipment
- Improved patient flow due to avoidance of repeated films
- Decreased cost of equipment service
- Ability to combine QA with office safety and radiation safety program to meet all of the regulatory agency requirements

Quality Assurance (QA) has four major steps:

1. Acceptance testing of new equipment that resolves any installation problems and ensures that it is operating within specifications (a good business decision)
2. Establishing baseline performance of the equipment
3. Diagnosis of changes in equipment performance before it becomes radiographically apparent
4. Verification of correction of causes of deterioration in equipment performance

Retake Analysis

California requires that a retake analysis be performed every 3 months. Using a relatively large sample will help see trends in the type of studies being repeated and the reason for the errors. This data is used to determine what additional training or equipment service might be required. If one does not learn from mistakes, one is bound to repeat those mistakes. The data collection can be combined with the X-ray log required by the state.

California Requirements of a Quality Assurance Program

I. Each facility shall have a Quality Assurance Plan and Manual that includes:
   A. List of names and qualifications of individuals responsible for:
      1. Supervision of the program
      2. Performing QC tests
      3. Repairing and servicing the equipment
   B. The program shall include at least the following:
      1. A brief description of the tests to be performed
      2. Frequency of the tests
      3. Limits or parameters of acceptability for each test
      4. Protocol for correcting each QC finding that is outside parameters
      5. Forms to be used for each test
      6. A list of equipment that includes:
         a. Homogeneous phantom
         b. Coarse wire mesh contract tool
         c. Thermometer
         d. Sensitometer
         e. Densitometer
         f. Step wedge
II. Each facility shall maintain QA and QC records.
   A. X-ray and ancillary equipment records for 3 years that include:
      1. Acceptance testing, performance evaluations, and radiation safety surveys
      2. Verification that the X-ray equipment is in safe working order, such as preventive service records
      3. Subsequent QC test results
   B. Service and repair logs and records
   C. Film processor records for 1 year that include:
      1. Processor control charts and films
      2. Processor maintenance records that include:
         a. Preventive maintenance
         b. Corrective maintenance
         c. Cleaning and chemical replacement
   D. All records shall be dated and initialed or signed by the person who performed the test
   E. All records shall be readily available for inspection by representatives of the Radiologic Health Branch (RBH) or designated agency.
III. Rules and regulations that must be adhered to in the darkroom and when performing radiography. See below.

Darkroom Quality Assurance (QA) Requirements

The darkroom QA routine is essential to the production of quality radiographs. These are the rules that must be adhered to.

1. No smoking, eating, or drinking in the darkroom.
2. Daily cleaning of the darkroom to keep it free of dust.
3. Daily cleaning of the countertops and processor feedtray.
4. Ascertain that hands are clean and dry before touching film.
5. Ascertain that the darkroom safelight is equipped with an appropriate filter and bulb combination.
6. Keep screens free of artifacts. Screens must be cleaned regularly (not less than monthly) with a screen cleaner recommended by the manufacturer of the screens.
7. Load only one film per cassette.
8. Handle film carefully (with clean and dry hands, and by the edges only) to prevent artifacts due to static electricity, fingerprints, crinkling, creasing, bending, or scratching.
9. Lock the darkroom door when processing films to so no one can open the door and expose the film or film bin to light.

Radiographic Quality Assurance (QA) Requirements

A systematic approach to the performance of radiographic technology is essential to production of quality radiographs. The following sequence shall be adhered to by X-ray personnel:

1. Measure the thickness of the patient with caliper.
2. Consult technique chart and record on the X-ray request form the technical factors and any accessory equipment such as filters needed to perform the radiograph.
3. Enter the appropriate technique into the generator.
4. Position the patient correctly, keeping patient to film distance to a minimum. Position equipment and film correctly.
5. Collimate beam to the area of clinical interest.
6. Give patient the appropriate breathing instructions and ask patient to hold very still.
7. Watch patient as exposure is made.

The equipment performance standards used in this book are the standards established by the California Department of Radiologic Health for general radiographic equipment. Most of these tests and standards have been met for many years by hospital-based radiology departments. Many are the same as any medical facility providing mammography. At the minimum, processor quality control, screen cleaning, and the radiographic quality control tests should be performed as recommended.

19.2 How to Do a Retake or Repeat Analysis

A repeated radiograph/X-ray is known as a retake. Reasons for a retake can be divided into (1) equipment and accessory failure, malfunction, or error, and (2) X-ray personnel error.

Equipment and Accessory Failure, Malfunction, or Error

Equipment and accessory failure, malfunction, or error are referred to as technical errors (or hardware errors), and include the following:

- Inaccurate kilovoltage (kVp) calibration
- Inaccurate milliamperage (mA) calibration

- Inaccurate timer calibration
- Dirty or damaged cassettes
- Improperly labeled or damaged grids
- Malfunctioning collimator
- Improper film storage
- Incorrect or inconsistent film processing

X-Ray Personnel Error

X-ray personnel errors include all of the following:

- Use of incorrect technical factors (kVp, mAs, distance)
- Incorrect positioning
- Failure to measure the patient with calipers
- Improper collimation
- Use of improper accessories such as grids, cassettes, and filters
- Improper handling of unexposed or exposed films
- Failure to communicate clearly to the patient to hold the breath or to hold still

Experienced X-ray personnel typically do not repeat more than 2% of the examinations while inexperienced or careless X-ray personnel repeat 10% or even more of all examinations taken.

Retakes not only unnecessarily contribute to patient radiation dose but also add to the expense of the films, X-ray personnel time, wear and tear on the equipment and accessories, as well as inconvenience to the patient.

Repeat Film and Retake Studies

Studies regarding retakes show that approximately 50% of retakes are due to error in exposure factors (resulting in films or radiographs that are either too dark or too light; that is, the film has incorrect density or shows poor contrast). Positioning errors account for approximately 25% of all retakes. Other reasons for retakes include:

- Motion (respiratory or other) (11%)
- Film processing errors (6%)
- Wrong film, wrong projection, multiple exposures (4%)
- Improper X-ray beam–film alignment (3%)
- Screen, cassette, grid errors (3%)
- Foreign objects (1%) and other reasons (2%)

The frequency of retakes by body areas under examination were as follows:

- Cervical spine: 7%
- Thoracic spine: 17%
- Lumbar spine: 8%
- Hips and pelvis: 8%
- Upper extremities: 8%

- Lower extremities: 5%
- Chest: 5%
- KUB/abdomen: 12%
- Ribs and sternum: 8%
- Skull: 5%
- GI tract: 15%
- Other examinations: 2%

The abdominal region X-ray examinations (KUB, abdomen, lumbar spine, hips, pelvis, and GI contrast studies) account for 25% of all diagnostic X-rays performed in the U.S., and repeated examinations account for nearly 40% of all retakes. These exams are high bone marrow and high gonad radiation exposure examinations; therefore, every effort must be made to keep repeat rates of these examinations to a minimum.

Supervisor Responsibilities

In most clinical settings, the chiropractic clinician will perform his/her own radiographs. This is different from the medical field where X-ray personnel position the patient, select the technical factors, collimate the beam, and expose and process the radiographs. In either case, the person who holds the Operator and Supervisor Permit is responsible for conducting the X-ray examination and the quality of the results.

The responsibilities of a Radiography Supervisor and Operator include all of the following:

1. Ensuring that X-ray personnel have appropriate authorization to use X-rays on human beings
2. Ascertaining that X-ray equipment is operated only by persons who have adequate instruction in safe operating procedures and who have demonstrated competence in the safe use of equipment [Section 30305 (b) (1), (2) and (3) CAC Title 17]
3. Ensuring that all X-ray equipment is in proper operating condition and appropriate for the procedures being performed
4. Enforcing the radiographic quality assurance standards

How to Minimize Film Retakes

The production of quality radiographs is a complex process and involves satisfactory X-ray equipment operating performance, adequate quality accessories, well-trained and conscientious X-ray personnel, and, above all, adequate supervision.

The performance of X-ray personnel is influenced by many factors. Rather than discuss the many variables that can cause a retake film, several generalizations are offered to the X-ray Supervisor as means to minimize retakes:

1. Employ only well-qualified X-ray personnel (holders of valid authorizations issued by the California Department of Health Services, Radiologic Health Branch) who respect their work and conscientiously follow their assigned duties.
2. Give counsel and assistance to X-ray personnel as needed. (Supervisors must understand the processes of radiologic technology.)
3. Secure good equipment and accessories adequate for the examinations at hand. This is especially true when radiographing children.
4. Recognize that X-ray personnel under pressure tend to take shortcuts and thus make careless errors.

5. Provide sufficient positioning aids such as radiolucent positioning sponges, sandbags, and lead blockers.

6. Supervise X-ray personnel activities closely and, if indicated, offer or provide for additional training.

7. Require X-ray staff to follow these steps:

    a. Measure the thickness of the patient with calipers.

    b. Consult the technique chart.

    c. Set the technique factors using the technique chart.

    d. Position the patient correctly.

    e. Instruct the patient to hold breath and hold still.

    f. Watch patient as film is exposed.

    g. Process the exposed film carefully.

Repeat Film/Retake Analysis

It is necessary to have an ongoing retake analysis program. In order to reduce retakes, it is essential to make an analysis of the type of films and projections that are being repeated and know the reason(s) why films are being repeated. This must be undertaken not only because of the monetary considerations, but most importantly in order to reduce patient radiation exposure.

Conducting retake analysis must be done judiciously and in such a manner as to minimize interference with the normal X-ray-taking activities. The data derived from the analysis should be used as an educational tool and not for disciplinary or personnel action. The analysis will demonstrate the strengths and weaknesses of the X-ray operation. Personnel with significantly high retake rates may need additional training or supervision. The analysis can also show problems with the equipment or technique charts that must be addressed with corrective action.

Repeat analysis data is captured on the examination log and includes the reason, film size, and projection that was repeated. On a quarterly basis, the total films and reasons for retakes are calculated and a percentage of repeats derived. The projection(s) repeated are also noted and if indicated, assessment made. The goal of the program is to keep the repeat rate at less than 5%. (See Table 19.1.)

Supervisors should remember that Section 25692 of the Health and Safety Code states the following: Any person who violates or aids and abets the violation of any of the provisions of this chapter or regulations of the department adopted pursuant to this chapter is guilty of a misdemeanor.

How to Perform the Retake Analysis

1. Design the X-ray procedure log in a manner that records the size and number of films used to take each patient's radiographic study. Because one is required by law to keep a log, make it as useful as possible. Also include codes for the reason for each retake and the view that was being repeated. (See Table 19.1.)

2. Monthly or quarterly, go through the log and total the repeats, procedures, film totals, and reason for the retakes. Look for trends in the totals. Using a Repeat Analysis Form (Table 19.2) total the retakes by reason and number of retakes.

3. Determine the percentage for each reason and the total retake rate. There should be less than 5 to 7% total retakes.

4. Other data that can be analyzed include retake costs in wasted film — one will know by size, how many sheets were wasted. One can also determine if there is a trend in the view that is being commonly repeated. Additional study or continuing education may be needed to improve the positioning or technique chart.

TABLE 19.1
P.C.C.W. X-ray Examination and Repeat Log

Date: _____   Clinic: _____

Reasons for Repeating an Exposure Codes

1. Overexposed (dark)	4. Processing Error	7. Motion (not respiratory)
2. Respiratory Motion	5. Film-Beam Alignment	8. Multiple exposures
3. Positioning Error	6. Underexposed (light)	9. Artifact (foreign object)

10. Screen error
11. Grid Error
12. Other (specify)

Exam	Patient Name	Age:	Number	Intern Name	Room Number	Repeat Film Size	Repeat View	Repeat Reason Code	Film Used						Routine Series					
									14 × 36	14 × 17	7 × 17	10 × 12	8 × 10	411 Series	412 Series	Ltd Cerv.	Ltd Thor.	Ltd Lumb.	Other Specific
1.																			
2.																			
3.																			
4.																			
5.																			
6.																			
7.																			
8.																			
9.																			
10.																			
11.																			
12.																			
13.																			
14.																			
15.																			
16.																			
17.																			
18.																			
Total																			

TABLE 19.2
Repeat/Reject Film Analysis Form

Facility TASMAN CLINIC   From: 07/01/96 THROUGH 09/30/96

A repeat analysis is done quarterly at each clinic. A copy of the analysis will be forwarded to Russell Wilson, CRT, at the Tasman Clinic and a copy sent to Dominic Scuderi, D.C., at the Benton Clinic.

Cause	Number of Films	Percent Repeats (%)	Percent Total Films (%)
1. Overexposed (dark)	2	13.33	0.39
2. Respiratory motion	0	0	0
3. Positioning error	2	13.33	0.39
4. Processing error	0	0	0
5. Film-beam alignment	3	20.0	0.58
6. Underexposed (light)	7	46.67	1.36
7. Motion non-respiratory	0	0	0
8. Multiple exposure	0	0	0
9. Artifact (foreign object)	0	0	0
10. Screen error	0	0	0
11. Grid error	0	0	0
12. Other	1 empty cassette	6.67	0.19
Total retakes	15	100	2.91
Total retakes:	15		
Total films:	516	144 exams	
Overall repeat rate:	2.91%		

19.3   Acceptance Testing of Radiographic Equipment

A major expense will be purchasing or leasing radiographic equipment for the office. One can easily spend more than $20,000 for equipment. Room modifications, electrical power, plumbing, and shielding can also be very expensive. With this scope of investment, it would be very prudent to have the equipment tested before using it on patients. At most chiropractic colleges, X-ray machines are loaned to the college for a year and then sold to alumni. This means that there is a continual process of removal and replacement of relatively new radiographic equipment. This author has yet to have a new machine pass all elements of acceptance testing on the 1st try. If the equipment is not tested, problems such as grid cut-off, poor kVp calibration, and inconsistent exposures would be left unchecked. Some of these problems could be passed on to the chiropractor who purchases the equipment.

Recently, this author did not have a kVp test cassette back from calibration by the manufacturer. The films were coming out dark, particularly at the upper kVp ranges. Service personnel tested the kVp using their ion chamber and with the oscilloscope; they assured me that everything was perfect. All of the technique charts stored in the machine were replaced and filtration on smaller patients was increased. This went on for over 9 months. The unit was sold and replaced. The technique charts were transferred to the new unit. The manufacturer's service personnel assured me that the unit was fine and that it would shoot just like the unit that was replaced. It did shoot just like the unit that was replaced. I tested the unit with my kVp cassette. The kVp was high by 11%. The kVp was recalibrated and tested again. This time it was only high at the upper ranges. It had to be adjusted twice before it was correct. The ion chamber that the service company used to check the kVp had not been recently calibrated. It gave them a false reading. The technique charts had to be reduced back to the initial settings. This also explained why, on a state inspection, this author's technique chart for the lateral lumbar spine was higher in radiation exposure that in previous inspections.

There have been similar problems with phototimer calibrations on new equipment. The problem defies physics. The kVp and mAs were in what appeared to be good calibration with linear exposures. Yet when using automatic exposure control, a higher mAs backup had to be set for small focal spot than for large focal spot. Again, the problem turned out to be kVp calibration. A less pragmatic person may not have persisted.

It will cost only a couple of hundred dollars to have the equipment tested and verified that it meets state and national safety standards. Then, if one starts to have problems, there will be an established baseline that one can use as a standard. One may be able to obtain some baseline technique charts produced by the person testing the equipment. Use someone who is trusted by both ideally the equipment seller and the equipment buyer.

As many of the parameters as possible should be tested. The limit will most likely be based on the equipment available. One does not need very expensive meters to adequately test equipment. With just the step wedge, densitometer, and nine pennies, one can test basic calibration of exposure and collimation. With a lead apron and densitometer, grid cut-off can be checked. To test shielding, however, very expensive meters are required. Most radiation physicist will have all of the tools needed to make a very complete evaluation of the equipment. Hospital-based medical radiology facilities must have their equipment tested at least every 2 years. Mammography equipment is tested more often.The purchase of an established practice will be not guarantee that the radiographic equipment is working properly. Ask to see past state inspection reports and preventive service reports as a minimum. See if there are technique charts and quality control tests available. If working technique charts and service records are not available, ask to see some of their recent films. It is highly advisable to have the equipment tested. This is similar to buying a used car: if the car will not pass the smog check, one should not buy it. Many of these tests will be discussed further in radiographic quality control testing (Chapter 22). It is amazing what one can do with an aluminum step wedge and some pennies. Today there is some very expensive test equipment that radiation health physicists use. One can find a physicist by contacting a local hospital or a state health department.

Recommended Tests	Parameters	Test Equipment
Collimation accuracy	Within 2% of SID	9 Pennies or collimation test tool
Tube centering	Within 2% of SID	9 Pennies or collimation test tool
Accuracy of exposure	Within 5%	Step wedge and densitometer, or rate meter
kVp	Within 5%	kVp test cassette or rate meter
Grid centering and perpendicularity	Within 2°	Grid centering test tool, or collimation and beam alignment test tool
Timer accuracy	Within 5%	Spinning top, timer test tool, or rate meter

Examples of Acceptance or Annual Survey Equipment and Tests

kVp Test

The Wisconsin kVp Test Tool uses multiple step wedges to measure kVp within 1 kVp in the 60- through 120-kVp ranges. After the exposures are made and film processed, a densitometer is used

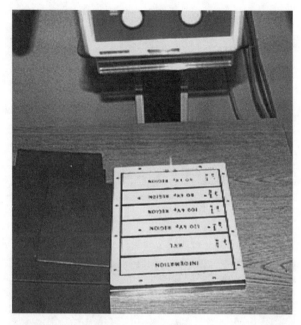

FIGURE 19.1
kVp test tool.

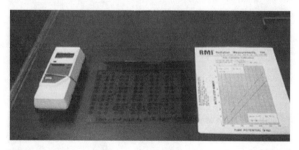

FIGURE 19.2
kVp test film.

to determine which steps match. The step is compared to the calibration chart to determine the actual kVp. (See Figures 19.1 and 19.2.)

mAs and Timer Accuracy

This test tool consists of a disk with two slits in it. It is driven by a motor at a rate of one revolution per second. A protractor is used to measure exposure time. It also has a step wedge to monitor mAs. (See Figures 19.3 and 19.4.)

Beam Perpendicularity and Grid Alignment

This tool will test collimation and the alignment of the beam to the film or grid. As long as the two steel balls are within the 1st circle, the unit is within 2° of perpendicular. (See Figures 19.5 and 19.6.)

Testing the focal spot will be discussed in the chapter covering radiographic quality control testing (Chapter 22.5).

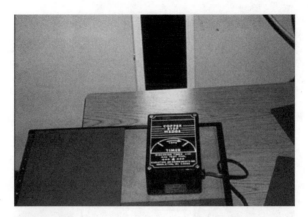

FIGURE 19.3
Timer test tool.

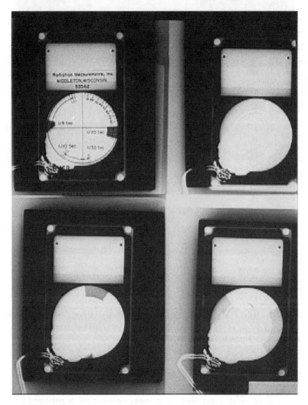

FIGURE 19.4
Timer test film.

19.4   Developing Technique Charts

The technical factors used to take the radiograph will have the greatest impact on both image quality and radiation safety. The most common reason for repeated films results from errors in the radiographic technique. If every facility that takes X-ray films on patients would accurately measure the patients and use good updated technique charts, over half of the unnecessary repeated exposures

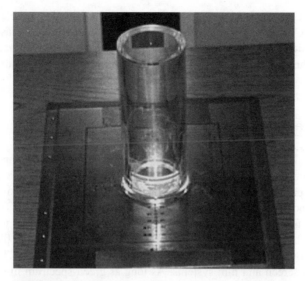

FIGURE 19.5
Beam perpendicularity test tool.

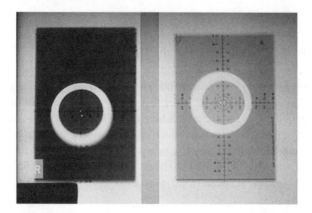

FIGURE 19.6
Beam perpendicularity test film.

could be avoided. The types of technique charts and how to use them were discussed previously. This section discusses how to produce and maintain technique charts. Equipment and film manufacturers will usually be willing to help establish the technique charts; the operator's ability to produce good-quality films with a particular product makes good business sense.

Radiographic Equipment Manufacturer

Sources for baseline technique-charts include the manufacturer of the X-ray unit or the film and screen manufacturer. Many years ago, this author obtained a book from General Electric Medical Systems on how to make technique charts and has used it many times to establish a starting point for the technique chart. The equipment manufacturer is an excellent source of help in starting a technique chart. The manufacturer can also be of assistance in reading tube limit and cooling charts. These limits are very important in terms of X-ray tube life. Any machine operated in proper calibration with a known screen and film relative speed value should use similar technical values. For a new unit, if one knows the RSV of the screens and generator type, existing charts can be converted. If the old unit had a bed X-ray tube or major calibration problems, conversion will probably not work. Changing the equipment from single phase to three phase or high frequency will require a reduction in the mAs by 0.50; this can be accomplished by reducing the exposure time and possibly changing to the small focal spot. This change will dramatically improve detail on the image.

Film Screen Manufacturer

Film suppliers will also help the user set up technique charts. Users will need to provide some techniques that they know will work well. Based on the provided technical factors, computer software is used to produce technique charts. Film manufacturers will recommend the optimum kVp for their film and screens. Many rare-earth systems lose speed below 60 kVp.

The screen and film used must be compatible. The film needs to react to the color spectrum that the screen phosphors produce. Green-sensitive film cannot be used with blue-emitting screens. For a mixed system, one may never be able to get consistent technique charts. Table 19.3 is included to illustrate matched screen and film systems. As long as green-spectrum film is used with green-spectrum screens, the system is considered matched. That is, a particular manufacturer's film does not always need to be used with that manufacturer's screens. The X-ray film market is very competitive now.

Charts from the Notes or from Another Facility

Although some charts are included in this chapter, it is impossible to guarantee that they will work for everyone. They are only examples of what this author would include on the technique chart. Any forgotten information (such as tube angulation and I.D. location) can be included on the chart. [Your X-ray unit type, screen and film combination, grid ratios, and filtration systems would need to match the cited equipment for all of the charts to work for your office.] For the charts given here, high-frequency generators with 10:1 103-line grids, film/screen RSV 400 for spinal work, and extremity screen film system speed of 80 were used. (See Table 19.5.)

Getting Started

Make sure that the processor and radiographic equipment is working properly before starting a technique chart. If one does not have a non-grid film holder for the Bucky, get one.

The radiographic equipment type (single phase, three phase, or high frequency) and the method used to enter technical factors into the machine will greatly impact technique chart design.

Units that only use focal spot, power level, mAs, and kVp will need only those factors on the chart. Units that have focal spot, mA and timer stations, and kVp will need that type of detail on the chart. With a perfect chart, there will be times when it will be necessary to change the exposure time. The author designs charts to use primarily the small focal spot and maximum power for the best geometric detail possible with the machine. Large or uncooperative patients may require shorter exposure times. The operator will need to know to change to the large focal spot to reduce the exposure time. The long exposure time will increase the chance of motion on the films. The most powerful office units available will not stop motion if the patient fails to hold his/her breath. Try to keep exposure time below 0.50 seconds to minimize motion.

The best technique charts will have a fixed kVp and variable mAs. The kVp is determined by the area of the body and the desired contrast scale. Many state radiation safety regulations will

TABLE 19.3
High-Frequency Generator with 400 Speed Rare-Earth Screen Combination

Cervical Spine Series

A-P Lower Cervical and Posterior Oblique
SID: 40 in.
Angle: 15° cephalad
kVp: 70
Film: 8 in. × 10 in. regular I.D. down

Lateral Cervical Spine
SID: 72 in. Non-Bucky
Angle: None
kVp: 70
Film 8 in. × 10 in. regular I.D. down

Part Size (cm)	mAs	Part Size (cm)	mAs
6	3	6	3
7	3	7	3
8	5	8	5
9	6	9	6
10	8	10	8
11	8	11	8
12	10	12	10
13	10	13	10
14	10	14	10
15	12	15	12
16	15	16	15
17	18	17	18
18	18	18	18

Cervical Spine APOM
SID: 40 in.
kVp: 78
Angle: 5° cephalad or none
Film: 8 in. × 10 in. regular I.D. down

Pillars or Fuchs Projection
SID: 40 in.
Angle: pillars 45° cephalad
kVp: 78
Angle: Fuchs None
Film: 8 in. × 10 in. regular I.D. down

Part Size (cm)	mAs	Part Size (cm)	mAs
6	3	6	6
7	3	7	6
8	5	8	10
9	6	9	12
10	8	10	14
11	8	11	14
12	10	12	20
13	10	13	20
14	12	14	25
15	12	15	25
16	15	16	30
17	18	17	35
18	18	18	40

TABLE 19.3 (continued)
High-Frequency Generator with 400 Speed Rare-Earth Screen Combination

Thoracic Spine Region

A-P Thoracic Spine SID: 40 in. Filter: Cervicothoracic 40 in. kVp: 74 Film: 7 in. × 17 in. regular I.D. down		Lateral Thoracic Spine SID: 40 in. Filter: Points per size kVp: 80 Film: 14 in. × 17 in. regular I.D. up		
Part Size (cm)	mAs	Part Size (cm)	mAs	Points
13–14	10	18–19	10	None
15–16	12	20–21	12	None
17–18	15	22–23	15	None
19–20	18	24–25	18	None
21–22	20	26–27	20	#1
23–24	25	28–29	25	#2
25–26	30	30–31	30	#3
27–28	35	32–33	35	#4
29–30	40	34–35	40	#4, #1
31–32	60	36–37	60	#4, #2
33–34	85	38–39	85	#4, #3
35–36	100	40–41	100	#4, #4

Swimmer's View SID: 40 in. kVp: 80 Film: 10 in. × 12 in. regular I.D. up		Ribs above Diaphragms SID: 40 in. kVp: 70 Film: 14 in. × 17 in. regular I.D. up	
Part Size (cm)	mAs	Part Size (cm)	mAs
18–19	15	13–14	5
20–21	18	15–16	6
22–23	20	17–18	8
24–25	25	19–20	10
26–27	30	21–22	12
28–29	35	23–24	15
30–31	40	25–26	18
32–33	60	27–28	20
34–35	70	29–30	25
36–37	85	31–32	30
38–39	100	33–34	35
40–41	125	35–36	40
		37–38	50
		39–40	60

TABLE 19.3 (continued)
High-Frequency Generator with 400 Speed Rare-Earth Screen Combination

Lumbar Spine

A–P or P–A Lumbopelvic
SID: 40 in.
kVp: 74
Film: 14 in. × 17 in. regular I.D. up

Oblique Lumbar Spine/A–P Sacral Base
SID: 40 in.
Sacral Base: 30° cephalad
kVp: 80   Oblique: No angle
Film oblique: 10 in. × 12 in. regular I.D. down
Film sacral base: 8 in. × 10 in. regular I.D. up

Part Size (cm)	mAs	Part Size (cm)	mAs
13–14	10	13–14	10
15–16	15	15–16	15
17–18	20	17–18	20
19–20	30	19–20	30
21–22	40	21–22	40
23–24	60	23–24	60
25–26	85	25–26	85
27–28	100	27–28	100
29–30	125	29–30	125
Change to 78 kVp		**Change to 84 kVp**	
31–32	100	31–32	100
33–34	125	33–34	125
35–36	150	35–36	150
37–38	200	37–38	200
39–40	250	39–40	250
41–42	300	41–42	300

Lateral Lumbar Spine
SID: 40 in. no angle
kVp: 90
Film: 14 in. × 17 in. regular I.D. up

Spot Lateral L5/S1
SID: 40 in. no angle
kVp: 100
Film: 8 in. × 10 in. regular I.D. up

Part Size (cm)	mAs	Part Size (cm)	mAs
14–15	10	14–15	10
16–17	12	16–17	12
18–19	18	18–19	18
20–21	20	20–21	20
22–23	25	22–23	25
24–25	30	24–25	30
26–27	35	26–27	35
28–29	40	28–29	40
30–31	50	30–31	50
32–33	60	32–33	60
34–35	85	34–35	85
36–37	100	36–37	100
38–39	120	38–39	120
40–41	170	40–41	170

TABLE 19.3 (continued)
High-Frequency Generator with 400 Speed Rare-Earth Screen Combination

Sacrum, Coccyx, SI Joints, and Lower Ribs

A–P Sacrum or Coccyx
SID: 40 in.
kVp: 76
Film: 8 in. × 10 in. regular I.D. up

Lateral Sacrum and Coccyx
SID: 40 in.
kVp: 90
Film: 10 in. × 12 in. regular I.D. up

Part Size (cm)	mAs	Part Size (cm)	mAs
13–14	10	14–15	10
15–16	15	16–17	12
17–18	20	18–19	18
19–20	30	20–21	20
21–22	40	22–23	25
23–24	60	24–25	30
25–26	85	26–27	35
27–28	100	28–29	40
29–30	150	30–31	50
		32–33	60
Change to 80 kVp		34–35	85
31–32	100	36–37	100
33–34	125	38–39	125
35–36	150	40–41	150
37–38	200		
39–40	250		
41–42	300		

Sacral Iliac Joints
SID: 40 in.
kVp: 80
Film: 8 in. × 10 in. regular I.D. up

Ribs below Diaphragm
SID: 40 in.
kVp: 74
Film: 14 in. × 17 in. regular I.D. up

Part Size (cm)	mAs	Part Size (cm)	mAs
15–16	15	14–15	12
17–18	18	16–17	18
19–20	30	18–19	25
21–22	40	20–21	30
23–24	60	22–23	35
25–26	85	24–25	40
27–28	100	26–27	60
29–30	125	28–29	70
		30–31	85
Change to 84 kVp		32–33	100
31–32	100	34–36	125
33–34	120	36–37	150
35–36	170	38–39	200
37–38	200	40–41	250
39–40	250		

require that the kVp be as high as possible to achieve the desired contrast. If the kVp is fixed, one is assured that the body part is properly penetrated and that contrast levels are fixed. The latitude of exposure is also broader. Even with a fixed kVp chart, larger body parts may need more kVp to properly penetrate the anatomy. To reduce exposure times, the kVp can be increased on large patients. Very frail or emaciated patients will require less kVp than normal.

The best technique chart will work only about 85% of the time. Experience with the equipment and judging patient habitus will help the user make adjustments to the technique when needed. As an example, a patient with more muscle will require an adjustment in filtration.

Supertech Radiographic Technique Chart Software

A very good computer program to generate fixed kVp technique charts is sold by Supertech. An exposure of a penetrometer is made for each type of film and screen combination used in the office. It is used to determine the correction factor for the machine and film. That factor is entered into the program and the mAs is computed, based on the machine output. The kVp can be changed, and various mA stations can be used, based on the setting that generator allows.

The program works similar to the slide rule that preceded it. There are additional correction factors for grid ratio changes, distance changes, screens, and added filtration. Initially, it may be rather cumbersome, but it certainly beats computing every technique by hand. The program is also very paper-hungry, as each chart prints as a full page.

The Supertech Slide Rule Technique Calculator

The Supertech X-ray Slide Rule Technique Calculator can replace the technique charts if one does not mind calculating technical factors before each exposure. It uses the pentrometer like the computer program mentioned previously. This is used to establish the master correction factor for the equipment. There are additional correction factors for grid ratio changes, distance changes, screens, and added filtration. This feature makes the Supertech and the Supertech Computer Program one of the best means to establish a technique chart. On a slow afternoon, the user could make a chart based on the range of measurements and views taken in the office.

Supertech also shows multiple technique choices using the mAs and kVp relationship. It does take longer to use than a technique chart, and not all views are identified. Many users feel that this unit is instrumental to their success in taking quality films. It cannot be overemphasized that the key to taking good radiographs starts with accurate measurement of the patient.

Nolan Accu-rad X-ray Calipers

There is an alternative to technique charts. Nolan Accu-rad X-ray Calipers will give the technical factors as soon as one measures the patient. The calipers will need to be calibrated for the output of the radiographic equipment and screen/film RSV. This makes the process very quick. It also has a built-in conversion scale for varying the source to image distance. The entrance skin radiation exposure for the oblique cervical spine can be reduced using a 48 to 60 in. SID.

The calipers use a point scale where constants such as grid ratio, SID, and screen speed are given point factors. These points are used for the calibration process to set the mAs scale. The patient body habitus is also given point factors. The patient factors are used to fine-tune the technique or to determine the need for point filtration.

The calipers use a higher kVp than normally recommended. This will make the films somewhat flatter in contrast. It will also significantly reduce the absorbed radiation exposure for the patient.

For each view, the scale will give five techniques at different kVp settings. Only the Nolan Accurad Calipers and the Supertech Calculator give the operator a choice of technical factors. This will give the user some control over contrast and exposure time.

Automatic Exposure Technique Charts

With increased computerization of radiographic equipment, the cost of automatic exposure control (AEC) has dropped. The cost reduction makes it possible for offices to buy it. It will generally pay for itself in about 2 years, with reduced film waste. Many major medical centers use this to reduce repeated studies due to poor technical factors. With AEC, an ion chamber is positioned between the grid and the film. As soon as a sufficient number of photons strikes the chamber, the exposure is automatically terminated.

An AEC chart should note which ion chamber should be activated. If the area of interest is in the center of the film, the center chamber is used to measure the exposure. This is true for spines and most extremity views. For the P-A chest, the lungs are monitored by the side chambers. The master density level should also be on the chart. This can be varied for body habitus and view.

The kVp should be the optimum kVp for the view. The operator needs to set a backup mAs for the view. This should be long or high enough to allow the ion chamber to terminate the exposure. It should not be set excessively high. If the backup mAs is too high, the exposure time will be longer than needed because as the mAs is increased, the exposure time will also increase. If the operator fails to turn on the AEC or selects the wrong chamber, the patient will get excessive and unnecessary radiation exposure. Based on the body habitus, the mAs might need to be increased.

AEC will work on most films taken with collimation slightly less than film size. It does not work for tightly collimated views or small body parts; nor will it work for Non-Bucky or tabletop films. Some manual techniques may still be needed. For cervical spine films, manual techniques are recommended.

AEC will significantly reduce retakes and provide consistent contrast from patient to patient. If the positioning is correct, the view should be technically superior to manually set technical factors. The unit will be able to better adjust exposure for patient habitus and unseen pathology by the operator. It will save time and money in the long run and will pay for itself many times over the life of the equipment.

Tables 19.3 to 19.6 are examples of technique charts. All are fixed kVp and variable mAs charts. An extremity chart (Table 19.5) and AEC chart (Table 19.6) are included as examples.

TABLE 19.4
Example of Chart for Use with the Nolan Filtration System

A-P Full Spine View   72 in. FFD   14 × 36 Lanex Regular

cm Range	mAs	kVp	Focal	Power	Point Filter Female	Point Filter Male
12 cm	38	80	Small	Full	3	2
13 cm	38	81	Small	Full	3	2
14 cm	38	82	Small	Full	3 + 1	2 + 1
15 cm	46	80	Small	Full	3 + 1	2 + 1
16 cm	46	81	Small	Full	3 + 1	2 + 1
17 cm	46	82	Small	Full	3 + 1	2 + 1
18 cm	55	82	Small	Full	3 + 2	2 + 2
19 cm	55	84	Small	Full	3 + 2	2 + 2
20 cm	79	80	Small	Full	3 + 3	2 + 3
21 cm	79	82	Small	Full	3 + 3	2 + 3
22 cm	79	86	Small	Full	3 + 4	2 + 4
23 cm	95	84	Small	Full	3 + 4	2 + 4
24 cm	95	86	Small	Full	3 + 4	2 + 4
25 cm	114	80	Large	Full	4 + 4	3 + 4
26 cm	114	82	Large	Full	4 + 4	3 + 4
27 cm	114	84	Large	Full	4 + 4	3 + 4
28 cm	137	80	Large	Full	4 + 4	3 + 4
29 cm	137	82	Large	Full	4 + 4	3 + 4
30 cm	137	84	Large	Full	4 + 4	3 + 4
31 cm	165	80	Large	Full	4 + 4	3 + 4

Filter sequence: 1. Lung or paraspinal filter
For APFS   2. Cervical-thoracic 72 in. or thyroid 72 in.
                    3. Skips space
                    4. Point filter per chart
                    5. Point filter per chart
Point filters for lateral lumbopelvic view:
   Added for patients with wide hips and narrow waist.
   Measure patient at tronchanters and at the umbilicus.
   Subtract umbilicus measurement from tronchanter measurement.
   Subtract 5 from the product. The resulting number is the needed point filter total.

TABLE 19.5
Extremity/Chest Radiographic Technique Chart

Fixed kVp Variable mAs Exposure Guide Room 1

Anatomy	Projection	Cassette EXT = Fine REG = Reg	Grid	SID or FFD	Focal Spot	kVp	Avg. Thickness (cm)	mAs −4 cm	−2 cm	Average	+2 cm	+4 cm	Avg. ESE (mR)/ Exposure
Upper Extremity													
Fingers	All	Ext	No	40 in.	S	60	2		1.2	1.4	1.7		6.3
Hand &	P-A & Obl.	Ext	No	40 in.	S	62	3–4		1.7	2	2.5		10.1
Wrist	Lat.	Ext	No	40 in.	S	64	6–8	2	2.5	3	4	5	15.8
Forearm	A-P & Lat.	Reg	No	40 in.	S	64	7–9	1.2	1.2	1.4	1.7	2	8.3
Elbow	A-P & Obl.	Ext	No	40 in.	S	60	7–8	3.5	4.2	5.1	6.1	7.4	25.9
	Lat.	Ext	No	40 in.	S	64	8–9	3.5	4.2	5.1	6.1	7.4	30.8
Humerus	A-P & Lat.	Reg	No	40 in.	S	64	9–11	2.9	3.5	4.2	5.1	6.1	33.6
Shoulder	A-P Int & Ext	Reg	Yes	40 in.	S	76	13–14	3.5	4.2	5.1	6.1	7.4	57.4
Clavicle	P-A & Tang	Reg	Yes	40 in.	S	72	13–14	3.5	4.2	5.1	6.1	7.4	46.6
AC joints	w & w/o wts	Reg	Yes	40 in.	S	70	13–14	3.5	4.2	5.1	6.1	7.4	42.9
Bi-lat AC jnt	w & w/o wts	Reg	No	72 in.	S	70	13–14	3.5	4.2	5.1	6.1	7.4	11.4
Scapula	A-P	Reg	Yes	40 in.	S	76	13–14	3.5	4.2	5.1	6.1	7.4	57.4
	Lat. (Tang.)	Reg	Yes	40 in.	S	76	13–14	7.4	8.9	11	13	15	116.5
Lower Extremity													
Toes	All	Ext	No	40 in.	S	60	3		1.4	2	2.5		6.4
Foot	A-P & Obl.	Ext	No	40 in.	S	60	6–7	2	2.5	3.5	4.2	5.1	20.7

	View		Grid	Distance	Screen	kVp	mAs						
OS calis	Lat.	Ext	No	40 in.	S	64	8–9	2.9	3.5	4.2	5.1	6.1	24.8
	Axial	Ext	No	40 in.	S	70	7	2.9	3.5	4.2	5.1	6.1	29.4
	Lat.	Ext	No	40 in.	S	60	7	2.9	3.5	4.2	5.1	6.1	24.8
Ankle	A-P & Obl.	Ext	No	40 in.	S	64	9	3.5	4.2	5.1	6.1	7.4	30.8
	Lat.	Ext	No	40 in.	S	60	7	3.5	4.2	5.1	6.1	7.4	25.3
Tib-fib	A-P & Lat.	Reg	No	40 in.	S	64	10–13	1.7	2	2.4	2.9	3.5	15.8
Knee	A-P	Reg	Yes	40 in.	S	70	12–13	2.9	3.5	4.2	5.1	6.1	42.9
	Lat.	Reg	Yes	40 in.	S	70	12–13	2.4	2.9	3.5	4.2	5.1	35.3
	Tunnel	Reg	Yes	40 in.	S	70	12–13	4.2	5.1	6.1	7.4	8.9	51.3
	Sunrise	Ext	No	40 in.	S	70	12–13	1.7	2	2.4	2.9	3.5	20.2
Femur	A-P & Lat.	Reg	Yes	40 in.	S	76	16–18	5.1	6.1	7.4	8.9	11	88.4
Hip	A-P & Frog	Reg	Yes	40 in.	S	76	20	8.9	11	13	15	18	138.1
Pelvis	A-P	Reg	Yes	40 in.	S	76	24	15	18	20	25	30	278.6
Misc.													
Chest	P-A	Reg	Yes	72 in.	L	110	24	1.7	2	2.4	2.9	3.5	16.2
	Lat.	Reg	Yes	72 in.	L	115	30	3.5	4.2	5.1	6.1	7.4	37.3

TABLE 19.6
Bucky Automatic Exposure Control Guide

Revised 10/03/96

Anatomy	View	FFD	kVp	mAs Backup	Focal Spot	Power	Ion Chamber	Master Density	Filters
T-spine	A-P	40 in.	76	50	S	Full	2	N	Thyroid
	Lateral	40 in.	80	100	S	Full	2	+1	Per size
	Swimmers	40 in.	80	120	S	Full	2	N	None
Chest	P-A	72 in.	110	5	S	Low	1	+1	None
	Lateral	72 in.	110	10	S	Low	2	+1	None
	Apical	72 in.	110	5	S	Low	1	N	None
Lumbar	L-P A-P or P-A	40 in.	76	100	S	Full	2 or 3	N	None
	Obliques	40 in.	82	100	S	Full	2 or 3	N	Lat. gonad
	Lateral	40 in.	90	150	S	Full	2 or 3	+1	Lat. gonad
	L5/S1 Spot	40 in.	100	150	S	Full	2 or 3	+1	Lat. gonad
	Sac. base	40 in.	82	100	S	Full	2 or 3	N	None
Full spine	A-P	72 in.	80	150	S	Full	3	N	Per size
Pelvis	A-P	40 in.	76	100	S	Full	2 or 3	N	None
Shoulder/scapula	A-P, Lateral	40 in.	70	50	S	Full	2	N	None
Hip	A-P & Frog	40 in.	70	50	S	Full	2 or 3	N	None
Knee	All	40 in.	70	20	S	Full	3	-1	None
C-spine	Lateral turn AEC off and use Non-Bucky holder and manual technique:								
manual tech. or	A-P, APOM, OBL	40 in.	75	50	S	Full	2	N	None

T-Spine Point Filter Chart

Lat (cm)	T-Spine
<26	None
26–27	#1
28–29	#2
30–31	#3
32–33	#4
34–35	#4 + #1
36–37	#4 + #2
>38	#4 + #2

A-P Full Spine Point Filters

UMB (cm)	Female	Male	
12–13	3	2	+ Thyroid and lung filter
14–17	4	3	+ Thyroid and lung filter
18–19	4 + 1	4	+ Thyroid and lung filter
20–21	4 + 2	4 + 1	+ Thyroid and lung filter
22–24	4 + 3	4 + 2	+ Thyroid and lung filter
25–31	4 + 4	4 + 3	+ Thyroid and lung filter

Lumbar Lateral Point Filters for Female Patients

Tronchanteric lateral measurement minus umbilical > 5 cm

Difference 5–6 cm	#1 Point filter
Difference 7 cm	#2 Point filter
Difference 8–9 cm	#3 Point filter
Difference 10 cm or >	#4 Point filter

Body part must be centered to cell
Cell #1 is upper side detector
Cell #2 is upper middle detector
Cell #3 is lower middle detector

Master Density Control Setting

Normal to small patient = N
Large flabby = +1 and double mAs back up
Large obese/muscular = +2 and increase kVp 6 to 10 and double mAs

Turn off AEC for
Non-Bucky work

Chapter 20

Darkroom and Film Storage Quality Control*

This chapter covers the proper environment for the storage of radiographic film. Image quality will be severely impacted if the film is outdated or has been improperly stored. The film can be fogged by heat, age, and light. Fogged films from improper storage will generally be dark because the film started out dark before it was exposed.

Film that is exposed is very sensitive to fog in the darkroom or being left in the X-ray room during another exposure. The darkroom must be light-tight. The safelight used must be designed for the film. The testing of the safelight is discussed in Section 20.2.

20.1 Specification for Film Storage and the Darkroom

The photographic process controls image quality/contrast, density, base-plus-fog, and with it, the patient radiation dose. The optical density (O.D.) range shall fall within 0.5 to 2.5 O.D. values.

Film and Chemical Storage

Test	Test Device	Performance Criteria	Frequency
Film and chemical storage	Visual inspection; thermometer, hygrometer	Chemical fumes present? Is radiation present? 65° ± 5°F 50% ± 10% humidity	Monthly

Photographic material should be stored at temperatures less than 75°F, preferably in the range of 60 to 70°F. Open packages should be stored in an area with humidity ranging between 40 and 60%. Photographic material should not be stored in areas where it can be exposed to radiation or chemical fumes. Film is sensitive to pressure damage; consequently, film should be stored on edge — never flat.

---

* The format for this chapter was adapted from *Syllabus on Radiography Radiation Protection*, State of California Department of Health Services, Sacramento, 1995. With permission from Edgar D. Bailey.

Photographic chemicals should be stored under conditions similar to film in closed containers. The lid, airtight, should be closed on storage containers. They should be in secondary containment. The containment should be checked for leaks and damage. Chemical and hazardous waste storage records shall be monitored monthly. Some local codes require a minimum of weekly testing.

Darkroom Conditions

Test	Test Device	Performance Criteria	Frequency
Darkroom conditions	Visual inspection	Is darkroom clean?	Monthly
	Thermometer	70° ± 5°F	
	Hygrometer if available	50% ± 10% humidity	

Major problems encountered in darkrooms are dust and dirt. The log of darkroom cleaning shall be monitored monthly. The same environmental conditions for film and chemical storage also applies to the darkroom. If the film and chemicals are stored in the darkroom, darkroom conditions and storage conditions can be combined.

Darkroom Fog

Test	Test Device	Performance Criteria	Frequency
Darkroom fog	Visual inspection, desnitometer step wedge, opaque material (cardboard)	<0.10 increase in density in 2 minutes No visible light leaks in the darkroom	Semiannually

Film fogging must be eliminated because it reduces film contrast in the mid-density range. Adequate time (15 to 20 minutes) should be spent in the darkroom before testing for darkroom fog to allow for dark adaption and to allow for visual inspection of the darkroom for visible white light (light leaks).

20.2   Darkroom Safelight and Light Leakage Testing

Frequency

Semi-annual or after change

Purpose

To test the safelight filter for deterioration or failure.
To assure that the film can be exposed to the safelight for at least 2 minutes with no increase in density or fog.
To find any light leaks in darkroom and correct them before film is exposed to light.

Materials Needed

8 in. × 10 in. rare-earth fine or detail; step wedge; densitometer; opaque material such as a piece of cardboard

Procedure

1. Center step wedge to the center of a 8 in. × 10 in. Extremity cassette at 40 in. FFD.
2. Expose film using 1.5 or 1.7 mAs and 80 kVp (Figure 20.1).
3. Turn off the safelight.
4. Enter the darkroom and close the door.
5. After eyes are accustomed to the darkness, check room for light leaks. This process can take up to 20 minutes.
6. Remove the exposed film from the cassette and cover one half of it with a piece of cardboard while lights are still off. Use one half piece of the cardboard that comes in the 8 in. × 10 in. film (Figure 20.2).
7. Turn on the safelight and expose the uncovered portion of the film for 2 minutes.
8. Process the film and read the step wedge densities with the densitometer.

Quality Criteria

At the step closest to 1.20 O.D., there should not be more than a 0.10 O.D. difference between the two halves of the film.

Corrective Action

1. Make sure the safelight is at least 48 in. from the countertop. If not, relocate the safelight and retest. This can be done until all locations are exhausted.
2. Make sure that the safelight is designed for type of film used. Orthographic film or film that reacts to green-spectrum light uses a different safelight filter than blue-sensitive film. If wrong, replace filter or unit.

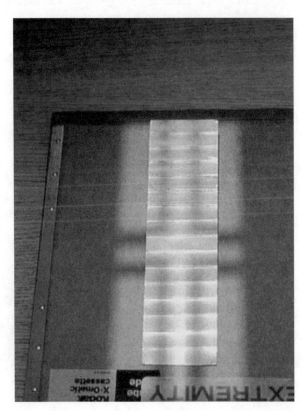

FIGURE 20.1
Safelight test film exposure.

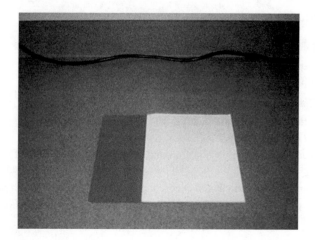

FIGURE 20.2
Safelight test film covered.

3. Relocate safelight farther from the work counter.
4. Check the bulb wattage to see if the wrong wattage was installed.

Safelight Test Examples

Figure 20.3 shows a properly working safelight. Some fogging is observed after 2 minutes, but it is not more than the 0.10 O.D. limit.

Figure 20.4 demonstrates a failed test. There is significant fogging of the film. The safelight was installed less than 48 in. from the work counter. The safelight was moved and a new filter installed. Figure 20.3 is the result of these changes. The darker side of the image is fogged.

Notice the effect that fog has on image contrast.

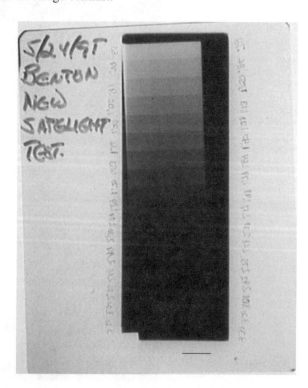

FIGURE 20.3
Safelight test film passed.

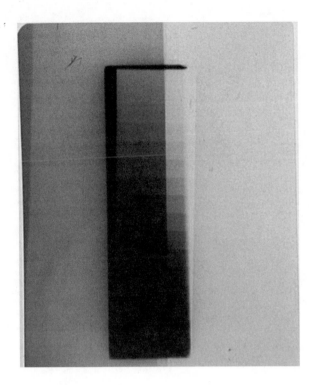

FIGURE 20.4
Safelight test film failed.

Chapter 21

Film Processing
Quality Control*

21.1 Principles of Automatic Processor Operation

The first automatic film processor was introduced by Pako in 1942. It took 40 minutes to process each film. It was a significant breakthrough because the manual process took 1 hour per film. Kodak introduced the 1st roller transport film processor in 1956. The processor was over 10 feet long, weighed 1500 pounds, and sold for $33,000 ($150,000 current dollars). In 1965, Kodak introduced the first 90-second processor with film and chemicals designed to dry in a 90-second cycle. It remains as the standard of the industry today. In 1990, an automatic processor with a cycle time of 30 seconds was introduced by Kodak. Currently, processors cost between $6000 and $25,000 (list price).

The automatic film processor consists of a film transport system, developer temperature control, replenishment and recirculation systems, fixer recirculation and replenishment systems, water flow control, and film dryer system. The film is manually inserted into the processor from the feed tray. The film is transported through (1) the developer rack, (2) the fixer rack, (3) the wash rack, and (4) the dryer section, and then (5) exits dry and ready to read. The film path is a serpentine route. This enables proper emulsion agitation and maximum chemical-to-emulsion coupling that produces the optimum speed and contrast. The developer produces the latent image exposed onto the film. The fixer essentially stops that development process and makes the resultant image permanent. Washing removes the chemicals to ensure proper drying and long-term archival.

Basics of Automatic Processor Operation

The modern automatic processor is divided into six functional systems. In order to make minor repairs and diagnose what may be wrong with the processor, it is important to understand the systems and what they control.

---

* The format for this chapter was adapted from *Syllabus on Radiography Radiation Protection*, State of California Department of Health Services, Sacramento, 1995. With permission from Edgar D. Bailey.

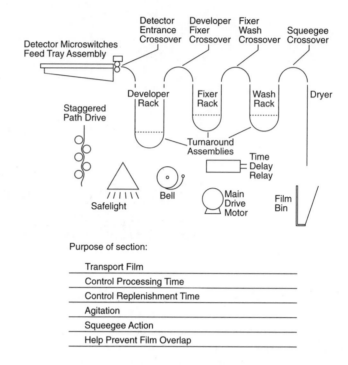

Purpose of section:

Transport Film
Control Processing Time
Control Replenishment Time
Agitation
Squeegee Action
Help Prevent Film Overlap

FIGURE 21.1
Roller transport system.

Roller Transport System

The roller transport system (Figure 21.1) is the drive system that takes the film through the chamicals and dryer, and then releases the finished film into the film bin. It controls the time that the replenishment pumps. When a film is far enough into the processor to leave the darkroom or feed another film into the unit, a bell, alarm, or light will come on.

Developer Recirculation System

The developer recirculation system (Figure 21.2) agitates the developer. This agitation and the serpentine path that the film takes through the developer tank promotes complete development of the film. Koadak processors use the water in the wash tank to help control the developer temperature. The heating and thermostat that control developer temperature are important parts of this system. The Kodak processor also filters the developer to keep the chemical cleaner.

Water Circulation System

The wash circulation system (Figure 21.3) cleans the film after it exits the fixer tank. Fresh water is fed into the processor to properly clean the film. Many processors use cool water to help regulate the developer and fixer temperature.

Fixer Recirculation System

The fixer stops development and clears the film (see Figure 21.4). The cleaning process removes silver ions from the film. The silver makes the used fixer hazardous waste.

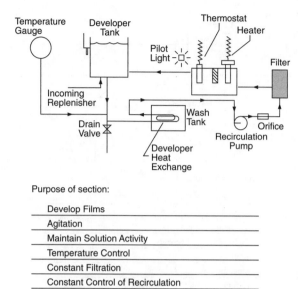

Purpose of section:

Develop Films
Agitation
Maintain Solution Activity
Temperature Control
Constant Filtration
Constant Control of Recirculation
Help Control Fixer Temperature

FIGURE 21.2
Developer recirculation system.

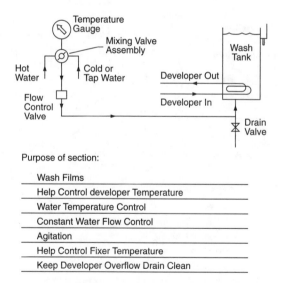

Purpose of section:

Wash Films
Help Control developer Temperature
Water Temperature Control
Constant Water Flow Control
Agitation
Help Control Fixer Temperature
Keep Developer Overflow Drain Clean

FIGURE 21.3
Water circulation system.

Developer and Fixer Replenishment System

The replenishment systems (Figure 21.5) add fresh chemicals to the processor tanks when films are being processed. This maintains solution activity and proper levels in the processor developer and fixer tanks. The rate of replenishment is based on daily activity.

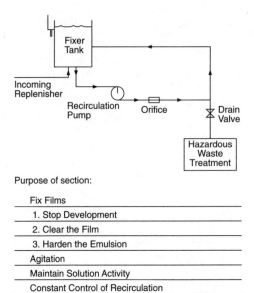

Purpose of section:

Fix Films
1. Stop Development
2. Clear the Film
3. Harden the Emulsion
Agitation
Maintain Solution Activity
Constant Control of Recirculation

FIGURE 21.4
Fixer recirculation system.

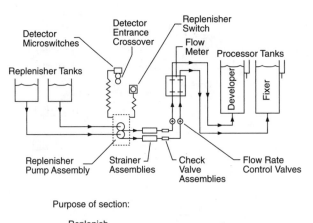

Purpose of section:

Replenish
To Maintain Solution Activity and Solution Level
Constant Straining
Control/Adjust Replenishment Rates
Check Replenishment Rates
Prevent Siphoning or Backflow of Replenisher

FIGURE 21.5
Developer + fixer replenishment system.

Dryer or Air Circulation System

This system (see Figure 21.6) dries the film. The heater is controlled by a thermostat that controls the temperature of the air. If possible, exhaust the hot air outside the darkroom to keep the air temperature in the darkroom cool. Some new processors use infrared lamps to dry the film and avoid the heat problem.

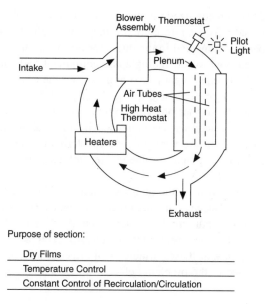

Purpose of section:

Dry Films
Temperature Control
Constant Control of Recirculation/Circulation

FIGURE 21.6
Air circulation/recirculation system.

Film Processing Chemicals

It is rare to find someone today mixing their own automatic processing chemicals. Most facilities order premixed working-strength chemicals from a film-processing service company. This factor significantly reduces the hazards of working with the developer and fixer.

The developer is mildly alkaline in nature and contains some harmful chemicals. It is slightly yellow in color and turns brown when oxidized. Great care should be taken if mixing one's own developer. Working Strength Rapid Processing Developer contains 2% hydroquinone, 1% potassium hydroxide, and 1% glutaraldehyde sodium bisulfite. These chemicals can cause skin and eye irritation in working strength. In bulk form, very good ventilation is required. Some people may be allergic to the developer. Sensitization can be minimized by the use of gloves when handling; and if skin contact occurs, use a nonalkaline-type hand cleaner and regularly clean work surfaces. Neither used nor unused developer is considered a hazardous waste; but as with most chemicals, water should be used to dilute the discharge into the sewer.

The fixer is acidic in nature and corrosive. It has a rather strong ammonia odor, even in working strength. The principal ingredients are 10% ammonium thiosulfate and 5% sodium thiosulfate. It remains clear in color but does crystallize. Remember that fixer coming from the processor contains silver ions removed from the unexposed portions of the film. Silver is very toxic to aquatic life and therefore requires special treatment before it can enter the environment. Unused fixer can be disposed into the sewer but water should be used to dilute the chemicals. The corrosive nature of the fixer will destroy pipes and even stainless steel. Work surfaces should always be clean to avoid corrosion.

Darkroom and Processor Quality Control

Processor and Darkroom Quality Control is the foundation of the Radiographic Quality Assurance Program. The daily testing of the processor and frequent testing of the darkroom environment is nothing new to radiography in hospitals and facilities that perform mammography. Organizations such as the American College of Radiology (ACR) and the Joint Commission of Accreditation of

Healthcare Systems (JCAHO) recognized that the quality of radiographic services depends significantly on the technical quality of its information. Since late 1976, the importance of monitoring the film processor has been documented in the quest for consistent film quality.

Previously, one learned how to test radiographic equipment and care for the screen system. One knows now that the X-ray equipment is operating within the established limits; and that each time an exposure is taken by a given technique, the density will be the same on the film; that the collimator is working properly so that one can collimate to the essential anatomy; and that the X-ray equipment has been serviced as recommended by the manufacturer. The parameters for operating the radiographic system are very important in terms of radiation exposure to operator and the patient. With modern equipment, problems are rare and, therefore, they are not the most important variables for image quality.

The most influential component in the imaging chain for final image quality is the darkroom and automatic film processor. Because of this, processor quality control is not only necessary, it should take top priority in any radiographic quality control program. Automatic film processing variables include (1) processing cycle time, (2) temperature, (3) chemical replenishment, (4) agitation, and (5) drying. A change in any of these variables will affect image quality. Quality control with very tight limits will alert one to the problem before it impacts image quality.

21.2   Processor Sensitometry

Processor quality control is based on sensitometry, which is the study and measurement of a film's response to exposure and processing. The characteristic or H & D curve is the traditional method of demonstrating the film's response. The sensitometer is a device that exposes the film to a repeatable series of graded light exposure. It has a light source that pulses light up through an optical step wedge, ranging from very light to very dark. Prior to sensitometers, a step wedge was exposed to X-rays and the film was processed to produce the steps of exposure. This adds the variables of X-ray generation into the control process. Today, it is highly recommended that the sensitometer be used for processor quality control.

The density of each step is measured using a densitometer. The densitometer's light source generates a calibrated amount of light that is focused with the help of a small-aperture diaphragm. The image to be measured is placed between the diaphragm and the densitometer's sensor arm. When the sensor is activated, it compares the amount of light emitted to the amount of light passing through the image on the film. The densitometer will display a number called an optical density unit that indicates the darkness of the film at the spot. The higher the number, the darker the film. After all the densities are measured, they are plotted on the vertical (y) axis of a graph against the log of their relative exposures (mAs) on the horizontal (x) axis. By connecting the points with a curve of best fit, the characteristic curve is constructed. The bottom or toe of the curve represents the low-density region of the image. The middle or straight line corresponds to the clinically useful density range. The shoulder or upper part is the high-density range of the image.

From the characteristic or H & D curve, certain properties of the image can be assessed, including base-plus-fog, speed, and contrast. The base-plus-fog is the lowest optical density value or lowest value of the curve. This value is used to monitor the overall fog level of the image. An increase in the value would show greater fog levels on the image.

The second property monitored is speed. Speed can be visually assessed by determining the proximity of the curve to the vertical or density axis. If the curve moves closer to this axis, it indicates an increase in speed, and vice versa. A specific speed index for the image can be determined by identifying the optical density value closest to 1.0 plus the base-plus-fog value. When the speed index step is determined, it can be used to monitor the speed index. When the optical density number increases, the speed has increased, and vice versa.

The third property monitored is contrast. Normally, one is more concerned about a film's overall or average contrast, or contrast index. Like speed, this can be visually assessed or specifically quantified. To visually assess contrast, examine the slope of the middle or straight line portion of the curve. To determine the average contrast or contrast index, take the difference between two specific values. The first value is the step closest to 0.25 plus base-plus-fog. The second is the step closest to 2.00 plus base-plus-fog. In formula form,

Step A (value of ~2.00 + base + fog) – Step B (value of ~0.25 + base + fog) = Contrast index

It would take too much time to daily produce the characteristic curve to monitor the photographic quality of the film. It would also be very difficult to see any changes each day. Therefore, once the steps that correspond to speed and contrast indexes are established, these properties can be monitored by daily monitoring of these specific steps. The unexposed film is monitored for the base-plus-fog level. By charting four spots on the film, one can establish that the film processor is operating within the standards of ±0.10 optical density changes from baseline.

Starting the Processor Sensitometry Program

There are several problems or factors that can play havoc with sensitometric information. The basis of quality control is to reduce all sources of variability. An automatic film processor's operating levels have a slight amount of inherent variability considered random and acceptable. This is indicated by the range of acceptable reading of ±0.10 optical densities. However, some sources of variability that may first appear as random are really due to variations in the process that produced and processed the sensitometric strip, called systematic variability. Steps must be taken to eliminate these variations.

The sensitometer should be set to the color spectrum of the film and screens used. Rare-earth or the Kodak Lanex and TMG films are green-sensitive, while the older high-speed and RP film systems are blue-sensitive. The battery that powers the unit should be changed annually. The densitometer must be calibrated each day. Both units need to have initial calibration to ensure accurate data. The films from the first week should not be graphed, but the numbers should be averaged to establish the operational baseline of the processor.

A control batch of film needs to be selected and stored in a separate film bin or location from the clinical film. This will minimize the variable exposure to the safelight that film in the clinical film bin receives. Using the same batch of film also eliminates manufacturing variations that are normal when comparing batches of film. Before the box of control film runs out, a new box should be selected and a sheet from the new box should be processed with the old batch to determine if new control values will need to be established.

To prevent differences in emulsion, both sides of the film are flashed with the sensitometer. The numbers are averaged to provide the most accurate reading. This also reduces the impact of bromide drag. Bromide ions are a byproduct of the development process. As the film's crystals develop, bromide ions are created and released into the gelatin that bonds the emulsion to the base. This inhibits the developer solution electrons from getting to the undeveloped film crystals. This results in decreased density on the trailing edge of the film. Even the flow of the developer as it recirculates in the tank and changes in temperature from replenishment can result in variances. These are minimized by routinely feeding the film into the processor the same way each day. It should be fed along the left rail of the feed tray.

Even the time of day can impact the results. The strip cannot be processed until the processor is warmed up to full operating parameters. The roller cleaning films should also have been run to clean any residual chemicals from the rollers. The water must be turned on and the water flow visually checked. The temperature of the developer, water, and fixer should also be within set parameters. These parameters should have been recorded on the Quality Control sheet. The developer temperature is also graphed with the sensitometry. Be sure to wash the thermometer probe tip between immersion in the developer and fixer tanks and after use.

Once the processor has been properly prepared, the rest of the darkroom environment must be evaluated. Periodically and after any bulb change, the darkroom safelight should be tested. It is important that the filter of the safelight match the film being used. Older RP type film used a Wratten 6B filter that will not protect the TMG type film. The newer filter, called the GBX-2 filter, will work with either film. It is very important that the wattage of the bulb in the safelight be checked, particularly if there is an increase in base + fog levels. The low wattage bulbs can be difficult to locate. The wattage of the beehive type filter should not exceed 15 Watts. The fluorescent filters should be replaced as a unit, with bulb and filter replaced as a unit. The darkroom should also be evaluated for proper temperature, ventilation, humidity, and any light leaks.

There are a couple of ways to test the safelight. One uses a step wedge exposed to X-ray and the other uses film exposed with the sensitometer. Both are valid means to test the light. In both cases, half of the film is masked with cardboard with the safelight off. The safelight is turned on and the film is left under the safelight for 1 minute. The film is processed, and readings from both sides of the film are made using the densitometer. There should be no more than a 0.05 optical density difference.

Ensure that the processor has been appropriately prepared

Daily

1. Check the level of chemicals in the fixer and developer tanks and replenishment tanks.
2. Check the water flow into the wash tank and that it is full.
3. Visually check the racks and gears for wear.
4. When the developer thermostat light begins to cycle on and off, check and record the developer, fixer, and water temperatures.
5. Close the cover of the processor and process three roller cleaning films.
6. Check all plumbing for leaks, particularly the line running to the tanks and tank level for the hazardous waste storage.

Semi-annual and Initial Setup

1. Check immersion or processing time of film.
2. Measure water flow rate.

Steps for ensuring proper processor operation

1. Ensure that the processor has been appropriately prepared (daily).
2. Ensure that the darkroom is safe (initial and semi-annual testing of the safelight).
3. Expose the control film with the densitometer.
4. Process the sensitometric control film.
5. Determine base + fog, speed, and contrast index values.
6. Record data on a processor control chart.
7. Analyze the results and take appropriate action.

21.3 Processor Sensitometry Problem-Solving

Now that one knows the basics of how to perform the daily processor quality control and generate and graph the sensitometry strips, one can begin to do some problem-solving using the data. It is impossible to review all of the situations that could result in unacceptable conditions; some of the more common occurrences are presented in Figures 21.7 to 21.12. Becoming an expert problem-solver requires experience looking at charts and an intimate knowledge of the particular film processor. It is very important to understand the basic function of each of the components in the processor in order to make an intelligent decision about what is causing the problem. The preventive cleaning of the processor can impact the sensitometry when fresh chemicals with starter are added. The date of cleaning should be marked with an asterisk. Trends on the control chart are as important as sudden changes that are outside the limits. Trends allow one to correct common problems before they become major ones.

Should the control film have readings that are outside acceptable limits, expose and process another strip to confirm the data. If the reading continues to be unacceptable, immediate action should be taken. If the reading is out of control by 0.10 O.D., repeating the strip after a few films are run may resolve the problem. It will also confirm if the problem is getting worse.

Chart 1: Normal Operating Control Chart

Chart 1 (Figure 21.7) demonstrates a processor operating within control limits. Note the control limits on the chart. For speed and contrast index, variances of ±0.10 O.D. are acceptable. With

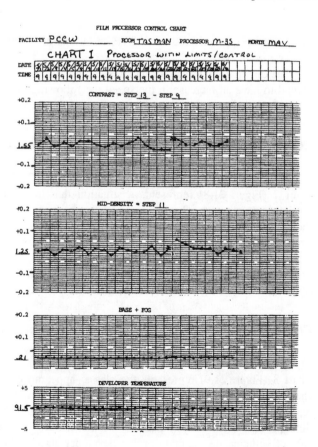

FIGURE 21.7

Chart 1: Normal operating control chart.

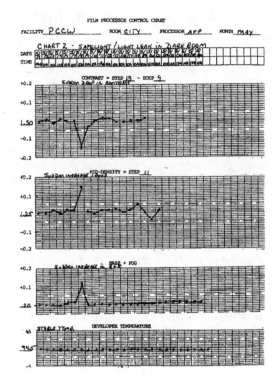

FIGURE 21.8
Chart 2: Sudden increases in B + F and speed with decrease in contrast and normal developer temperature.

base-plus-fog now referred to as B+F, the limits are ±0.05 O.D. The control limit for developer temperature is ±0.5°.

The day that the processor received its monthly preventive service is marked with a star. It is normal to have an increase in the speed the following day due to fresh chemicals. If the increase is too high, the service company can add more developer starter to properly season the developer.

Chart 2: Sudden Increases in B+F and Speed with Decrease in Contrast and Normal Developer Temperature

Chart 2 (Figure 21.8) represents a situation that may arise occasionally and produces classic sensitometric changes. The processor has been operating within control limits. Suddenly the strip shows a sharp rise in B+F, a rise in speed, and a sharp drop in contrast with no change in developer temperature. The most likely cause is unsafe darkroom conditions because the combination is characteristic for film fog. Because it is a sudden change, a darkroom safelight problem should be examined first. The bulb may have been changed and the wrong wattage bulb installed or the filter adjusted. If the safelight is correct, look for a white light leak into the darkroom.

Chart 3: Gradual Decline in Speed and Contrast with normal B+F and Developer Temperature

Chart 3 (Figure 21.9) represents the classic appearance of problems with replenishment of the chemicals. The gradual decline in speed and contrast with normal B+F and developer temperature represents under-replenishment of the developer. A prime factor in replenishment is the volume of films processed each day. When the volume of films is very low, the normal replenishment rates are not sufficient to maintain proper developer activity. Developer chemicals lose free electrons

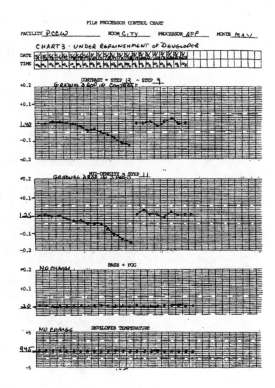

FIGURE 21.9

Chart 3: Gradual decline in speed and contrast with
normal B + F and developer temperature.

to the air when the developer sits idle, causing exhaustion. A slight increase in replenishment rates
may be warranted to see if it will even out the chart.

The best way to avoid this problem is to run two or three 14 in. × 17 in. films each day. Roller
cleaning film and outdated film work great. Do not reuse rejected film because it will have some
residual fixer on the film; the residual fixer will eventually contaminate the developer. Keep the
processor turned off when not needed. The recirculation of the chemicals will speed the oxidation.

Chart 4: Gradual Rise in Speed and Contrast, Followed by a Sudden Drop in Speed, Contrast, and Developer Temperature

Chart 4 (Figure 21.10) is used to demonstrate two common problems. If under-replenishment results
in a gradual decrease in speed and contrast, it is logical that over-replenishment will result in an
increase of speed and contrast. This can happen after the processor has been cleaned and the tanks
filled with fresh chemicals. It is recommended that the replenishment rates be checked with each
cleaning of the processor. If the volume of films has been very high, the replenishment can be too
high for the volume. The brand and type of film used will significantly impact the effects of
replenishment on the Quality Control Program. Kodak TMG type film is very stable, and it takes
dramatic changes in replenishment to affect its image quality. It is recommended that rates not be
decreased as long as the chart is within limits. If the chart is high on a Friday, the chart will probably
be correct on Monday after a weekend of inactivity. If the speed is routinely high, a minor reduction
in the replenishment rate may correct the problem and save some money. There are other factors
that can cause the speed to increase. A slower transport speed can keep the film in the developer
too long. Development of the film is controlled by developer temperature, activity of the chemicals,
and the total time spent in the developer. If a new box of control film has been opened, a new batch
may be a little faster than the last batch. The operator should consider increasing the aim or baseline
speed index if everything tests good.

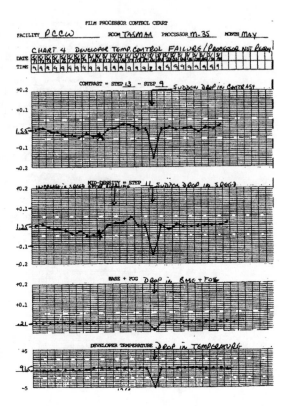

FIGURE 21.10
Chart 4: Gradual rise in speed and contrast, followed by a sudden drop in speed, contrast, and developer temperature.

The other problem is demonstrated by the sudden drop in speed, contrast, and developer temperature. Normally, this film should not have been processed because the processor was not properly prepared. This is indicated by the developer temperature being out of limits. Because one also checks water and fixer temperatures, any fluctuation in developer temperature before the strip is run will probably never occur. It could indicate that the water is too cold, a failure in the developer recirculation system controls, or someone has turned the temperature control knob. In the example, once the control thermostat was replaced, the processor returned to normal operation. The problem could have been a failure of the developer heater. The most likely reason for these readings is that the processor quality control film was processed before the developer had completely warmed up. It is important to know how long it takes the processor to reach normal operating temperature. Most processors will have either an LED that flashes on and off when the temperature is correct or a thermometer. The built-in thermometer should be tested occasionally for accuracy. Never use a mercury-filled thermometer in a processor; if broken, it will severely contaminate the chemicals.

If the speed index reading comes out low, run a couple more cleaning films. Repeat the test after waiting an additional 30 minutes. If the processor has a button that allows manual replenishment, pump a couple of cycles of fresh developer into the processor.

Chart 5:   Repeated Increases in Speed, Contrast, and Developer Temperature

Chart 5 (Figure 21.11) demonstrates a processor not in control. The problem is with the water flow or temperature. The water in the wash tank regulates the heating of the developer. The water flow

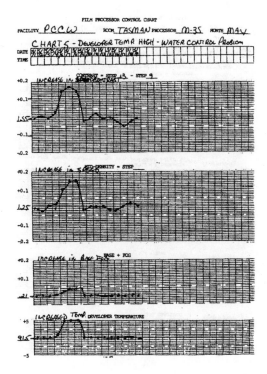

FIGURE 21.11
Chart 5: Repeated increases in speed, contrast, and developer temperature.

is controlled by a control valve or regulator in the processor. If this unit fails or the water pressure is too low, the flow of water into the tank can be too low to maintain proper developer and wash water temperatures. The water control valve should be tested semi-annually. If this problem occurs, it should be immediately tested. The Bay Area water is high in mineral content and can result in deposits that obstruct the flow of water. This can be avoided by water filters, but they are seldom used in clinical practice.

Chart 6: A Processor that Continues to Fall Out of Limits and Everything Has Been Checked

Chart 6 (Figure 21.12) shows a processor with the speed very erratic, the contrast extremely low and off the scale, and some variation in B+F with the developer temperature within limits. The developer replenishment is set to factory specifications and water and fixer temperatures are normal. The first clue is the extended periods of non-operation demonstrated by the dates that quality control was performed. This processor was located in a very low-volume office. On the days after cleaning, the processor was fine. After sitting idle for 10 days, it was out of limits.

Remember that the developer loses its free electrons when sitting idle. This will happen even more quickly if the processor is turned on. The replenishment of the developer is usually activated by films being fed into the processor. This is called volume replenishment. Most modern processors can be converted to timed or flood replenishment. Although this will probably result in more chemicals being used, the processor will stay within limits and function as a stable unit. This will also prevent chemical buildup on the roller assemblies. One notes that all of the problems that sensitometry demonstrates involve developer, replenishment, or temperature control.

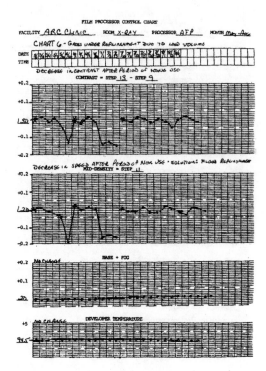

FIGURE 21.12
Chart 6: A processor that continues to fall out of limits and everything has been checked.

Fixer, Wash Water, and Processor Quality Control

The only time when the fixer will impact actual image quality is when it gets into the developer and contaminates the developer. This is usually the result of a film jam in the processor. When contamination occurs, the developer filter and all chemicals must be drained and the processor cleaned. Contaminated developer may be cream in color and will generate films that are pink due to the inhibition of the development process and stopping action of the fixer.

If the replenishment of the fixer is wrong, the films will not adequately dry. Fixer can also be contaminated by the developer or wash water. This will result in the films being dark and grainy due to the continued developing process.

Fixer and washing of the film is tested semi-annually using a hypo test kit. The residual fixer on the film is measured by the stain resulting from the test kit. If the fixer and wash functions are within limits, the films will have good archival properties.

Occasionally, someone will forget to turn on the water feeding the processor or the water may be shut off. This will eventually result in the developer overheating. The lack of water will also not stop the fixing process. The films will suddenly be very dark and even brownish-black in color. Processing should be stopped until the developer temperature is back within limits.

Care and Cleaning of the Processor

A clean processor rarely jams and rarely produces artifacts on the film. The daily cleaning of the feed tray and darkroom counter will reduce scratches and other artifacts on the processed film. The daily cleaning of the crossover racks will reduce buildup of chemicals on the rollers and provide an opportunity to check them for cracking of the rollers. Visually checking the drive gears for wear will reduce the chance of film jams.

After the unit has warmed up, the processing of two roller transport cleaning films will provide a final cleaning of the rollers before quality control and clinical films are processed. These films are tacky and will remove any emulsion flecks or dry chemicals missed by washing the rollers.

Conclusion

A systematic approach to processor quality control will have the greatest impact on image quality found in a Radiology Quality Control Program. The monitoring of control charts and daily quality control will demonstrate trends before they shut down the department. Monitoring is also a great tool for problem-solving when dates of service, chemical delivery, and cleaning are documented.

When processor and radiographic quality control are combined, optimum quality can be achieved on a consistent basis. Good and consistent technique charts can be produced. With the practice of sound radiographic technique, patient and staff exposures to radiation can be significantly reduced.

One will be able to spend more quality time with patients and be less likely to get behind schedule due to retakes. By practicing sound sequencing of the radiographic exam, one will be less likely to make an error. By monitoring errors, one will be able to determine one's strengths as well as the areas that may require further training or reading.

Costs will be reduced because less film and chemicals will be wasted. If a film does come out poorly, one will be able to correct the technique with confidence that it is a result of patient habitus and not a malfunctioning processor or X-ray machine. One will be able to take pride in one's radiographic services, and the patient will be happy with the service.

21.4   Control Limits for Processor Quality Control

Processor quality control (QC) is performed by processing a freshly exposed sensitometric strip and reading the strip with a densitometer. The objective of processor QC is to test the processor and chemicals with the same film normally used in the processor. The sensitometric strip should be exposed to sensitometric light of the same color as the light emitted by the intensifying screens. It is never exposed to X-rays.

Control charts are the key to the processor QC program, because they allow for the perception of trends, both slow and rapid changes, in the areas being monitored.

A processor QC program shall monitor the following:

* Base-plus-fog density
* Speed or mid-density (optical density nearest 1.0 plus base-plus-fog level)
* Contrast or density difference (calculated by subtracting the step closest to 0.25 + base + fog from the step closest to 2.00 + base + fog. Often, these steps will be two above and two below the speed step)

Processor Sensitometric Evaluation

Test	Test Device	Performance Criteria	Frequency
Processor sensitometry evaluation	Sensitometer; densitometer; control film	Base + fog ± 0.05 Speed ± 0.10 Contrast ± 0.10	Daily before processing the first patient's films

Processor QC shall be carried out at the beginning of the day, after sufficient time has elapsed for the processing chemicals temperature to reach their operating level and all systems have stabilized. The stand-by controls and the developer heater light shall have cycled off. This may require up to 30 minutes.

Developer Temperature

Test	Test Device	Performance Criteria	Frequency
Developer temperature	Thermometer	±0.5°F	Daily

The developer temperature shall be within ±0.5°F of the manufacturer's recommended developer temperature for the film and processor being used. If the processor has a built-in thermometer, the recording of the reading meets this standard. If used, the built-in thermometer accuracy shall be monitored monthly.

Tank Level Check, Clean-up Films, Cleaning of Crossover Rollers

Test	Test Device	Performance Criteria	Frequency
Tank level checks, clean-up films, and clean cross-over rollers	Visual inspection; clean-up films	Full tanks; no scratches on films; are crossover rollers clean?	Daily

Part of the morning QA routine is to check that the tanks in the processor are full. A low level could indicate a replenishment problem. Before processing the sensitometry strip, two 14 in. × 17 in. roller cleaning films will be processed. These films should be totally clear. Never use reject films, as small amounts of fixer will be put in the developer, causing contamination.

At the end of the workday, the crossover rollers can be removed, cleaned with warm water and a damp, soft cloth, and dried. The cover of the processor should be left open about 2 in. so that moisture and chemical fumes do not accumulate and cause corrosion.

Cleaning and Preventive Maintenance of Processor

Test	Test Device	Performance Criteria	Frequency
Cleaning and preventive maintenance	As suggested by manufacturer; check of fixer and developer replenishment rates	As indicated by manufacturer	Monthly

On a monthly basis, the film processor shall be cleaned, developer filter changed, and replenishment rate for developer and fixer verified by personnel trained to maintain film processing equipment. The replenishment rates shall be set to factory specifications.

Wash Water Temperature

Test	Test Device	Performance Criteria	Frequency
Wash water temperature check	Thermometer	±5°F	Daily

The wash water is used to regulate the heat exchange from the developer heater and fixer temperature. If the water is too cold, greater energy will be required to keep the developer at the proper operating temperature. The fixer temperature may also be too low.

Fixer Temperature

Test	Test Device	Performance Criteria	Frequency
Fixer temperature	Thermometer	±5°F	Daily

This is part of the daily processor quality control program. Major temperature changes will impact the proper fix of the image. Always wash the thermometer after testing the fixer temperature. Checking fixer temperature is a California QC recommendation.

Processor Stand-by Unit

Test	Test Device	Performance Criteria	Frequency
Verify function of the processor stand-by unit	Visual inspection	Units maintains the developer temperature with drive off	Daily

When films are not being processed frequently, the stand-by unit places the processor in the stand-by mode, which turns off the drive system and dryer blower and reduces water flow. The developer temperature and dryer heat level are maintained at the operating temperature. In the stand-by mode, the developer temperature is monitored to assure the stand-by unit is functioning.

Water-Flow Meter Accuracy

Test	Test Device	Performance Criteria	Frequency
Flow meter accuracy	Stopwatch and graduated cylinder	±5%	Quarterly

The water-flow meter that controls the volume of water being replenished when the processor is operating was calibrated when the processor was installed. The calibration should be checked quarterly.

Film Fixer Retention

Test	Test Device	Performance Criteria	Frequency
Fixer retention of the processed film	Hypo test kit	<2 $\mu g/cm^2$ retained thiosulfate	Semi-annually

To assure proper archival ability of radiographic film, fixer retention is monitored. A few drops of the test solution are applied to one emulsion of the film in an unexposed area. The stain left on the film when dry is visually compared to a chart. It will determine the amount of thiosulfate ion on the film after wash and dryer function. The replenishment rate of the fixer is set based on this test.

Processor Transport Time

Test	Test Device	Performance Criteria	Frequency
Processor transport time	Stopwatch	±3%	Annually

The processor transport time is measured, using a stopwatch, from the instant the leading edge of the film enters the entrance roller until the leading edge exits the last roller in the dryer section of the processor. If not within 3% of specification, it can be adjusted to restore correct transport time.

21.5 Morning Darkroom and Processor Cleaning and Tests

Frequency

Daily

Purpose

To ensure that the processor is functioning properly
To ensure that there is no dirt that can get on films and result in artifacts
To ensure proper film transport in processor with no processor artifacts

Materials Needed

Thermometer
Densitometer
Sensitometer
Clean, lint-free towels

Procedure Before the First Case

1. Wipe down countertops and processor feed tray with damp cloth.
2. Complete hazardous waste checklist.
3. When processor is warmed up, check and record developer temperature. Limit is 0.5° (Figure 21.13).
4. Check and record wash water temperature. Limit is 5° (Figure 21.14).
5. Does the processor go into stand-by mode if so equipped?
6. Check and record fixer temperature (Figure 21.15). Limit is 5°. Rinse thermometer probe in water.
7. Run three 14 in. × 17 in. cleaning films through processor. Films should be clear films from the discard box or preferred special transport cleaning film.
8. If developer temperature is correct, expose an 8 in. × 10 in. film with sensitometer (Figure 21.16).

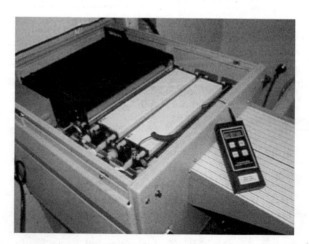

FIGURE 21.13
Check developer temperature.

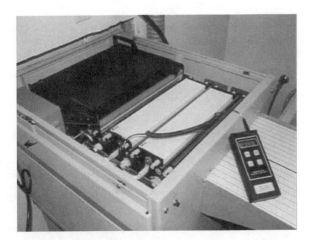

FIGURE 21.14
Check fixer temperature.

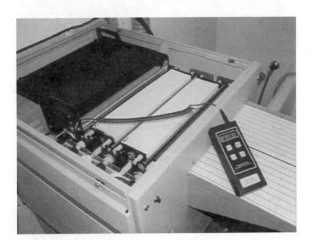

FIGURE 21.15
Check water temperature.

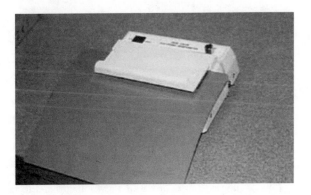

FIGURE 21.16
Test film exposed with senitometer.

9. Process the film with film to left rail (Figure 21.17).

10. Read the appropriate steps with densitometer. They are speed, base + fog, and density difference (Figure 21.18). Graph the reading on the processor control graph (Figure 21.19).

11. If processor is within operating parameters, proceed with day's case load.

12. Warm up X-ray units as assigned. Safety check locks and note any problems.

13. Record all data on the I.O.D. QC Log and initial.

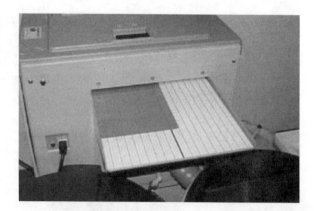

FIGURE 21.17
Test film processed.

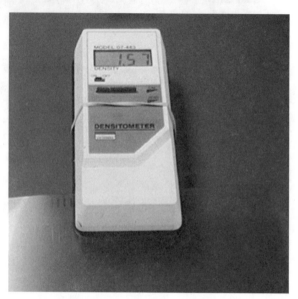

FIGURE 21.18
Test film reading with densitometer.

Quality Criteria for Film Processing: ±0.10 O.D. from Standard for Speed and Contrast Index and ±0.05 for Base + Fog

1. If speed too high, consider the following:
    High developer temperature: recheck developer temperature
    Water not running: recheck water flow or if water is turned on
    Decrease developer replenishment
    Fogged film: compare base + fog readings
2. If speed is too low, consider the following potential causes:
    Low developer temperature: wait a few minutes and recheck; consider thermostat problem
    Increase replenishment of developer
    Very cold water
    Developer recirculating problem
    Contaminated or oxidized developer
3. If base + fog is out of range, consider the following:
    Film outdated or improperly stored
    Wrong film or sensitometer setting

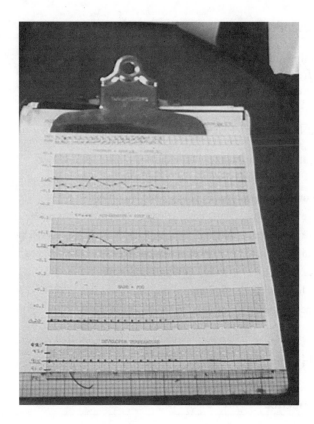

FIGURE 21.19
Results graphed.

    Safelight
    Developer temperature or over-replenishment
    Contaminated chemicals
4. If the contrast index is outside the limits, consider the following:
    Change in developer temperature
    Change in water temperature
    Change in developer replenishment
    Contaminated developer

21.6   Evening Darkroom and Processing Quality Control

Frequency

Daily

Purpose

To ensure artifact-free film processing by keeping rollers clean
To provide a systematic approach to monthly cassette care
To ensure that the X-ray department does not run out of chemicals

Materials Needed

Screen cleaning supplies
Clean, lint-free towel
Access to long, deep sink

Procedure Performed Prior to Closing X-ray Department

1. Check fresh chemical tanks; alert radiology staff if level is low.
2. Clean a couple of cassette screens. All screens need to be cleaned monthly.
3. Shut down processor, unplug power, and turn off water.
4. Remove lid and evaporation cover from crossover roller assemblies for developer and fixer tanks.
5. Remove developer to fixer crossover rack and fixer to wash water rack.
6. Wash in warm water with towel, drain, and then dry rollers and racks.
7. Replace racks and evaporation covers in processor.
8. Put lid back on process but leave it open at least 2 in.
9. Document performance of tests on QC log and Cassette Cleaning logs.

21.7   Hypo Estimator Testing

Materials Needed

> Kodak HT-2 Hypo Test Kit
>
> Sheet of white paper
>
> Tissue
>
> 8 in. × 10 in. Processor quality control test film

The Hypo Estimator test is a relatively simple method of estimating the amount of thiosulfate ion retained on the processed film. This will help determine the quality of film washing in the processor. Kodak manufactures and sells a kit with instructions, a strip used to read the results of the test, and two bottles of test solution (Figure 21.20).

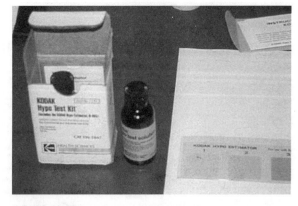

FIGURE 21.20
Hypo test equipment.

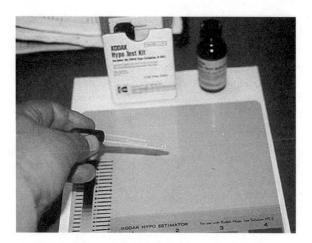

FIGURE 21.21
Hypo testing.

The test solution can be made by carefully combining:

Water	750 ml
28% Acetic acid	125 ml
Silver nitrate	7.5 g
Water:	To make 1 liter

Store solution in a brown screw-top bottle away from light. The test kit should be stored away from strong light sources and handled with care. Make sure than none of the test solution gets on clothing or on films. It will permanently stain the film or clothing black.

Procedure

1. Place one drop of test solution on a clear area of the emulsion side of a recently dried sheet of film. Position the drop away from the sensitometric exposed portion of the film. With double emulsion film, a drop on both sides of the film is ideal. Make sure the spots are not superimposed (Figure 21.21).

2. Allow the solution to stand for 2 minutes; then blot off any excess solution with the tissue.

3. Place the film on the sheet of white paper. Place the Estimator on top of the exposed film. Immediately compare the stain density to the patches on the Kodak Hypo Estimator. If the stains are not immediately interpreted or the solution is left on the film longer than 2 minutes, the results will not be accurate and will read high.

Test Interpretation

Test spots matching the patches on the Hypo Estimator correspond approximately to the following hypo contents:

Density of Stain	Estimated Thiosulfate Ion (g/m^2)
1	0.01
2	0.02 (Quality Control Standard)
3	0.05
4	0.12

Excessive Hypo retention indicates that the film is not being adequately washed. It will indicate that too much fixer is getting into the wash water, or the wash water is not being exchanged fast enough.

The properly installed processor will have adequate continuous flow of water into the wash tank. Excessive Hypo in the wash water will also indicate that the wash water will need to be treated as hazardous waste in many areas of the country.

Chapter **22**

Radiographic Quality Control Testing*

22.1 Radiographic Equipment Quality Control Limits

Conventional radiography systems have many elements, each of which is subject to variability or change in time. The more important elements in this system include:

- Kilovoltage (kVp)
- Milliamperage (mA)
- Exposure time
- X-ray beam filtration
- Collimation
- Focal spot size
- Grid (type, uniformity, and alignment)
- Intensifying screens
- Cassettes
- Radiographic film
- Darkroom conditions
- Photographic processor and chemicals

Each of the elements in the system can drift or degrade such that the image quality may be degraded. Therefore, in order to carry out operations in a cost-effective manner, it is essential to measure and control all of the appropriate variables in the radiographic chain. The costs of equipment to measure the performance of many of the X-ray systems are prohibitive for the small clinical practice; therefore, it is more cost effective to hire a Radiation Health Physicist to perform many of the annual tests, acceptance tests, and tests after replacement of major components such as the X-ray tube.

---

* The format for this chapter was adapted from *Syllabus on Radiography Radiation Protection,* State of California Department of Health Services, Sacramento, 1995. With permission of Edgar D. Bailey.

The appropriate QC tests shall be performed, after the repair or replacement of any component of the X-ray system, prior to using the equipment on human beings if such repairs and/or replacement may affect the following:

- Image quality
- Exposure timer accuracy
- Milliampere-seconds (mAs) linearity
- Kilovolt peak (kVp) accuracy
- Skin entrance radiation dose
- Focal spot size

There are some radiographic equipment tests that can be performed by staff that can monitor the performance of radiographic systems. These tests are performed semi-annually or more often, if indicated.

Light Field and X-ray Field Alignment and X-ray Beam Perpendicularity

Test	Test Device	Performance Criteria	Frequency
Light field and X-ray field alignment and beam perpendicularity	Alignment template and perpendicularity test tool and tape measure	±2% of the source to image distance (SID)	Semi-annually or after the change of the collimator light bulb

The center of the X-ray field must be perpendicular with, and aligned to the center of the image receptor to within 2% of the SID. The SID indicator must be accurate to within 2%. The alignment of the center to the field is not the only concern. The edges must also be accurate to within 2%. Nine pennies can be substituted for the collimation template. A penny is about 0.8 in. in diameter. This is the control limit for a 40 in. SID. This is a very large error and this author feels that the light and beam should match.

X-ray Beam, Grid Centering

Test	Test Device	Performance Criteria	Frequency
X-ray beam and grid centering	Homogeneous phantom, lead strips, and densitometer	Lead strips should be centered; density uniform to ±0.10 O.D. perpendicular to the anode-cathode axis	Semi-annually

The X-ray beam must be perpendicular to the grid and centered to the X-ray film to obtain uniform density over the film.

Exposure Linearity Reproducibility (basic test performed by staff)

Test	Test Device	Performance Criteria	Frequency
Linearity	Step wedge and densitometer	±5%	Semi-annually

Reproducibility means that the kVp and mAs can be changed, the original technique reset, and the resulting radiograph will be of the same density ±5%. A minimum of three exposures are made to determine the average and range.

Semi-annual Radiographic Tests Performed by the Health Physicist or Qualified Radiographer

The following tests shall be performed by a qualified radiographer or, when necessary, a Radiation Health Physicist or state inspector at least semi-annually and after replacement of the X-ray tube or other major component of the radiographic system.

Test	Performance Criteria	Frequency
Filtration (HVL) Wisconsin kVp cassette or ion chamber	Meet regulatory requirements of Title 17 CAC, Section 30308 (a) (3)	Annually
Focal spot size RMI focal spot test tool	NEMA Standard XR-5	Annually
Kilovoltage (kVp) Wisconsin kVp cassette or ion chamber	±5%; ±2% over range of 60 to 100 kVp	Annually
Exposure linearity and mAs linearity using a step wedge and densitometer	± 5%	Semi-annually
Radiation dose reproducibility using a phantom and densitometer	± 5%	Annually
Radiation dose (exposure) per film using TLDs and phantom	Based on a properly exposed A-P lumbar film	Annually

22.2 Collimator Accuracy and Beam Centering Testing

Frequency

Semi-annual or after replacement of collimator light bulb or service

Materials Needed

Collimator field alignment test tool
Beam perpendicularity test tool

or

9 pennies and ruler or tape measure
X-ray grid

Performance Criteria Limits

Beam cannot be larger or smaller than 2% of FFD, or cannot be more than 0.80 in. off at any part of the exposed film

Procedure Without Beam Alignment Test Tool (Figure 22.1)

1. Set focal film distance (FFD) to 40 in. Bucky.
2. Center film to horizontal light tape 8 in. × 8 in. grid to center of cassette (optional).
3. Set collimator field to 5 in. square.
4. Arrange pennies at center of ray, each corner of field and horizontal and vertical lines of the collimator.
5. Make exposure at 1 mAs and 60 kVp.
6. With ruler, mark center of ray, and horizontal and vertical axes of the beam.

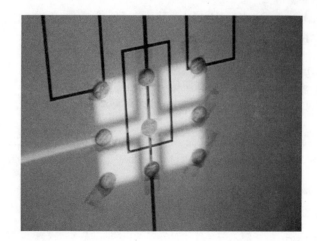

FIGURE 22.1
Collimator testing.

Procedure With Beam Alignment Test Tool (Figures 22.2 through 22.5)

1. Set FFD to 40 in. Bucky.
2. Center 8 in. × 10 in. film to beam.
3. Collimate beam to size of box on alignment test tool with vertical and horizontal line aligned with beam.
4. Tape perpendicularity test tool to Bucky at center of field (central ray).
5. Make exposure at 1 mAs and 60 kVp.
6. Process and measure beam size.

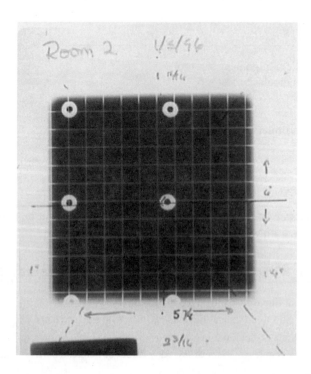

FIGURE 22.2
Collimator test film.

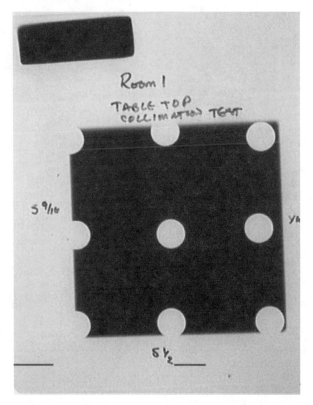

FIGURE 22.3
Collimator test film.

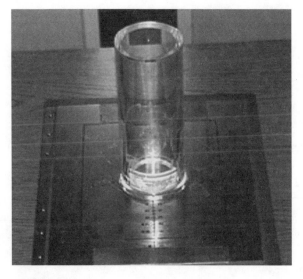

FIGURE 22.4
Beam perpendicularity test tool.

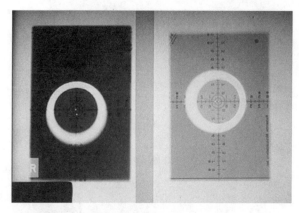

FIGURE 22.5
Beam perpendicularity test film.

22.3   Grid Cut-off and Perpendicularity Testing

Frequency

Semi-annual

Materials Needed

Neutral density phantom
(Block of lucite 14 in. × 17 in. × 2 in.) or lead apron
Screen contact test tool
14 in. × 17 in. Cassette

Criteria

X-ray exposure should be equal perpendicular to the cathode of the X-ray tube or within 0.10 O.D.

Technique

5 mAs, 60 kVp for screen contact test tool; 10 mAs, 70 kVp for apron at 40 in.

Procedure (Figure 22.6)

1.   Tape the screen contact test tool to the front of a 14 in. × 17 in. cassette, or drape apron over Bucky. The apron or a piece of Lucite is the most accurate test tool.
2.   Set FFD at 40 in. and put cassette in the Bucky.
3.   Collimate to film size.
4.   Expose and process the film.
5.   Read the density exposure with the densitometer to right and left of the central ray. If the grid is properly aligned, the readings should be equal or within 0.10 O.D.

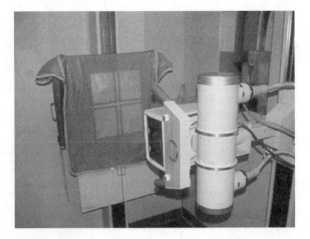

FIGURE 22.6
Grid alignment test at 40 in.

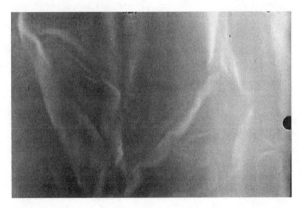

FIGURE 22.7
Grid alignment test film. (Note image lighter on one side: indicates grid cut-off due to alignment problem.)

22.4   Linearity of Exposure Testing

Frequency

Semi-annual or if problem is suspected

Materials Needed

Step wedge
Densitometer
14 in. × 17 in. cassette
Lead blockers

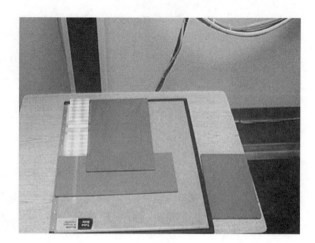

FIGURE 22.8
Exposure linearity test procedure.

Performance Criteria

Density readings must be within 5% of baseline. Make six exposures on the 14 in. × 17 in. film.

Procedure (Universal AP-300 or AP-500 or machine with mAs settings and variable time settings) (Figure 22.8)

1. Set a baseline technique at a 40 in. FFD.
2. Make exposure of step wedge.
3. Change technical factors and then reset original baseline technique.
4. Make second exposure; repeat step 2 for a third exposure.
5. Select time option and change exposure time for three more exposures.
6. Process the film and read the density of a step closest to 1.20 O.D.
7. Compare reading of same step for all other exposures.

Exposures 1 through 3 will evaluate exposure tracking or linearity across mA, time, and kVp. Exposure 4 through 6 will test mAs tracking or linearity.

Procedure (Universal MP-300 or MP-500)

Steps 1 though 5 are the same as AP-500 units.
6. Select low power and make exposure.
7. Select medium power and make exposure.
8. Select high power and make exposure.
9. Process film and read the density closest to 1.20.
10. Compare reading of same step for other exposures.

Evaluation will be the same as for AP-500.

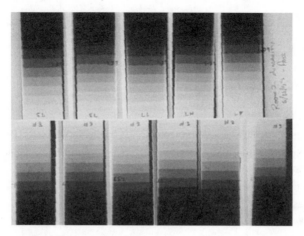

FIGURE 22.9
Exposure test passed (proper calibration).

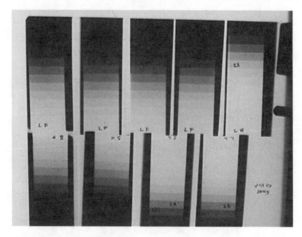

FIGURE 22.10
Exposure test filed (note: lighter images indicate poor calibration).

22.5   Focal Spot Size Testing

Frequency

Semi-annual, or if problem is suspected

Materials Needed

RMI Focal Spot Test Tool, NEMA Star Focal Spot Test Tool, or Pin Hole Camera
Detail or fine speed cassette
Lead blocker

Performance Criteria

Focal spot should be within 15% of advertised size

Procedure (Figure 22.11)

1. Set SID at 40 in. to a tabletop.
2. Place 8 in. × 10 in. Extremity cassette on table. Cover one half of cassette with lead blocker.
3. Set RMI Focal Spot Test Tool on cassette with the rivets aligned with the anode and cathode of the tube. Collimate to half of the film or tool size.
4. Set exposure factors for small focal spot and make exposure.
5. Cover the exposed portion of the cassette and repeat test with large focal spot. Use left marker to indicate large focal spot.
6. Process the film.

Interpretation of Results (Figure 22.12)

Look at the patterns of three vertical and horizontal bars. This test dramatically demonstrates the difference in detail with the large and small focal spots. 1.0 mm focal spot should resolve 11 line pairs per millimeter. 2.0 mm focal spot should resolve 5 line pairs per millimeter.

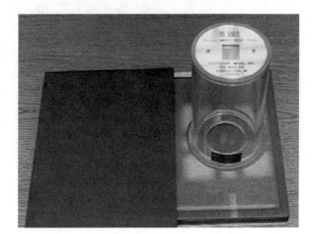

FIGURE 22.11
Focal spot size test.

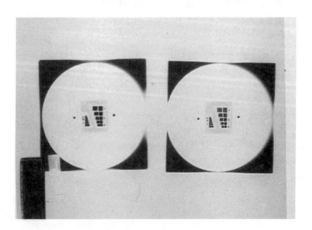

FIGURE 22.12
Focal spot test film.

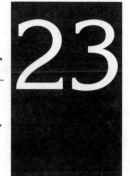

Chapter **23**

Accessory Quality Control Testing*

23.1   Accessory Quality Control Testing Limits

Accessory quality control involves testing of cassettes, intensifying screens, radiographic film, grids, and lead aprons and shields. These are the last variables in radiography that have not been evaluated under other portions of this plan. Typically, the accessories receive the most wear and tear from daily use and are the most prone to failure. Cassettes and screens require the most preventive care with monthly cleaning.

Screen-Film Contact

Test	Test Device	Performance Criteria	Frequency
Screen-film contact	Coarse copper mesh	Visual inspection: no areas of poor contact/blurring	Semi-annually

Screen Cleaning Record Check

On a quarterly basis, the cassette cleaning records will be reviewed to ensure that all of the cassettes were cleaned as required.

Grid Uniformity

Test	Test Device	Performance Criteria	Frequency
Evaluation of any clip or tape on stationary grids	Homogeneous phantom	Uniform film density of 1.20 ± 10 O.D. perpendicular to the anode-cathode axis	Annually

---

* The format for this chapter was adapted from *Syllabus on Radiography Radiation Protection,* State of California Department of Health Services, Sacramento, 1995. With permission of Edgar D. Bailey.

Screen-Film-Cassette Speed Matching

Test	Test Device	Performance Criteria	Frequency
Screen-film-cassette speed matching	Standard (comparison) cassette	Densities within 0.05 O.D. for all cassettes of the same speed/type	Annually

Lead Apron and Gonadal Shield Test

Test	Test Device	Performance Criteria	Frequency
Safety check via radiography of lead aprons and gonadal shields	X-ray unit, cassette and aprons	Radiographs should not detect any tears or holes in protective area of aprons and shields	Semi-annually

23.2 Screen Cleaning

Frequency

Monthly

Purpose

To ensure that there are no dirt artifacts on the radiographs

Materials Needed

Kodak Screen Cleaner
2 in. × 2 in. or 4 in. × 4 in. Non-sterile gauze pads
Cotton balls as a last-resort substitute for gauze pads
Sharpie black felt tip pen

Procedure

1. Remove good film from cassette and put it into the film bin.
2. Dampen a gauze pad with Kodak Screen Cleaner. If cassettes other than Kodak are used, follow the recommendations of the screen manufacturer.
3. Wipe one screen at a time with the damp gauze pad.
4. After cleaning, wipe each screen with a dry pad.
5. Allow screens to completely air dry.
6. If necessary, rewrite the cassette number on the screen next to the I.D. cutout with a Sharpie.
7. Reload the cassette with film and return the cassette to operation.

23.3   Screen Contact and Speed Match Testing

Frequency

Semi-annual

Purpose

To monitor the condition of cassettes and assure that all cassettes used have good screen film contact

Materials needed

X-ray machine
Screen-film contact test tool with coarse wire mesh
View box
Densitometer when checking speed matching

X-ray Technique

Lanex Regular cassettes 2 mAs, 50 kVp
Lanex Fine cassette (Extremity) 5mAs, 50 kVp

Procedure (Figure 23.1)

1. Set a tabletop or floor FFD of 40 in.
2. Collimate to film size.
3. Put screen contract test tool on top of the cassette.
4. Expose cassette with appropriate technique.
5. Process the film.
6. Either clean the cassette or reload film.
7. View film standing 72 in. from view box.
8. Record results in the screen contact test log.

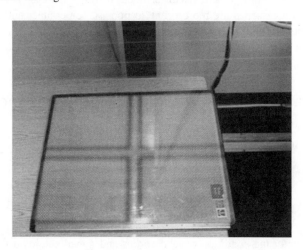

FIGURE 23.1
Screen contact test procedure.

FIGURE 23.2
Failed test film.

Quality Criteria

Look at areas of loss of detail of the wire mesh and density differences.

1. If none present, return cassette to service.
2. If poor contact is seen, clean screens and repeat the test.
3. If poor contact is still present, determine if it is in an area where essential clinical data would be present.
4. If the defect is where essential clinical data may be present, remove cassette from service.

By numbering each cassette next to the I.D. blocker and on the back of the cassette, the operator can quickly find cassettes with artifacts or dirty screens. Older and cassettes other than Kodak X-omatic cassettes are more prone to poor screen contact and light leaks. By reading the density of exposure with the densitometer, the speed of the cassettes can be compared. Old screens will take more exposure to produce the image.

23.4   Apron and Gonad Shield Testing

Frequency

Semi-annual

Purpose

To monitor the condition of lead aprons and gonad shields used for patient radiation protection

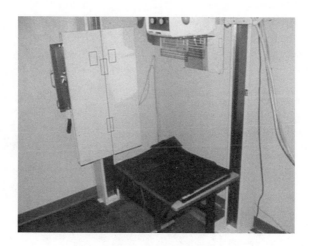

FIGURE 23.3
Apron test.

Materials Needed

X-ray machine
14 in. × 17 in. Regular speed cassette
View box
Lead aprons and lead shields

Technique

70 kVp and 2 mAs for Non-Bucky exposure
70 kVp and 10 mAs for Bucky exposure

Procedure: Half apron, small shields (Figure 23.3)

1. Place unexposed cassette on table. Center the tube to the film with a 40 in. SID.
2. Place the half apron or other shields on top of cassette. Pay close attention to the center of the shield.
3. Make the exposure and process the film.

Procedure: Coat-type full apron with 14 in. × 36 in. Bucky

1. Hang apron over Bucky.
2. Set SID at 40 in. to Bucky and place Bucky tray in upper slots.
3. Put 14 in. × 17 in. cassette in Bucky tray and expose the film.
4. Move Bucky tray to lower slots and expose second film.
5. Process both films.

Evaluation of the Test Film

1. Any cracks in the lead will show up on the film. If the cracks are in the area that would cover the gonads, the apron or shield will need to be replaced. (See Figure 23.4.)
2. If the film is significantly exposed, the apron may not be of adequate lead equilivancy. Lead gonad shields must be 0.5 mm lead equilivancy.

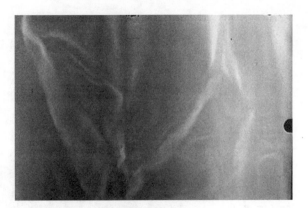

FIGURE 23.4
Apron test film.

Methods to Protect Aprons and Increase Their Useful Life

1. Never fold the apron.
2. Store flat or hanging on an apron rack.
3. Do not use lead blockers for extremity views.
4. Protect aprons from heat and direct sunlight if plastic covered.

Chapter **24**

Film Artifact Identification and Problem-Solving*

Most artifacts on the radiographic films are the result of improper film handling in the darkroom or problems with the processor. If the film is carelessly handled in the darkroom, the base of the film may be crinkled. This will cause an artifact on the film. If the film is handled by the edges with both hands, this artifact can be avoided. Wet, greasy, or dirty hands can smudge the film or actually make fingerprints on the film. These are easily avoidable artifacts. The person processing the film must have clean, dry hands. The countertop and feed tray of the processor should be cleaned daily.

Scratches

Dirt on the countertop of feed tray will produce random scratches on the film. Likewise, if film is dropped on the floor, scratches are likely to happen. If unexposed film is dropped on the floor when reloading the cassette, do not put the film in the cassette. Save it to be used as a cleaning film or process it.

Scratches that run the length of the film or come and go on the film require a little more detective work. Think about how the film travels through the processor. Are the scratches in the same direction as the film travel? How far apart are the scratches? Are there any missing films from a previous study? The answer to these questions will help solve the source of the artifacts.

1. Parallel scratches that are evenly spaced across the film and run in the same direction as the film travels through the processor are generally caused by the metal or plastic turnaround or guide shoes in the crossover rack or at the bottom of the rack of rollers in the tanks. Black scratches happen in the developer or entrance area of the processor. Scratches that are clear generally occur in the fixer or wash racks or tanks. Proper cleaning of the processor can help avoid these scratches if they are the result of chemical buildup on the film. These scratches will generally result in a service call for the processor.

2. More random but equidistant scratches can be caused by a film being stuck in the processor. If the film wraps around a roller, it will scratch the film when the edge of the film comes in contact with the new film. It may also cause the film to turn off its true path through the processor and make a more diagonal scratch. A clue to this type of problem is if the film exits the dryer diagonal to transport but was properly

* The format for this chapter was adapted from Lam, R.W., *Processor Quality Control for Radiographers, Home Study Reference NM 904*, American Society of Radiologic Technologists, Albuquerque, NM 1994. With permission of ASRT.

fed into the processor; there is a film stuck in the processor. This is why it is so important to feed the film the same way each time and against the feed tray film guide.

3.   Scratches or artifacts that resemble tractor or tank treads are the result of the film getting so crooked in the processor that it gets into the chain drive of the processor racks. One reason for this may be that the film was not properly fed into the processor. This also can be caused by a broken spring or rack roller or a film stuck in the processor. If no film is stuck, service on the processor will be required.

4.   When the processor jams due to misfeed or mechanical problems, multiple scratches and other damage will result. Use gloves and wear eye protection when clearing the jam. Remember that the developer will also stain clothing, and one does not want to get any chemicals in eyes. Run multiple cleaning films after the jam is cleared to get any loose emulsion out of the chemicals and ensure proper operation. Only after ensuring that the processor is operating properly can one repeat the damaged films. If the machine continues to jam, call for service. Remember that bad or overly diluted fixer will cause jams. It will also cause the film to scratch easily.

Crinkle Marks

The most common artifact on films is the crinkle mark. It is a crescent-shaped mark that results from bending the emulsion during loading or unloading of the film. If the film is handled with one hand pinching the emulsion, a bend in the emulsion will result. Proper handling of the film will avoid this artifact. Use both hands to handle the film without bending the film.

Partly Exposed or Fogged Film Artifacts

Dark densities on the film are areas of fogging of the film. Fogging can result from chemicals, light, or stray radiation. If the cassette is left in the room during an exposure, the scatter radiation can fog the film. This may appear as an area of gradual darkness or uniform darkness on the film. Light leaks in the darkroom or a faulty safelight can cause fog on the film. The cover being left ajar on the processor can also cause film fog. These are all operator-avoidable problems.

If the film is not completely in the processor, and the light is turned on or the darkroom door opened, an image of the entrance rollers will appear on the film. This can be avoided by listening to the beep or tone that is heard when the time delay relay activates the bell or buzzer. This ensures that the film is completely in the processor.

If there is a problem with the film transport system of the processor caused by a jam, stuck film, or broken gear, the film may stay in the developer too long. This will cause a chemical fog on the film. The pattern will be consistent with the direction of travel. There may also be scratches associated with the hesitation of the film.

Developer on the crossover rollers or faulty squeegee springs in the processor can add dark or fogged areas to the film. Proper cleaning of the crossover racks and the use of roller cleaning films can help avoid this artifact.

If a portion of the film is totally black or the area has the appearance of black spots on the edge of the film, this is a result of a light leak in the cassette. The cassette popping open in the room can also produce this artifact. The potential of light exposure to the unexposed film because the top is left off the box and the film bin opened in white light must also be considered. The 14 in. × 36 in. film does not fit into the film bin. It is easy to forget to replace the lid on the box. The 14 in. × 36 in. cassettes are also prone to light leaks because of their size and relative weakness.

If the film is improperly placed in the cassette with an edge outside the cassette, a light leak will occur. There will also be an imprint of the edge of the cassette in the film and evidence of poor screen contact.

A light leak in the darkroom or a faulty safelight can actually cast a shadow of one's hand on the film. A uniform fog on the film is usually caused by the safelight. The safelight and darkroom should be checked every 6 months and after replacement of the bulb. If area modifications or air conditioning workers have moved ceiling panels, check the darkroom. It is prudent to caulk around the ceiling of the darkroom.

"The Tree"

If the relative humidity is too low and clothing becomes prone to generating static electricity, one can get a static discharge on the film. It will have the appearance of a tree or lightening strike in black. Proper air conditioning and no carpeting in the darkroom can help avoid this artifact.

Spots

There are two types of spots that can appear on the film. The spots will either be white or black. Black spots are the result of the film getting wet or contaminated prior to processing. Flecks of emulsion from a previous processor jam adhering to the film during processing will make a black spot. If the level of the fixer is too low and the fixer is foaming, this too will cause a black spot as the stopping of the development process will be uneven if air bubbles keep the fixer from stopping the process.

The most common cause for white spots is dirty screens. With single-emulsion film, one often see areas where the emulsion is removed from the film during processing. This is generally blamed on a dirty processor, but any manufacturing defect on the film will also cause this problem. Proper cleaning and service of the processor can eliminate it as the source. Monthly cleaning of the screens will reduce the chance of artifacts on the film. Cassettes and screens will not last forever; after about 10 years, one should consider replacement.

Patient-Generated Artifacts

In the cervical spine, wet or heavily moussed or braided hair will cast an artifact on the film. Ideally, one should wait until the hair is dry before doing cervical spine or skull X-rays. Jewelry and hairpins are the most common artifacts in cervical and skull films. Wigs will also produce an artifact, as will gum and contact lenses.

Clothing such as T-shirts or sweatshirts with writing on them may cast the writing onto the image. If the clothing is wet, artifacts will be present. Do not roll the sleeve or pant leg up for elbow or knee films, as the rolled cloth will cast an artifact on the film.

Proper gowning instructions are very important. Verification that the patient has properly changed is also important. Necklaces and earrings will also produce artifacts. With older patients, do not forget to ask about dentures. For female patients, the brassiere must be removed for thoracic and lumbar studies. With paper gowns, the belt and sometimes the underwear will produce artifacts if they are too tight. A roll appearance will be seen where the elastic is around the waist. Even the belt used to hold the gonad protection will produce artifacts on the film.

Body jewelry is typically not removable but will definitely show up on films. Becuase they cannot be removed, just note them on the film.

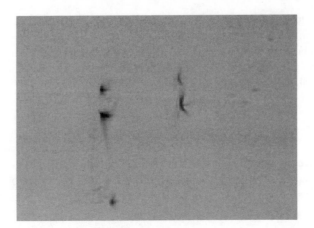

FIGURE 24.1
Crinkle artifact.

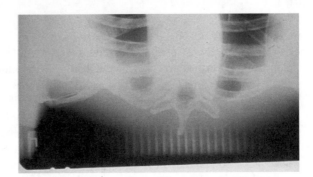

FIGURE 24.2
Film exposed by darkroom door opened.

Darkroom, Film Handling, and Processor Artifacts

1. Crinkle mark artifact (Figure 24.1).

2. Lights turned on or darkroom door opened (Figure 24.2) before film was completely in processor. Always listen for the beep.

3. Cassette opened in white light. Could be a faulty cassette latch or operator error. Could also happen when someone opens the darkroom door (Figure 24.3). Always lock door when processing films.

4. Pattern produced when top of film box is left off and door opened (Figure 24.4). Severe example would be total exposure of film.

5. The hazy appearance is the result of two films being fed into the processor at the same time, or a roller problem in the developer tank where the second film catches the first. Only one side of the film is developed. (Figure 24.5.)

6. Black artifacts on film are the result of dirty crossover or rollers above the chemical level. If the squeegee rollers do not remove the developer, the developer will dry on the rollers and produce the artifact. (Figure 24.6.) Clean processors with clean rollers will avoid this artifact.

7. Another example of two films being developed on top of each other (Figure 24.7). Only one side was developed.

8. Static tree results from a static electrical discharge (Figure 24.8).

9. Half of this film stayed in the developer too long (Figure 24.9). This can result from a jammed processor or loss of power to the film drive. If the film is fed down the middle, the processor may not sense it and go into standby mode.

10. Cassette light leak from hinge failure or one of the latches was not closed (Figure 24.10). This can happen with old cassettes when the felt has worn out.

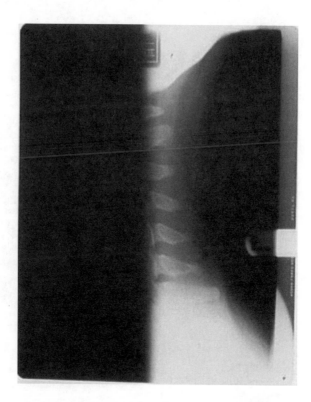

FIGURE 24.3
Cassette not closed or popped open.

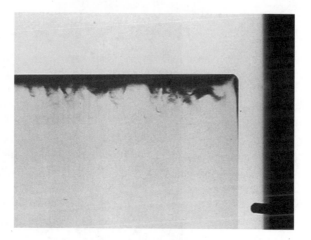

FIGURE 24.4
Film exposed to light.

Patient-Generated Artifacts

1. Hair. This patient was wearing dreadlocks (Figure 24.11). Patient was asked to put hair up for next image (Figure 24.12).

2. Gowning error: Patient did not remove brassiere (Figure 24.13). Lateral view of same patient (Figure 24.14).

3. Gowning error: Wet hair and metallic artifact from rubber band in ponytail (Figure 24.15). Earring also seen.

4. Gowning error: Hairpins (Figure 24.16).

5. Gowning error: Patient is wearing necklace (Figure 24.17).

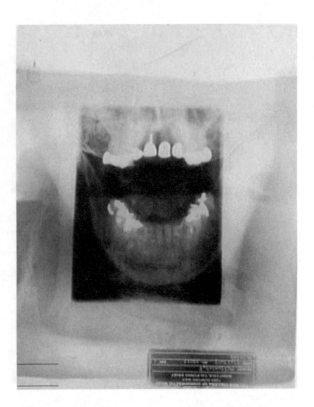

FIGURE 24.5
Kissing imaged film fixed.

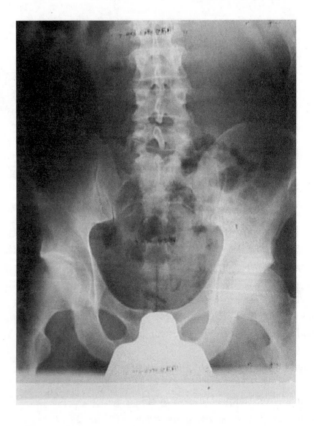

FIGURE 24.6
Dirty rollers artifact.

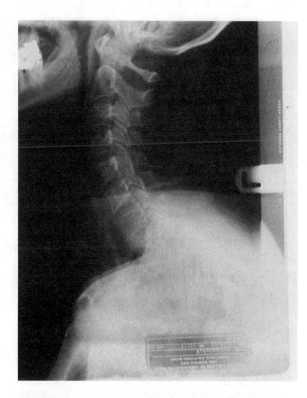

FIGURE 24.7
Kissing film artifact.

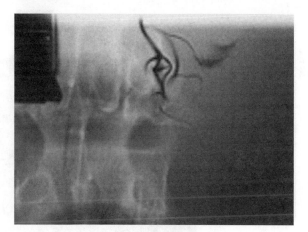

FIGURE 24.8
Static tree artifact.

6. Positioning error: Patient left arm next to Bucky down to side (Figure 24.18). Check the patient positioning before taking film.

7. Positioning error: Patient has arms crossed over chest on P-A view (Figure 24.19). Check patient position before taking films.

More Student Mistakes

1. Earrings, earrings, earrings (Figures 24.20 and 24.21).

2. Note the artifact in the upper thoracic spine in Figure 24.22. A patient flash card dropped into the cassette. It could be clearly read on the film. Of course, it was not the correct patient's card!

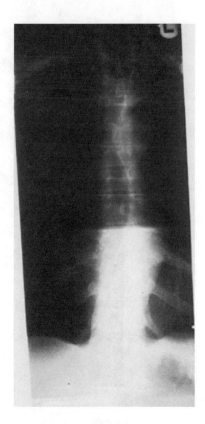

FIGURE 24.9
Film jammed in developer.

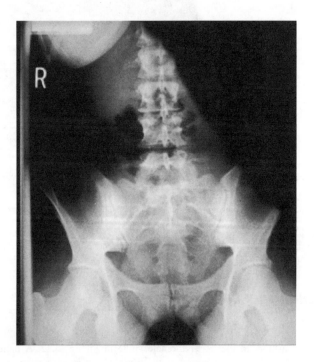

FIGURE 24.10
Cassette light leak.

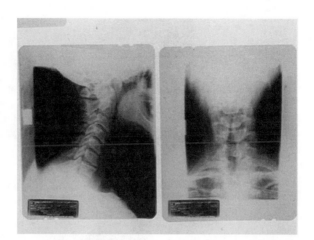

FIGURE 24.11
Dreadlock artifact.

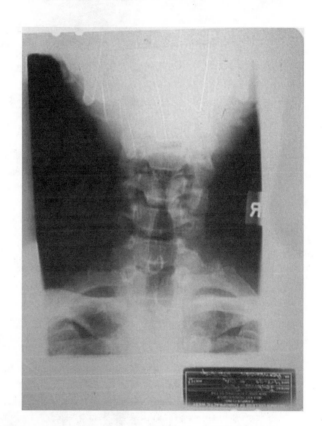

FIGURE 24.12
Same patient with hair up.

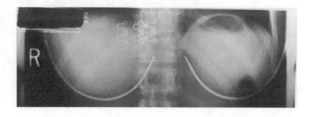

FIGURE 24.13
Bra in P-A view.

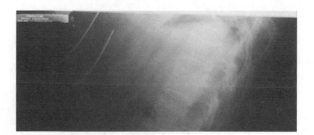

FIGURE 24.14
Bra in lateral view.

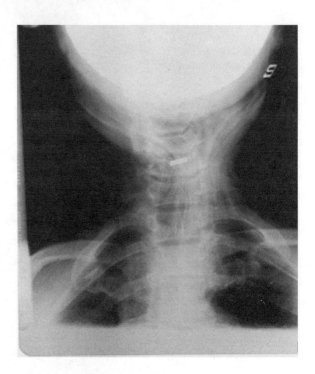

FIGURE 24.15
Wet hair and hairband metallic artifact.

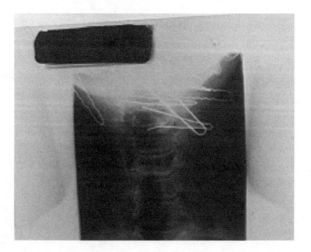

FIGURE 24.16
Bobby pins in hair.

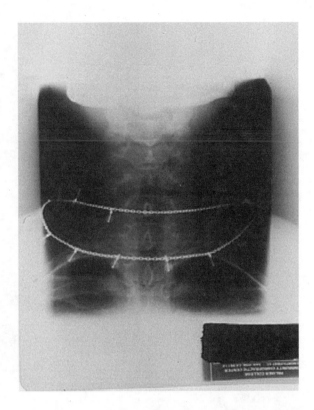

FIGURE 24.17
Necklace left on patient.

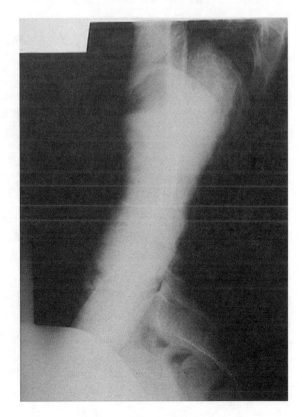

FIGURE 24.18
Arm left down on lateral lumbar view.

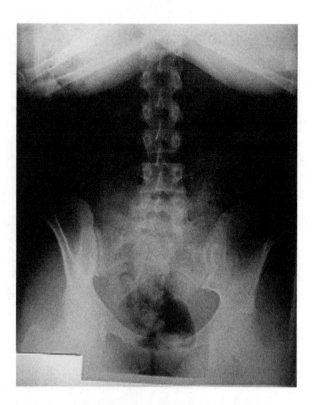

FIGURE 24.19
Arms across chest on P-A lumbar view.

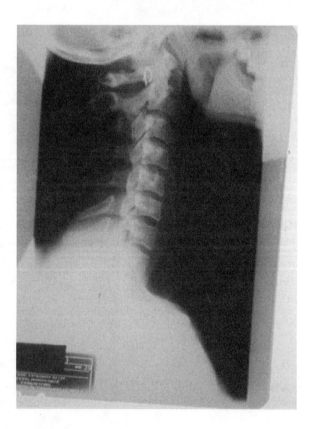

FIGURE 24.20
Earring on lateral C-spine view.

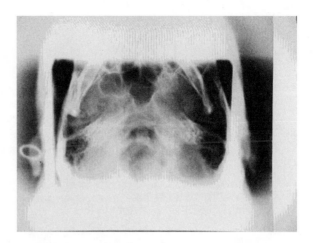

FIGURE 24.21
Earring on basilar view.

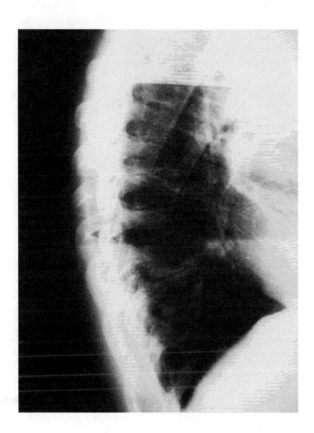

FIGURE 24.22
Flash card in cassette.

Review of Basic Radiographic and Quality Control Concepts

Quality Assurance and Quality Control

Quality Assurance (QA) includes Quality Control (QC) testing, preventive maintenance and corrective maintenance for problems found with the QC testing and the repeat film analysis. It also includes training and policies to control the variables of radiography. QA is required by state regulations and is designed to keep the patient and staff exposure to radiation as low as possible by finding problems before they cause repeat films.

Quality Control (QC) includes photographic and darkroom tests; accessories testing such as grids, lead aprons, and gonadal shields; cleaning and testing of the cassettes and screens; and radiographic testing of collimation, linearity of exposure, and calibration.

Photographic and darkroom QC testing consists of testing the processor with sensitometry; monitoring processing chemical temperatures; and preventive cleaning of the darkroom counters, film processor feed tray, and crossover racks. These tests are done daily. Semi-annually, the safelight in the darkroom is tested for fogging.

Accessory QC includes the cleaning of the cassette screens at least monthly with screen cleaner that contains an antistatic solution. Semi-annually, the cassettes are tested for screen film contact and exposure speed consistency.

Radiographic QC includes the semi-annual testing of beam alignment and collimator accuracy, kVp accuracy, and mAs linearity. The collimator should be checked when the lamp is replaced as well as semi-annually. There should be no change from the previous tests or exposures for the equipment to pass any of these tests.

Film Processing and Sensitometry

Processing chemical replenishment is controlled by the film transport system. The film passing through the entrance rollers will open a switch that detects the film and turns on the pumps to replenish the developer and fixer. The replenishment rate is controlled by the settings on the pump.

The switch also activates the time delay relay that will cause an audible tone that alerts the operator as to when he/she can leave the darkroom or feed a new film into the processor. The processor also contains a standby unit that keeps the chemicals and dryer at proper operating conditions, but reduces power use by turning off film transport and the dryer fan and reduces water flow.

The developer temperature is critical for consistent image quality. A change of 1° can be seen on the sensitometry film. The temperature is controlled by the incoming wash water to cool the developer, a thermostat set to the optimum temperature that controls a heater that warms the developer. The temperature of the developer is monitored daily.

Water flow problems will result in temperature fluctuations in the fixer and developer. The lack of water results in a brownish color image that will be dark. This is the result of the fixing action not being stopped by the wash water and developer overheating.

Factors that impact the film quality include the freshness or activity of the developer controlled by replenishment, the temperature of the developer, and the time the film stays in the developer controlled by the film transport speed.

Problems with under-replenishment of the fixer will cause film transport problems or jams in the wash or dryer sections of the processor. It will also cause the film to be prone to scratches and flecking of the emulsion. The film will not have good retention or archival properties.

The developer condition is monitored by the use of film sensitometry. A sensitometer is used to expose the film to a reproducible varying intensity of light of up to 21 steps. The film is processed in the same manner each day. The density exposure (O.D.) is measured using a densitometer. The base-plus-fog resulting from the darkroom and processing with no other exposure is monitored. The speed defined as an exposure of 1.00 O.D. plus the base-plus-fog is monitored. The contrast index or density is also monitored. These numbers are graphed daily as part of processing quality control.

The temperatures of the fixer and wash water are also checked and recorded daily. The daily monitoring of the processing parameters will demonstrate problems long before they degrade the film quality to a point that repeat films are required.

Common problems revealed by sensitometry include both under- and over-replenishment of the developer, chemical contamination, and light leaks or safelight problems long before they can cause retakes. Under-replenishment of the developer is represented by a gradual drop in speed and contrast with normal developer and water temperature. Over-replenishment results in an increase in speed and contrast that eventually stabilizes. Processor cleaning and chemical changes show these properties also. An increase in the base-plus-fog and speed with a drop in contrast with no change in temperatures demonstrates a darkroom or film storage environment problem. A light leak or safelight problem must be considered.

Processing Chemistry

The state of California requires employers to ensure that their staff knows about the hazards that they may encounter in the workplace. The material safety data sheet and labels on containers provide this data about chemicals. The employee or student working in a radiology department must understand the hazards and contents of the processing chemicals and abide by the handling rules. Film processing results in silver ions being deposited in the fixer and in the fixer processing tank. Silver is a heavy metal that is harmful to the environment, particularly to fish and marine plants. The used fixer is therefore a hazardous waste that must not be poured down the drain.

Neither fresh developer nor fixer are toxic to the environment and can be safely poured down a drain when diluted with water. Developer will stain clothing and contains harmful chemicals that require caution when handling, pouring, or mixing. A safe darkroom requires good ventilation. Developer turns brown when oxidized or used. It is alkaline in nature. Fixer will remain clear but has a distinct smell of ammonia and acetic acid. Fixer is rather corrosive. The characteristic of the chemicals are important in cleaning up a spill of used chemicals from the processor.

The fumes from processing chemicals are controlled by keeping air-tight lids on the storage tanks. This also reduces oxidation of the developer. Some people are allergic to these chemicals and should avoid exposure. Whenever handling chemicals, eye protection and gloves must be used. Spills on clothing should be avoided. Hydroquinone is the most hazardous component of film processing chemistry. It can be absorbed through the skin; thus, gloves are very important when working with the developer.

Retake Analysis

The principal reasons for retake or repeat films is overexposure (dark) or underexposure (light) films. This can be avoided by the systematic use of technique charts and accurate measurement of the patient. Exposure errors result in over 50% of repeat films. Positioning errors account for only about 25% of repeats. Most retakes are found in the exams of the torso and result in unnecessary gonadal and blood-forming organ exposure.

Properly trained operators rarely take repeat films. By measuring properly, setting the correct technical factors, accurately positioning the patient, and giving appropriate breathing and motion instructions, most repeats can be avoided. The operator must watch the patient before and during the exposure to avoid motion or breathing errors. These factors, when combined with a good quality control program, will significantly reduce radiation exposure to both the operator and the patient. It will also reduce costs for the operator as film, power, and supplies are expensive.

Basic Positioning Concepts

1. Collimation for extremities is generally done to include skin side to side or to slightly less than film size, whichever is smaller. Three borders should be seen on the film as proof of collimation. Collimation that is so tight that essential information is missed results in repeat exposures to the patient. Collimation greater than film size is unnecessary radiation exposure to the patient. Therefore, in order to understand collimation, one must know what the proper image should contain.

2. One will generally measure the patient where the central ray enters the patient.

3. Lead blockers are used to shield the exposed film from scatter radiation and as a guide for the operator to avoid double-exposing the film. They should be outside of the primary beam. They are not needed for grid or Bucky views because the grid cleans up the scatter radiation.

4. Extremity cassettes are not used in a Bucky due to the slow speed and excessive radiation needed to make the radiograph.

5. Extremity cassettes are used for extremities that measure less than 10 cm.

6. When doing Non-Bucky work, start by centering the cassette to the vertical central ray. Position patient over the area of film that is within the beam. The vertical central ray is the only fixed position with the tube stand.

7. Basic radiographic positions are designed to have the central ray pass straight through the joint space of clinical interest. The central ray will therefore be perpendicular to the area of interest. The film will be parallel to the area of interest.

Common and Not So Common Tube Angulations

Angle	Views
5° cephalad	A-P and lateral knee recumbent; APOM for anterior weight-bearing patients; P-A patella
10° cephalad	A-P foot
10° caudal	A-P coccyx; lateral scapula
15° cephalad	A-P cervical spine; posterior oblique C-spine; A-P sacrum zanca view of AC joints; axial view of toes and A-P clavicle; P-A axial scaphoid; A-P thumb if palm obscures view of trapezium
15° caudal	Anterior oblique C-spine; P-A axial clavicle; Caldwell sinuses; outlet view
20° cephalad	P-A ulnar flexion; apical lordotic chest
25° caudal	Schuller's view of TMJ
30° cephalad	A-P sacral base view
30° caudal	Towne's projection of skull; apical shoulder view; tunnel view of knee

Radiation Safety

1. Collimation is to the area of interest or slightly less than film size, whichever is smaller.

2. Patients shall not be held by the operator or radiographer except in emergencies as a last resort when all other methods of immobilization will not work. When necessary, a lead apron and gloves shall be used along with dosimetry. The person holding the patient shall not be in the primary beam path.

3. X-ray equipment shall be operated only by a properly licensed radiographer or operators in the state of California. The State Department of Radiologic Health requires the person wishing to operate or possess radiographic equipment to pass a test covering radiation safety, quality assurance, and operational skills.

4. Gonadal shielding shall be used except when it will obscure the area of clinical interest.

5. The highest possible kVp and lowest possible mAs shall be used to produce a radiograph of adequate contrast and density and diagnostic value.

6. All nonessential personnel must leave the X-ray room during the exposure. Those in the room other than be patient shall be behind the operator's barrier.

7. The door to the X-ray room shall be closed during the radiographic exposure.

8. The highest possible film/screen speed system shall be used to produce film of satisfactory detail or resolution.

9. When taking X-rays of the upper extremities, the lower extremities should never be placed under the table. They should be shielded with the lead apron.

10. The safest time to expose a female of child-bearing age is within 10 days of the onset of menses. The diagnostic value of the exam must be weighed against the potential risks of exposure to a fetus at other times. When possible, female patients may be turned P-A to reduce exposure to the ovaries.

11. The benefit of radiography must be greater than the risks associated with exposure to radiation before any X-ray test is performed.

12. The operator shall always stand completely behind the leaded barrier. The operator should monitor the patient through the window provided. The X-ray room must be designed to not allow the operator to make an exposure outside the control booth. This may mean relocating the exposure control buttons.

Technique Charts and Technique Changes

Benefits of Fixed kVp and Variable mAs Technique Charts

1. Provides optimum contrast and penetration of the body part being studied
2. Provides some latitude in exposure
3. Provides consistent control of scatter radiation
4. Provides a reduction in radiation exposure because the optimum kVp is typically higher than the factors found on other types of charts; the higher the kVp, the less ionizing effects on the body

When and How to Make Adjustments to the Technical Factors

1. Adjustments for body habitus: Most technique charts are designed for normal patient builds. If the patient has more adipose tissue or is extremely muscular, the technique needs to be increased. If the patient is extremely thin or is known to have pathologic conditions that result in mineral or tissue loss, the technique may need to be decreased 6 to 10 kVp. Each step in the technique chart is usually a 30% increase in density.

   a. Increased body fat: leave the kVp the same but increase mAs 40 to 80%. This can also be done by increasing anatomical measurement by 2 to 4 cm.

   b. Increased muscularity: increase kVp by 6 to 10 kVp and mAs by 20 to 40%. Edema and additive pathologic factors will also require this type of technical factor adjustment.

2. Adjustment for film/screen type or relative speed value:

80 speed to 400 speed:	Divide mAs by 5
400 speed to 80 speed:	Multiply mAs by 5
100 speed to 400 speed:	Multiply mAs by 0.25
400 speed to 100 speed:	Multiply mAs by 4
400 speed to 200 speed:	Multiply mAs by 2
200 speed to 400 speed:	Multiply mAs by 0.50

3. Generator type:

   Single phase to three phase or high frequency: multiply mAs by 0.50

   High frequency/three phase to single phase: multiply mAs by 2

4. Adjustment of contrast by changing technical factors:

   To reduce mAs 25%, increase kVp by 8% (longer scale of contrast)

   To reduce mAs 50%, increase kVp by 15% (longer scale of contrast)

   To increase mAs 100%, decrease kVp by 15% (shorter scale of contrast)

   In the range of 60 to 90 kVp, a change of 10 kVp is equal to 15%

5. Technique adjustment for change in film size and collimation:

   To convert from 14 in. × 17 in. to 10 in. × 12 in., multiply mAs by 1.25

   To convert from 14 in. × 17 in. to 8 in. × 10 in., multiply mAs by 1.40

6. Converting a non-grid technique to a grid or Bucky technique:

   Grids should be used when the body part is larger than 10 cm. They are also used when the kVp is above 70 kVp. The multiplier factors can also be used to convert a technique from non-grid to grid and depends upon the grid ratio.

   Non-Bucky to 5:1 grid ratio, multiply mAs by 2

   Non-Bucky to 6:1 grid ratio, multiply mAs by 3

Non-Bucky to 8:1 grid ratio, multiply mAs by 4

Non-Bucky to 10:1 grid ratio, multiply mAs by 5

Non-Bucky to 12:1 grid ratio, multiply mAs by 6

7. Inverse Square Law: If the FFD is reduced by one half, one will need to reduce the mAs by a factor of 4. If one doubles the distance, increase the mAs by a factor of 4.

Appendix 2

Review to Assist in Interpretation of Radiography with Common Film Marking Lines

This appendix is not intended to be a definitive source of information for the interpretation of radiographic series. It is provided as a review of information previously presented in other courses to assist in the viewing of films. It has information covering some of the more common roentgenometric and X-ray listings and pathologies that can be seen on the films.

An important part of the evaluation of films will be the assessment of the technical quality of the films. Pay close attention to artifacts and shielding seen on the films. Determine how to avoid the artifacts and improve shielding.

1. Evaluate patient positioning to determine what can be done to improve the next series. Look for rotation of the patient, improper centering, and the presentation of the anatomy on the film. Is the patient identification box out of the area of clinical interest? Was the correct film size used?

2. Look at the exposure of the film. If the image is light, it is underexposed due to the mAs or kVp being set too low. This could be due to incorrect measurements, inaccurate technique charts, incorrect breathing instructions to the patient, or improper SID. Was the patient obese or very muscular? A common source of error is the operator lifting the exposure button before the generator has completed the exposure. If one can visualize some bony detail, the kVp was probably correct and a repeated film would use more mAs.

3. If the film is too dark, the mAs was probably too high or filtration was not used. Getting A-P and lateral measurements mixed up, or not using additional filtration, are also common causes for dark films. Patient habitus, age, and pathologic processes can also result in dark films.

4. If the film is dark and lacks contrast, too much kVp was used. The image may appear to be flat. High kVp and lack of filtration are the common causes.

5. Evaluate the collimation of the view. Are three unexposed borders observed on the film? Was essential anatomy cut off? Are anatomical markers visible on the film?

This technical evaluation is an important learning tool if mistakes are noted and corrective action taken on subsequent studies. The remainder of this appendix reviews pathologic and items seen on films.

Items to be observed when viewing films

Alignment	Bones	Cartilage and Joints	Soft Tissue
Curves	CAMP	IVD	Swelling
Antero	Cortex	Spacing	Edema
Retro	Articular surface	Erosion	Calcifications
Spinous process	Medulla	Eburnation	Organomegaly
Rotation	Periostium	Calcification	Gas or fecal pattern
	Density/color	Vacuum phenom	Atrophy
	Trabeculation	Exostoses	Aortic calcifications
	Geodes	Disc calcification	Gall stones
	Block vertebrae		Renal stones
	Codfish/biconcave		Prostate calcifications
	Vertebrae		Uterine fibroids
	Box vertebrae		
	Ivory vertebrae		

APOM	A-P Cervical Spine	Lateral Cervical Spine
Anterior arch	Cervical rib	Position of Atlas
Posterior arch	Uncinate process	Os odontiodeum
Transverse Process C-1	Tracheal deviation	Agenesis of dens
Dens fracture	Spina bifida	Dens fracture
Os odontiodeum	Calcified nodes	Spinous process fracture
Agenesis of dens	Calcified carotid artery	Osteophytes
Lateral mass	Calcified thyroid	Hyper- or hypolordotic curve
Superior articular process of C-2	Osteophytes	Occipitalization
Paramastoid process	Missing pedicle	Block vertebrae
		Bent stick deformity (hypermobility)
		Pons posticus
		Hypoplasia or absence of C-1
		Posterior arch
		Kypholordosis (goose neck)

Cervical Oblique View	A-P Lumbar/Thoracic Spine	Lateral Lumbar/Thoracic Spine
Intervertebral Foramen	Excessively white	Spinous fracture
Bony margins	Blacker	Limbus
Disc spaces	Vertical stripes	Avulsion fracture
Facet orientation	Butterfly vertebrae	Calcified aorta
Laminae	Body height	Spondylolysis
	Missing pedicle	Spondylolisthesis
	Spina bifida	Discogenic spondy
	Transverse process fracture	Anterolisthesis

Tropism	Degenerative spondy
Aortic calcifications	PARS fracture
L5/S1 structural instability	Compression fracture
AS	Osteophytes
Osteophytes	Hyperlordotic/hypolordotic
Sprengel's deformity	Scheuermans
Cervical rib	Schmorels nodes
Hemivertebrae	Kissing spinous
	Costa vertebral joints

Lumbar Oblique	A-P Lumbo/Sacrum	Lateral Lumbar/Sacrum
Eye: pedicle	Increase or decreased density at lower 1/3 SI joint	Ephysis
Nose: transverse process	Check L4 is at iliac crest	Femoral capititus
Ear: superior articular process	Sacralization	Ishio pubic
Leg: inferior articular process	Lumbarization	Growth centers
Neck: pars	Tropism	Schmorels nodes
Body: lamina	Common iliac calcification	Pars fracture
Tail: opposing transverse process	Degenerative hip	Lumbar instability
RPO: R LAO-R	Protrusio acetabulum	
Foraminal occlusion	Pubis symphisis	
Collar: pars fracture	Pelvic growth centers	

When studying a radiograph, look for what is the same side to side and what is different. One's knowledge of radiographic anatomy is very important. One should have a working diagnosis of the patient from patient history and physical examination. What are the radiographic signs of the diagnosis?

Roentgenometric and X-ray Listings

Cervical Spine

Cervical lordotic curve		35–45°
ADI	Distance between the posterior aspect of the anterior tubercle and the anterior surface of the odontoid.	1–3 mm adults; 1–5 mm children
Weight-bearing gravitational line	Apex of dens to the body of C-7 Ant. or Post. Weight-bearing.	Should fall through C-7
Neural Canal		C-1 (16-22-31) C-2 (14-20-27) C-3 (13-18-23) C-4 to C-7 (12-17-22)
George's line	Posterior vertebral body alignment = Antero or Retro.	Should be no breaks in the line
McGregor's line	Posterior superior margin of the hard palate to most inferior surface of occiput. Measure height of dens.	<8 mm males <10 mm females
Retropharyngeal and retrotracheal soft tissue space	Measure from anterior inferior body to airspace.	C-1 10 mm C-2 5 mm C-3 7 mm C-4 7 mm C-5 to C-7 20 mm

| Approximation of spinouses on extension | 1. A template is made by outlining the cortical margins drawn from the neutral lateral on a clear piece of film or transparency.
2. Angular motion in degrees and translation (in mm) are measured on the posterior-inferior aspects of each vertebra at all levels. The template is used to determine which segments are fixed.
3. The fixed segments are outlined onto the template. This will determine which levels have hypomobility. | Stair-step effect of bodies on flexion (1–2 mm per level).
Rocking effect of the vertebral bodies should be seen on both flexion and extension.
The spinouses should fan on flexion. |
| Quantitative measurements of instability | | Gooseneck deformity
Translation of posterior body >3.5 mm
A difference of segmental angulation greater than 11°
X = upper segment
Y = lower segment
(Y-(-X) > 11° |

Thoracic Spine

Thoracic kyphosis	Superior endplate T1 to inferior endplate T12	Age	Male	Female	
		<10	21	24	
		<20	25	26	
		<30	26	27	
		<40	29	28	
		<50	30	33	
		<60	33	41	
		<70	35	42	
		<80	41	45	
Cobb's angle	Superior endplate and inferior endplates of first and last tilted vertebrae	<5°			Gives larger measurement than Risser-Ferguson method analysis
George's lines	Posterior body alignment	Should be no breaks in the line			
Risser-Ferguson angle	1. Draw upper end vertebra. 2. Draw apical vertebra. 3. Draw lower vertebra. 4. Connect line from upper to apical. 5. Connect line from lower to apical. 6. Measure angle.	Mild to moderate scolioses is less than 50°.			Higher inter-examiner reliability compared to Cobb-Lipman method in mild to moderate scolioses. Best used in multidisciplinary settings.

Lumbo Pelvic Series

George's lines	Posterior vertebral body alignment line = antero or retro	Should be no breaks in line
Lumbar lordosis	Superior endplate at L1 to inferior endplate of L5	50 to 60°
Ferguson's angle	Lumbar gravity line from L3 passes to L5	Through the sacral base Ant = AWB (hypolordosis) Post = PWB (hyperlordosis)
Ferguson's line	Vertical from center of L3 body to sacrum	Should touch anterior 1/3 sacrum
Femur head height	Measure height of femur heads and compare	Should be same height
Lumbosacral angle	Superior endplate of sacrum and inferior endplate of L5	10–15°
Ulmann's line	Right angle to anterior margin of the sacral base	L5 should be touching or posterior
Cobb's angle	Superior endplate and inferior endplate of first and last tilted vertebrae	<5°

Lumbo Pelvic Series

Lumbosacral disc angle	Line that is horizontal that meets a line drawn from the sacral base	29–41-56°
Pelvic tilt		
Neural canal		
Lumbar instability	Line drawn across adjacent vertebral body endplates. Distance from the point of intersection to the posterior inferior body margin is measured.	<1.5 mm >1.5 mm possible nuclear, annular or posterior ligamentous damage

Pelvis A-P

Osteitis pubis	Widening of the symphysis pubis greater than 10 mm with irregular margins and sclerosis	Football, soccer, rugby, and running injury

Hip Series

Shenton's line	Inferior margin of superior pubic ramus to under surface of femoral neck	Smooth curve, no breaks
Ilio femoral lines	Lines from outer surface of ileum to the superior femoral neck	Symmetrical B/L

Acromioclavicular Joint

Normal A-C joint measurements	AC joint measurement Males 3.3 mm Females 2.9 mm	Acromiohumeral joint space 7 mm 9 mm 11 mm Coracoidclavicular distance 1.0 to 1.3 cm
Grade 1 sprain (mild)	A-C joint measurement 3 mm to 8 cm	Within normal limits
Grade 2 sprain (moderate)	1.5 cm	>25–50%
Grade 3 sprain (severe)	>1.5 cm	Apparent dislocation of the distal end of clavicle

Shoulder

Axial relationship of shoulder use A-P external rotation view	1. Draw line bisecting and parallel to humeral shaft. 2. Draw line from the superior aspect of the greater tuberosity to the junction of the humeral head and the proximal diaphysis.	Male avg.: 60° Female avg.: 62°
Glenohumeral joint space	4–5 mm average	Increased space may be result of posterior dislocation

Elbow

Radiocapitellar line from lateral view	1. Draw line parallel and bisecting the long axis of the radius. 2. Line parallel to the anterior cortex of the distal humerus to the middle 1/3 of the capitelum.	1. Line should bisect the center of the capitellum. 2. Line should not be disrupted. If either is disrupted, a fracture or dislocation may exist.
Axial alignment from A-P view	1. Draw line bisecting humeral shaft. 2. Draw line bisecting the shaft of the ulna. 3. Draw line along the articular surfaces of the trochlea and capitelum.	Humeral head to ulnar shaft angle and carrying (angle lines 1 and 2): 154–178°; avg.: 169° Ulnar line and humeral line angle (lines 2 and 3): 72–99°; avg.: 84° Humeral line (lines 1 and 3): 72–95°; avg.: 85°

Common Radiography Terms, Rules, and Rare-Earth Screen and Film Combination Chart

Terms

Anterior-Posterior view (A-P view): Patient is positioned with posterior surface next to film. The X-ray tube is in front of the patient. The beam passes from the anterior portion of anatomy through the posterior body part, then on the film. This is typically the true anatomical position. The lead anatomical markers are turned so one can read them.

Artifact: Any density on a radiograph that is caused by something not belonging to the part being X-rayed.

Axial plane: The plane that runs perpendicular to the vertical axis of the body. Most computed tomography images are in the axial projection.

Beam: A unidirectional flow of electromagnetic radiation (X-ray). **Primary X-ray beam:** The part of the radiation that passes through the window, collimating device of the X-ray tube. Also called useful beam.

Bucky: A device that contains a tray for holding the cassette and a fixed or moving grid. A true Bucky has a moving grid that uses the motion to remove any grid lines. (Non-moving grids are used at Palmer.)

Caliper: Ruler marked in inches and centimeters with arms used to accurately measure the thickness of the part being X-rayed. All radiographic measurements are in centimeters. The caliper is the key to proper technique selection.

Cassette: A light-tight film holder that contains the intensifying screens used to produce the radiographic image. Two types are used in the clinic. Regular cassettes using Lanex Regular Screens have black edges and are used for routine radiography. Extremity cassettes have gray edges and are used for extremities less than 10 cm thick. The Regular cassettes and current film is a 400 speed system. The Extremity cassette and same film is an 80 speed system.

Caudal Tube Tilt: The X-ray tube is angled toward the feet the prescribed number of degrees.

Central Ray: Refers to the center of the useful X-ray beam. This is where the vertical and horizonal beam intersect or the center of the cross hairs.

Cephalad tube tilt: The X-ray tube is angled toward the head the prescribed number of degrees.

Collimation: The beam should be restricted to the part being studied. Ideally, at least three borders should be seen on the film, as recommended by state law.

Collimator: The beam-limiting device containing lead shutters that restrict the beam and radiation to the part being radiographed. The use of the collimator is called collimation.

Compton Effect or Scatter: The interaction between an incoming X-ray photon and a loosely bound outer-shell electron of the irradiated object. The photon surrenders some of its kinetic energy to dislodge the electron from its orbit. It then continues in a different direction. This accounts for most of the scatter radiation produced in radiography.

Contrast: The photoradiographic property affecting image visibility, or the measurable or observed difference between adjacent radiographic densities. It is divided into two specific types. *Subject Contrast* is related to the X-ray exposure latitude and *Film Contrast* is related to the film, processing, and screen latitude.

Coronal plane (mid): The middle of the body as viewed in the lateral position. A slice of the body in the lateral projection is a coronal plane.

Density: The quantity of blackness appearing on the radiographic image. Density can be measured on a densitometer and perceived visually. The optimal density range for radiography is from 0.25 to 2.00 Optical Densities (O.D.).

Detail: The sharpness of the structure lines or contour lines of radiographic image on the processed film.

Developer: A liquid chemical compound that reacts with the exposed silver crystals in the emulsion, turning them black. Developer will stain clothing and can cause skin or eye irritation. Developer is the most hazardous of the processing chemicals as it contains hydroquinone and potassium hydroxide. In working strength, the hazards are minimal but some people may be allergic.

Distortion: Unequal magnification of different portions of the body being X-rayed.

Dose: The amount of ionizing radiation of absorbed per unit of mass. Absorbed dose is measured in rads. There are 100 rads in a gray (Gy). Dose equivalent is the product of the absorbed dose in tissue, quality factor, and other necessary modifiers at the area of interest. It is measured in rem and the Seivert. 1 rem = 0.01 Sv. In X-ray and gamma radiation, a rad equals a rem.

Emulsion: The sensitive layer of X-ray film that contains the silver compound suspended in a layer of gelatin. (The film at Palmer has two layers of emulsion.)

Entrance skin dose: The level of exposure to ionizing radiation that the skin of the patient receives from a given X-ray exposure. This dose is computed in mR.

Exposure: The actual taking of a radiograph. The generation of electromagnetic radiation.

Film Speed: A computed log relative exposure number needed to produce a density of 1.0 above gross fog; used in processor quality control to monitor the operation of the automatic processor.

Filter/filtration: Material placed in the useful or primary beam to absorb the preferentially soft or less-penetrating radiations. The appropriate use of filtration prevents the patient from receiving unnecessary radiation. The minimum filtration of the X-ray tube is 2.5 mm of aluminum. Added filters called Nolan Filters are used to equalize exposure and reduce unnecessary exposure by up to 85%.

Fixer: Fixer is used to clear any silver crystals that did not react to the exposure. It also bonds the exposed crystals to the emulsion. It has an ammonia odor and is acidic in nature. Its odor is the result of sulfur dioxide and acetic acid. Prior to use in the processor, it is not toxic to the environment. The clearing of the film results in silver being deposited in solution. Silver is a heavy metal and classified as toxic waste. Used fixer can never be poured down a drain.

Grid: A device that contains strips of lead that is used to reduce or eliminate scatter or off-focus radiation. This scatter radiation is the result of the X-rays being absorbed by the patient's tissues. This can result in a fogged film. The lead strips absorb the scatter radiation before it can react with the intensifying screen.The efficiency of the removal of the scatter radiation is determined by the grid ratio and number of lines per inch. (At Palmer, the grids in the vertical film holders are 10:1 ratio and the other grids are 5:1 ratio.) Grids must be handled with extreme care. Dropping or bending them will destroy them.

Grid cut-off: The loss of image detail resulting from misalignment of the X-ray beam and the grid lines.

Half-value layer: The thickness of a specified substance/material (usually aluminum or copper for X-rays and lead for shielding) that, when introduced into the path of a given beam, will reduce the exposure by one half.

Heel effect: The heel effect refers to the unequal intensity of the X-ray beam. The intensity is higher on the cathode side of the beam and less intense on the anode side of the beam.

Inverse Square Law: The intensity of the radiation is inversely proportional to the square of the distance from the source.

Kilovolt peak (kVP): A unit of maximum or crest value of electrical potential difference between the anode and cathode of the X-ray tube. Kilovolt peak (kVp) determines the penetrating ability of the X-ray and refers to the "quality" of X-rays.

Latitude: The property of an X-ray film to have a great number of units of density produced within certain long relative exposure numbers. Longer latitude films have lower contrast.

Linearity of exposure: The X-ray machine's ability to reproduce the same exposure.

Magnification: The ratio of image size to object size. The image may be larger than, smaller than, or equal to the object; so magnification can be greater than, equal to, or smaller than 1. Magnification is usually generated by increasing the object to film distance without changing the focal film distance. It makes geometric unsharpness unless the focal spot is very small.

Milliampere (mA): The electron current (measured in milliamperes) flowing across the X-ray tube from the cathode to the anode.

Milliampere second (mAs): The product of multiplying the mA times the duration of the exposure measured in 2nds. mAs is a measure of the "quantity" of X-rays.

Oblique: The turning or rotation of the body or part being X-rayed from A-P or P-A the prescribed number of degrees. If not otherwise stated, an oblique projection is 45°.

Operator's station: The area where the control panel for the X-ray equipment is located; it is either in a separate room or behind a barrier that will intercept the useful beam and any scatter radiation.

Phantom: An object used to simulate the absorption and scatter characteristics of the patient or used to simulate positioning and imaging of a human being.

Posterior-Anterior view (P-A view): The patient or part being X-rayed is positioned with the anterior surface next to the film. The X-ray tube is behind the patient. The lead anatomical markers are pronated or turned backward for any P-A film.

Quality: A term used to describe the penetrating power of X-rays and is related to the energies of the photons in the useful beam.

Quality Assurance: A management tool that includes policies and procedures designed to optimize the performance of the facility personnel and equipment. QA includes quality control, administration, education, and preventive maintenance methods.

Quality Control: Quality control (QC) refers to routine monitoring of performance and interpretation of equipment function and corrective action taken when needed.

Quantity: A term used to describe the number of photons in the X-ray beam.

Rad: The rad is a unit of absorbed dose; 1 rad is the dose corresponding to the absorption of 100 ergs per gram. The Gray (Gy) is the SI unit of absorbed dose.

Radiograph: A film produced by the action of X-rays transmitted through the patient.

Radiography: Utilizing ionizing radiation, the technique involves making shadow images on photographic emulsions. The image is the result of differences in the attenuation of the radiation as it passes through the objects in its path.

rem: The rem is a special unit of any quantities expressed as dose equivalent. The dose equivalent in rems is equal to the absorbed dose in rads multiplied by the quality factor (1 rem = 0.01 Sievert). For X-ray and gamma radiation, 1 rem = 1 rad.

Repeat/Retakes: Additional radiographs taken because of technical or mechanical errors. They result in increased radiation exposure to the patient and operator, and should be avoided.

Resolution: The process or capability to distinguish closely adjacent optical images.

Sagittal plane: A plane that runs vertically from the anterior to posterior part of the body. The *mid-sagittal plane* lies at the center of the body, running anterior to posterior.

Scatter radiation: Radiation that, during passage through matter, has deviated in direction. It also has been modified by a decrease in energy.

Secondary radiation: Radiation that serves no useful purpose. It includes tube or collimator leakage and scatter radiation.

Sensitometer: An instrument used to expose film to precisely controlled steps of increasing light intensity.

Sensitometric curve: The visual line graph produced by plotting density–radiation dose relationships of photographic films. Also called the characteristic or H & D curve.

Source to Image Distance (SID): The distance measured along the central ray from the center of the front of the source (focal spot) to the surface of the image detector (film). Also called FFD.

Source to skin distance (SSD): The distance measured along the central ray from the source (focal spot) to the skin of the patient. Also called FSD.

Step wedge (penetrometer): A device consisting of different density filters shaped in a step-like form where each step of filter differs in density by the square root of 2. Used for testing linearity of exposures and base calibrations.

Target: Material at which the electrons from the cathode in an X-ray tube are aimed in order to produce X-rays.

Target to film distance (TFD): The distance from the X-ray tube target (anode) to the film, measured in inches or centimeters.

Important Rules in Radiography

Ten Day Rule: The safest time to X-ray a female of child-bearing age is during the first 10 days after the onset of her menstrual cycle. Females of child-bearing age must always be asked if the X-rays to be taken are within this time frame. When in doubt, the clinical necessity of the X-ray must be weighed against the possibility of pregnancy. Routine X-rays should be delayed until there is no chance of pregnancy.

Fifteen Percent Rule: An increase or decrease of the kVp by 15% will have the same effect on the X-ray film as if the mAs was doubled or halved.

Rule of Ten: Within the mid-range of kVp selection, a change of 10 kVp will double or halve the density.

Reciprocity Law: A properly calibrated X-ray generator will produce the same density on the film for a given mAs despite different mA and time selections.

Density is directly proportional to mAs: A 10% change in mAs will produce a 10% change in density. It generally takes a change of 25% to be visually perceived.

mAs to kVp relationship for adjusting contrast:
1.   To reduce mAs 25%, increase kVp 8%.
2.   To reduce mAs 50%, adjust kVp by 15%.
3.   To increase mAs 100%, reduce kVp 12%.

Modern Rare-Earth Screen and Film Combinations

Kodak	Kodak Film (Green)	Speed	Kodak Film (Green)	Speed
Lanex Fine (single screen)	T-Mat Green (TMG-1/CSG-1	80	T-Mat Green High (TMH-1)/CSG-2	160
Lanex Fine (dual screen)	T-Mat Green (TMG-1/CSG-1	100	T-Mat Green High (TMH-1)/CSG-2	200
Lanex Medium	T-Mat Green (TMG-1/CSG-1	300	T-Mat Green High (TMH-1)/CSG-2	600
Lanex Regular	T-Mat Green (TMG-1/CSG-1	400	T-Mat Green High (TMH-1)/CSG-2	800
Lanex Fast	T-Mat Green (TMG-1/CSG-1	600	T-Mat Green High (TMH-1)/CSG-2	1200
Konica				
KR	Konica/Kodak Green 1	400	T-Mat Green High (TMH-1)	800
KR	Konica/Kodak Green 1	600	T-Mat Green High (TMH-1)	1200
Sterling	Blue-sensitive film			
Quanta Rapid/Quanta III	CRONEX 4	800	CRONEX 10 T	400
Quanta Fast Detail/Quanta II	CRONEX 4	400	CRONEX 10 T	250
Quanta Ortho/Quanta V	Konica/Kodak Green 1	400	T-Mat Green High (TMH-1)	800
Agfa Gevert	Gevert/Konica/Kodak		Gevert/Konica/Kodak	
Ortho-Fine (single screen)	HTA/Green 1/TMG-1	80	STH/Green 2/TMH-1	160
Ortho-Medium	HTA/Green 1/TMG-1	300	STH/Green 2/TMH-1	600
Ortho-Regular	HTA/Green 1/TMG-1	400	STH/Green 2/TMH-1	800
Ortho-Fast	HTA/Green 1/TMG-1	600	STH/Green 2/TMH-1	1200
Fuji	Fuji Film		Fuji Film	
HR-Medium	HRG-1	200	HRH	300
HR-Regular	HRG-1	400	HRH	600
HR-Fast	HRG-1	600	HRH	900
3M				
Trimax-2	Imation XDA	100		
Trimax-6	Imation XDA	300		
Trimax-8	Imation XDA	400		
Trimax-12	Imation XDA	600		
Trimax XM	Imation XDA	1200		

The light spectrum of the film and screens must match to get the proper speed.

The higher speeds will result in more quantum mottle or noise on the image.

All of the above systems are green light sensitive except the Sterling Quanta Rapid and Fast Detail screens.

Index